Compressive Neuropathies of the Upper Extremity

Dean G. Sotereanos
Loukia K. Papatheodorou
Editors

Compressive Neuropathies of the Upper Extremity

A Comprehensive Guide to Treatment

Springer

Editors
Dean G. Sotereanos
Orthopaedic Specialists - UPMC
University of Pittsburgh
Pittsburgh, PA
USA

Loukia K. Papatheodorou
Orthopaedic Specialists - UPMC
University of Pittsburgh
Pittsburgh, PA
USA

ISBN 978-3-030-37288-0 ISBN 978-3-030-37289-7 (eBook)
https://doi.org/10.1007/978-3-030-37289-7

This Springer imprint is published by the registered company Springer Nature Switzerland AG
The registered company address is: Gewerbestrasse 11, 6330 Cham, Switzerland

I would like to dedicate this book to my coauthors and coeditor, Loukia Papatheodorou, for contributing their hard work and time to make this book a success. Time is a surgeon's most valuable asset. It is a great honor to have had all of the coauthors give their time on my behalf.

I would also like to thank my wife, Donna, and my children, Alexis and Stella, for allowing me the time to practice what I love.

Dean G. Sotereanos, MD

Preface

There has been an evolution in the diagnosis and management of compressive neuropathies of the upper extremity over the past few decades. However, the ideal treatment is not yet established, and management of complications remains a challenge. Given the high incidence and the socioeconomic consequences of compressive neuropathies, especially in young and active patients, this book is intended to serve as a modern reference and practical resource for the orthopedic, plastic, or general surgeon interested in treating these unique maladies providing our patients with the most effective and highest quality care.

This book presents the current state of the art in the diagnosis and surgical management of compressive neuropathies of the upper extremity by experts in the field. It provides new and comprehensive coverage of diagnosis of primary and recurrent compressive neuropathies of the upper extremity including electrodiagnostic and ultrasound findings in correlation with the clinical findings. The chapters describe the latest, cutting-edge management of carpal tunnel syndrome, cubital tunnel syndrome, ulnar nerve syndrome, radial tunnel syndrome, pronator teres syndrome, thoracic outlet syndrome, and suprascapular nerve entrapment as well as revision carpal and cubital tunnel surgical treatment options. A step-by-step description of the surgical procedures along with intraoperative photos and detailed illustrations allows/helps the operating surgeon to successfully perform these techniques for primary or revision treatment. Surgical pearls, pitfalls, and controversies are discussed to enhance reader comprehension and learning promoting optimal outcomes and minimizing complications.

We would like to express our deep appreciation to all contributing authors for their efforts sharing their time and expertise. We are grateful to Kristopher Spring, senior editor, for his support and advice, and we wish to thank all of those who helped to put this project together.

Pittsburgh, PA, USA

Dean G. Sotereanos
Loukia K. Papatheodorou

Abbreviations

A

AANEM	American Association of Neuromuscular & Electrodiagnostic Medicine
ADM	Abductor digiti minimi
AIN	Anterior interosseous nerve
AP	Anteroposterior
ALS	Amyotrophic lateral sclerosis
APB	Abductor pollicis brevis
APL	Abductor pollicis longus
ASMT	Anterior submuscular transposition

B

BMRC	British Medical Research Council
BR	Brachioradialis

C

CAL	Coracoacromial ligament
CC	Coracoclavicular
CMAP	Compound motor action potential
CNAP	Compound nerve action potential
CMT	Charcot-Marie-Tooth
CRPS	Complex regional pain syndrome
CSA	Cross-sectional area
CT	Computed tomography
CTQ	Carpal Tunnel Questionnaire
CTS	Carpal tunnel syndrome
CUTS	Cubital tunnel syndrome

D

DASH	Disabilities of the arm, shoulder, and hand (score)
DCBUN	Dorsal cutaneous branch of the ulnar nerve
DSBUN	Dorsal ulnar hand

E

ECRB	Extensor carpi radialis brevis
ECRL	Extensor carpi radialis longus
ECU	Extensor carpi ulnaris
ECTR	Endoscopic carpal tunnel release
EDC	Extensor digitorum communis
EDM	Extensor digiti minimi
EDQ	Extensor digitorum quinti
EIP	Extensor indicis proprius
EMG	Electromyogram
EPB	Extensor pollicis brevis
EPL	Extensor pollicis longus
ETE	End to end
ETS	End to side

F

FCR	Flexor carpi radialis
FCU	Flexor carpi ulnaris
FDI	First dorsal interosseous
FDP	Flexor digitorum profundus
FDS	Flexor digitorum superficialis
FPB	Flexor pollicis brevis
FPL	Flexor pollicis longus

H

HFPF	Hypothenar fat pad flap
HGF	Hepatocyte growth factor

I

IPJ	Interphalangeal joints
IPPN	Inflammatory pseudotumor of peripheral nerve

L

LABC	Lateral antebrachial cutaneous
LABCN	Lateral antebrachial cutaneous nerve
LACN	Lateral antebrachial cutaneous nerve

M

MABC	Medial antebrachial cutaneous
MBACN	Medial brachial and antebrachial cutaneous nerve
MBC	Medial brachial cutaneous
MCN	Musculocutaneous nerve
MCPJ	Metacarpophalangeal joints
MCP	Metacarpophalangeal
MEPP	Miniature end plate potential
MHQ	Michigan Hand Questionnaire
MICTR	Minimal incision carpal tunnel release
MIMS	Medial intermuscular septum
MIS	Minimally invasive surgery
MN	Median nerve
MNAP	Motor nerve action potential
MPNST	Malignant peripheral nerve sheath tumors
MRI	Magnetic resonance imaging
MUAP	Motor unit action potential

N

NCS	Nerve conduction study
NCV	Nerve conduction velocity

O

OCTR	Open carpal tunnel release
ODM	Opponens digiti minimi

P

PCB	Palmar cutaneous branch
PCBMN	Palmar cutaneous branch of the median nerve
PET	Positron emission tomography
PIN	Posterior interosseous nerve
PINCS	Posterior interosseous nerve compression syndrome

PL	Palmaris longus
PNST	Peripheral nerve sheath tumor
PQ	Pronator quadratus
PS	Pronator teres syndrome

R

RDN	Radial digital nerve
RS	Radial styloid
RSD	Reflex sympathetic dystrophy
RTS	Radial tunnel syndrome

S

SBRN	Superficial branch of the radial nerve
SETS	"Supercharged" end-to-side transfer
SHGC	Spontaneous hourglass constriction
SNAP	Sensory nerve action potential
SSEP	Somatosensory evoked potentials
SST	Simple Shoulder Test
STS	Soft tissue sarcoma

T

TCL	Transverse carpal ligament
TENS	Transcutaneous electrical nerve stimulation
TF	Trigger finger
TOS	Thoracic outlet syndrome
TSCAI	Two small cross aligned incisions

U

UA	Ulnar artery
UN	Ulnar nerve
US	Ultrasonography
UTS	Ulnar tunnel syndrome

V

VAS	Visual Analog Scale
VCL	Volar carpal ligament
VEGF	Vascular endothelial growth factor

W

WALANT	Wide-awake local anesthesia no tourniquet
WFR	Wrist-to-forearm ratio
WMSN	Wartenberg's migrant sensory neuritis

Contents

1 **The Basics of Electrodiagnostic Testing Carpal Tunnel and Cubital Tunnel Syndrome** ... 1
George A. Small

2 **Ultrasound Anatomy of the Median and Ulnar Nerves** ... 11
Antonios Kerasnoudis, Min-Suk Yoon, Georgios Barmpalios, and Aaron I. Venouziou

3 **Diagnosis and Clinical Presentation of Carpal Tunnel Syndrome** ... 27
John R. Fowler

4 **Standard Open Carpal Tunnel Release** ... 37
Hannah H. Lee and Robert J. Goitz

5 **Carpal Tunnel Release with Two Small Cross-Aligned Incisions** ... 43
Konstantinos N. Malizos, Antonios Koutalos, Fotis Papageorgiou, Anna Ziogou, and Marianthi Papanagiotou

6 **Endoscopic Carpal Tunnel Release** ... 53
Aaron I. Venouziou and Antonios Kerasnoudis

7 **Complications of Carpal Tunnel Release** ... 61
Panagiotis Giannakopoulos, Konstantinos Kourkoutas, and George Kasimatis

8 **Revision Carpal Tunnel Surgical Options** ... 75
Travis Littleton, Cassidy Costello, and Mark Baratz

9 **Hypothenar Fat Pad Flap: Surgical Technique** ... 85
James W. Strickland and Gary M. Lourie

10 **Tumors and Tumor-Like Lesions Mimicking Peripheral Neuropathies** ... 89
Zoe H. Dailiana and Vasileios A. Kontogeorgakos

11 **Clinical Presentation and Diagnosis of Cubital Tunnel Syndrome** ... 103
Claudius D. Jarrett

12 **In Situ Decompression of Cubital Tunnel** ... 111
Thomas Hughes

13 Endoscopic Ulnar Nerve Release 121
Margaret Woon Man Fok, Tyson Cobb, and Greg Bain

14 Subcutaneous Transposition of the Ulnar Nerve 131
Natalie H. Vaughn, Brittany E. Homcha, and Alexander H. Payatakes

15 Submuscular Transposition of the Ulnar Nerve 145
Maureen A. O'Shaughnessy and Marco Rizzo

16 Minimal Medial Epicondylectomy 155
Loukia K. Papatheodorou, Dimitrios G. Vardakas, and Dean G. Sotereanos

17 Revision Cubital Tunnel: Surgical Options 161
Aikaterini G. Bavelou, Efstratios G. Papanikos, Panayotis N. Soucacos, and Zinon T. Kokkalis

18 Nerve Transfers for Neuropathies of the Median and Ulnar Nerve 169
Joshua Allan Gillis and Steven L. Moran

19 Ulnar Tunnel Syndrome (Guyon Canal) 185
Elizabeth P. Wahl and Marc J. Richard

20 Radial Tunnel Syndrome - Posterior Interosseous Nerve Compression Syndrome 195
Ioannis K. Sarris and Ilias D. Alafropatis

21 Pronator Teres Syndrome: Anterior Interosseous Nerve Compressive Neuropathy 209
Konstantinos Anagnostakos, Nikolaos P. Zagoreos, and Nickolaos A. Darlis

22 Lateral Antebrachial Nerve Entrapment 217
Filippos S. Giannoulis, Nikolaos G. Papoulidis, and Anastasia V. Krexi

23 Wartenberg's Syndrome 225
Efstratios D. Athanaselis, Ioannis Antoniou, and Sokratis E. Varitimidis

24 Thoracic Outlet Syndrome 231
A. Lee Osterman and Matthew S. Wilson

25 Vein Wrapping of Peripheral Nerves: Surgical Technique 247
Loukia K. Papatheodorou and Dean G. Sotereanos

26 Cervical Radiculopathy Mimicking Carpal Tunnel Syndrome 253
Gurpreet Surinder Gandhoke and Raymond F. Sekula

27 Suprascapular Neuropathy 259
Christopher M. Treat and Christopher C. Schmidt

Index 277

Contributors

Ilias D. Alafropatis, MD 3rd Orthopaedic Department, Papageorgiou General Hospital, Aristotle University of Thessaloniki Medical School, Thessaloniki, Greece

Konstantinos Anagnostakos, MD Bioclinic Athens, Athens, Greece

Ioannis Antoniou, MD University Hospital of Larissa, Larissa, Greece

Efstratios D. Athanaselis, MD University Hospital of Larissa, Larissa, Greece

Greg Bain, MD Department of Orthopaedic Surgery, Flinders University, Adelaide, South Australia

Mark Baratz, MD Department of Orthopaedic Specialists, University of Pittsburgh Medical Center (UPMC) Passavant, Pittsburgh, PA, USA

Georgios Barmpalios, MD Department of Radiology, Iatriki Diagnosi Private Imaging Centre, Serres, Greece

Aikaterini G. Bavelou, MD Department of Orthopaedics, University Hospital of Patras, Patras, Greece

Tyson Cobb, MD Shoulder Elbow wrist and Hand Center of Excellent, Davenport, IA, USA

Cassidy Costello, BA Department of Community Medicine, University of Pittsburgh Medical Center (UPMC) Passavant, Pittsburgh, PA, USA

Zoe H. Dailiana, MD Department of Orthopaedic Surgery, Faculty of Medicine, University of Thessaly, Larissa, Greece

Nickolaos A. Darlis, MD Metropolitan Hospital, Athens, Greece

Margaret Woon Man Fok, MBChB (Otago) Department of Orthopaedics and Traumatology, Queen Mary Hospital, The University of Hong Kong, Hong Kong, China

John R. Fowler, MD Department of Orthopaedics, University of Pittsburgh Medical Center, Pittsburgh, PA, USA

Gurpreet Surinder Gandhoke, MD Marion Bloch Neuroscience Inst, Saint Luke's Hospital of Kansas City, Kansas, MO, USA

Panagiotis Giannakopoulos, MD Hand, Upper Limb and Microsurgery Center, Athens Medical Center, Athens, Greece

Filippos S. Giannoulis, MD, PhD Hand, Upper Extremity and Microsurgery Department, KAT Hospital, Athens, Greece

Joshua Allan Gillis, MD Maine General Medical Center, Department of Plastic Surgery, Augusta, ME, USA

Robert J. Goitz, MD Department of Orthopaedic Surgery, University of Pittsburgh Medical Center, Pittsburgh, PA, USA

Brittany E. Homcha, MD Department of Orthopaedics, Penn State Health Milton S. Hershey Medical Center, Hershey, PA, USA

Thomas Hughes, MD Department of Orthopaedic Surgery, UPMC Passavant Hospital, University of Pittsburgh, Pittsburgh, PA, USA

Claudius D. Jarrett, MD Division of Orthopaedic Surgery, Wilmington Health Associates, Wilmington, NC, USA

George Kasimatis, MD, PhD, FEBOT, FEBHS Athens Medical Center, Athens, Greece

Antonios Kerasnoudis, MD, PhD Department of Neurology, St. Luke's Hospital, Panorama, Thessaloniki, Greece

Zinon T. Kokkalis, MD, PhD Department of Orthopaedics, University Hospital of Patras, Patras, Greece

Vasileios A. Kontogeorgakos, MD, PhD Department of Orthopaedic Surgery, Attikon University Hospital, National and Kapodistrian University of Athens, Athens, Greece

Konstantinos Kourkoutas, MD Hand, Upper Limb and Microsurgery Center, Athens Medical Center, Athens, Greece

Antonios Koutalos, MD Department of Orthopaedics & MusculoSkeletal Trauma, University of Thessaly, Larissa, Greece

Anastasia V. Krexi, MD Hand, Upper Extremity and Microsurgery Department, KAT Hospital, Athens, Greece

Hannah H. Lee, MD, PhD Department of Orthopaedic Surgery, University of Pittsburgh Medical Center, Pittsburgh, PA, USA

Travis Littleton, MD University of Pittsburgh Physicians, University of Pittsburgh Medical Center (UPMC) Passavant, Pittsburgh, PA, USA

Gary M. Lourie, MD The Hand and Upper Extremity Center of Georgia, Atlanta, GA, USA

Konstantinos N. Malizos, MD Hand Unit – Department of Orthopaedics & Musculoskeletal Trauma, University of Thessaly Medical School, Larissa, Greece

Steven L. Moran, MD Division of Plastic Surgery & Department of Orthopedic Surgery, Mayo Clinic, Rochester, MN, USA

Maureen A. O'Shaughnessy, MD Department of Orthopaedic Surgery, University of Kentucky, Lexington, KY, USA

A. Lee Osterman, MD Philadelphia Hand Center, King of Prussia, PA, USA

Fotis Papageorgiou, MD Department of Orthopaedics & MusculoSkeletal Trauma, University of Thessaly, Larissa, Greece

Marianthi Papanagiotou, MD Department of Orthopaedics & MusculoSkeletal Trauma, University of Thessaly, Larissa, Greece

Efstratios G. Papanikos, MD Department of Orthopaedics, University Hospital of Patras, Patras, Greece

Loukia K. Papatheodorou, MD Orthopaedic Specialists - UPMC, University of Pittsburgh, Pittsburgh, PA, USA

Nikolaos G. Papoulidis, MD, MSc Hand, Upper Extremity and Microsurgery Department, KAT Hospital, Athens, Greece

Alexander H. Payatakes, MD Department of Orthopaedics, Bone and Joint Institute, Penn State Health Milton S. Hershey Medical Center, Hershey, PA, USA

Marc J. Richard, MD Duke University Medical Center, Department of Orthopaedic Surgery, Durham, NC, USA

Marco Rizzo, MD Department of Orthopedic Surgery, Mayo Clinic, Rochester, MN, USA

Ioannis K. Sarris, MD, PhD 3rd Orthopaedic Department, Papageorgiou General Hospital, Aristotle University of Thessaloniki Medical School, Thessaloniki, Greece

Christopher C. Schmidt, MD Department of Orthopaedic Surgery, University of Pittsburgh Medical Center, Pittsburgh, PA, USA

Raymond F. Sekula Jr., MD Department of Neurological Surgery, University of Pittsburgh Medical Center (UPMC) Presbyterian, Pittsburgh, PA, USA

George A. Small, MD Department of Neurology, Allegheny General Hospital, Pittsburgh, PA, USA

Dean G. Sotereanos, MD Orthopaedic Specialists - UPMC, University of Pittsburgh, Pittsburgh, PA, USA

Panayotis N. Soucacos, MD, PhD Orthopaedic Research and Education Center (OREC), Attikon University Hospital, University of Athens, School of Medicine, Department of Orthopaedics, Athens, Greece

James W. Strickland, MD St. Francis Hospital, Indianapolis, IN, USA

Department of Orthopaedics-Emeritus, Indiana University School of Medicine, Indianapolis, IN, USA

Christopher M. Treat, MD Hillcrest Medical Center, Tulsa, OK, USA

Dimitrios G. Vardakas, MD General Hospital of Ioannina "G. Hatzikosta", Department of Orthopaedic Surgery, Ioannina, Greece

Sokratis E. Varitimidis, MD University Hospital of Larissa, Larissa, Greece

Natalie H. Vaughn, MD Department of Orthopaedics, Penn State Health Milton S. Hershey Medical Center, Hershey, PA, USA

Aaron I. Venouziou, MD Division of Upper Extremity Surgery, Orthopaedic Department, St. Luke's Hospital, Panorama, Thessaloniki, Greece

Elizabeth P. Wahl, MD Duke University Medical Center, Department of Orthopaedic Surgery, Durham, NC, USA

Matthew S. Wilson, MD Orthopaedic Hand Surgery, Thomas Jefferson University Hospital, Philadelphia Hand to Shoulder Center, Philadelphia, PA, USA

Min-Suk Yoon, MD, PhD Department of Neurology, EVK Hattingen, Hattingen, Germany

Nikolaos P. Zagoreos, MD Metropolitan Hospital, Athens, Greece

Anna Ziogou, MD Department of Orthopaedics & MusculoSkeletal Trauma, University of Thessaly, Larissa, Greece

The Basics of Electrodiagnostic Testing Carpal Tunnel and Cubital Tunnel Syndrome

1

George A. Small

Though carpal tunnel syndrome and cubital tunnel syndrome are the thrusts of this chapter, it is worth reviewing the basic anatomy of nerve to understand the types of pathology that give way to these syndromes, and determine prognosis for recovery. Endoneurium, perineurium and epineurium surround the axons of somatic peripheral motor and sensory nerves (Figs. 1.1 and 1.2). Endoneurium is the direct supporting structure around individual axons. Perineurium forms a looser tissue barrier over bundles of nerve fibers. Epineurium, the outermost surrounding nerve structure, envelops multiple nerve bundles itself. Diffusion of chemical constituents can occur across perineurium more readily than across endoneurium.

The spinal nerve roots can merge with the outermost supporting structure of peripheral nerves, but the lack of endoneurial collagen at the nerve root level can explain why some disease processes selectively involve the root. in some disease states, contributing to cubital tunnel syndrome and carpal tunnel syndrome. This is quite important, as chemical processes that affect the nerve roots via chemical diffusion from the cerebrospinal fluid through which the roots initially traverse will generally not occur directly across named peripheral nerves more caudally, where the 'blood nerve barrier' resists many extracellular tissue constituents.

Nerve trunks contain myelinated and unmyelinated fibers. In myelinated fibers, individual Schwann cells envelop their thick, fatty-rich cell membranes around axons to form the myelin sheath. The nodes of Ranvier, located between adjacent Schwann cells, represent gaps along the myelinated fibers on myelinated axons. This structure facilitates myelinated nerves conducting action potentials with high velocity. Many cases of cubital tunnel syndrome and carpal tunnel syndrome occur in patients with diffuse demyelinating processes that render the anatomical distinction between unmyelinated and myelinated fibers important. Both cubital tunnel syndrome and carpal tunnel syndrome are much more prevalent in patients with primary diffuse disorders of axons or myelin themselves, such as those who suffer from severe kidney failure, uncontrolled diabetes, or chronic alcoholism and inherited myelin disorders such as the family of Charcot-Marie-Tooth (CMT) diseases. Such individuals are much more likely to suffer from cubital or carpal tunnel syndrome, particularly with any extra traumatic provocation.

If myelin is damaged alone, it can readily regenerate (neuropraxia). If axon continuity is transgressed completely (axontmesis); however, reinnervation of muscle served by nerve is less reliably predicted- and therefore the focal

G. A. Small (✉)
Department of Neurology, Allegheny General Hospital, Pittsburgh, PA, USA
e-mail: George.Small@ahn.org; gsmall@wpahs.org

D. G. Sotereanos, L. K. Papatheodorou (eds.), *Compressive Neuropathies of the Upper Extremity*,
https://doi.org/10.1007/978-3-030-37289-7_1

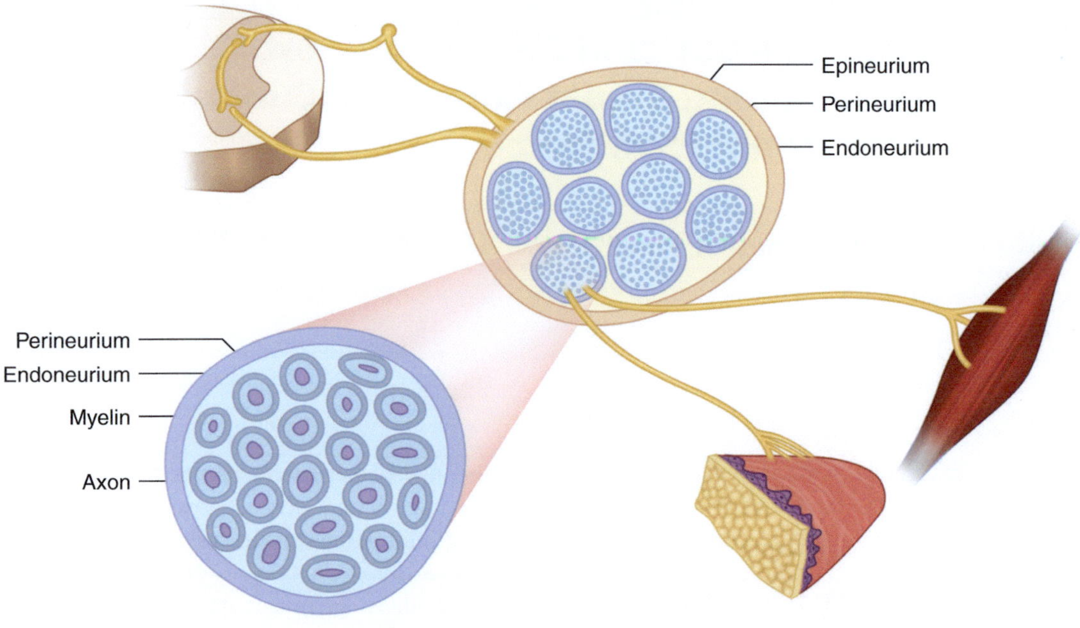

Fig. 1.1 Schematic of basic anatomy of the nerve

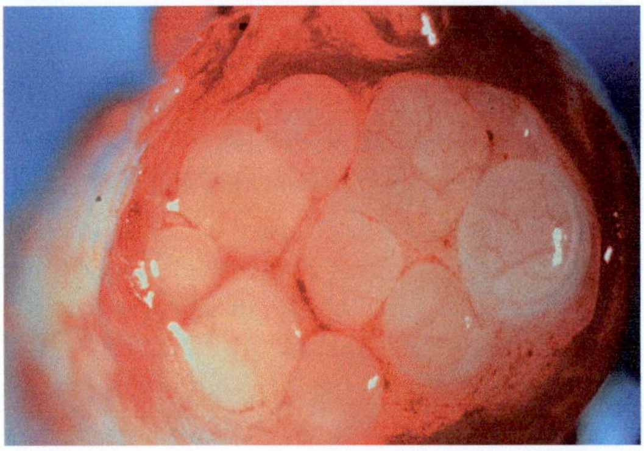

Fig. 1.2 View of basic anatomy of the nerve

demyelination which occurs with traumatic entrapment of nerve which does not involve the axon but does compress myelin has a much better prognosis. This reversible type of pathology causes 'conduction block' of nerve action potentials. This is true of any entrapment syndrome in any nerve throughout the body, and is especially true of cubital tunnel syndrome and carpal tunnel syndrome.

The carpal tunnel, through which the median nerve passes at its distal extent, is surrounded by tendons, bones and connective tissue. The dorsal surface is bounded by the tendons of the muscles to the extensor digitorum communis, extensor indicis proprius, extensor pollicis longus and extensor carpi radialis brevis muscles. On the ventral, or palmar boundary is the abductor pollicis longus muscle (APL) laterally, and the transverse carpal ligament, and muscles to the little finger. Within the carpal tunnel, which is bounded itself by a sheath of connective tissue is the median nerve itself and the tendons of the flexor pollicis longus, flexor digitorum profundus, as well as flexor digitorum sublimis muscles. The bones on the dorsum of the hand surrounding the carpal tunnel include the hamate, capitate, trapezium and trapezoid. This entire area, subject to a lifetime of chronic flexion and extension as well as crowding of tendons and connective tissue is the site of median nerve compression resulting in the carpal tunnel syndrome.

The median nerve arises from the lateral and medial cords of the brachial plexus. It is a mixed nerve (meaning it contains motor and sensory fibers). These fibers are derived from the C6, C7, C8, and T1 roots. It supplies muscles of the thenar eminence of the hand, but also cutaneous sensory fibers of the skin over the lateral aspect of the thenar eminence, and the index and middle fingers, as well as the tips of the terminal phalanges. It also serves sensation on the medial half of the ring finger. The sensory fibers of the middle finger are derived from the C7 nerve root, the lateral cord of the brachial plexus, as well as the middle trunk. The surface of the index finger receives sensory fibers from the C6 and C7 nerve roots through the lateral cord and upper and middle trunk of the brachial plexus. There is much variance to the sensory innervation of the fingers mentioned. There are no muscles in the proximal arm innervated by the median nerve proper. It traverses the arm alongside the humeral bone and enters the forearm between the heads of the pronator teres muscle- which it supplies with motor fibers along with the flexor carpi radialis, palmaris longus and flexor digitorum superficialis muscles. It gives rise to a pure motor branch, the anterior interosseous nerve, which innervates the flexor pollicis longus, pronator quadratus, and flexor digitorum profundus muscles to digits one and two. The remainder of the median nerve descends in the forearm and goes through the carpal tunnel along with the tendons previously mentioned. It first branches off a recurrent thenar nerve, and then branches to the lumbrical 1 and 2 muscles of the hand. The recurrent thenar nerve innervates the abductor pollicis brevis and the lateral half of the flexor pollicis brevis and opponens pollicis muscles. Generally, although carpal tunnel syndrome results in sensory abnormalities, the symptoms do not include such abnormalities of the lateral portion of the thenar eminence, as the sensory branch to that area does not go through the carpal tunnel. This is why anesthesia of the lateral portion of the thenar eminence, along with other sensory symptoms, may suggest a more proximal process, either in the median nerve or at the plexus or root levels, or even the brain or spinal cord. Other entrapment syndromes of the proximal median nerve at the antecubital fossa and in the forearm, resulting in an almost pure motor anterior interosseous nerve syndrome exist, but are not the subject of this chapter.

As in all medical issues, history is paramount. Carpal tunnel syndrome usually presents with nocturnal paresthesias in any combination of the lateral 3 digits of either hand, more commonly the dominant one [1]. Causes of the nocturnal predominance is not clear, but may relate to the patient being more aware of the symptoms when the distractions of the day are at a minimum. Occurring frequently upon awakening in the morning and although the patient may insist he does not sleep on the arm in question- ALL people twist and turn at night and may compress the forearm, upper arm, or wrist during sleep, thus increasing the risk of compressing the median nerve in the narrow carpal tunnel. Weakness alone is rarely the presenting symptom of carpal tunnel syndrome, as sensory nerve fibers are more prone to chemical and physical injury than motor nerves. Many an amyotrophic lateral sclerosis (ALS) victim has been referred to the electromyographer's attention with a wasted, atrophic hand, without sensory symptoms. Carpal tunnel syndrome occurs in the dominant hand in the vast majority of cases and electrophysiologically can found to be bilateral in 15% of the time, even if the side not in question is asymptomatic. This is why bilateral electrophysiologic testing for carpal tunnel syndrome is so important, both to delineate the severity of the process on the side which is the subject of the patient's complaint, and as a baseline for further potential therapy in the less, or non-symptomatic side.

As alluded to above, history of glucose intolerance, uremia, hypothyroidism and hand or wrist trauma is of paramount importance to know. Some patients suffer from carpal tunnel syndrome, denying a history of diabetes, are found on examination to have it by their surgeon or neurologist, even prior to their PCP or endocrinologist making the diagnosis. Diabetes is the most common accompanying medical problem occurring when carpal tunnel syndrome is diagnosed. Diabetes causes both hypoxemic damage to nerves in the body as well as direct hyperglycemic damage to both axon and myelin. A glucose tolerance test or hemoglobin A1c should be tested in all patients with carpal tunnel symptoms, as well as tests of thyroid and renal function.

Along with a detailed history of any accompanying medical problems, as well as determining that the predominant symptoms affect the lateral portion of the hand up to and perhaps including the medial 4th digit, examination of the patient with carpal tunnel syndrome generally begins with inspection. Isolated atrophy of the lateral thenar eminence is a clinical key that the problem is originating in the median nerve at its distal extent at the carpal tunnel. Accompanying forearm atrophy can be seen with more proximal median nerve problems. If indeed there is atrophy of the lateral thenar eminence (abductor pollicis brevis [APB] muscle), then inspection of other C8 and T1 innervated muscles is paramount to rule out a lesion at these nerve root levels or the lower trunk of the brachial plexus.

Weakness of the distal tips of digits 2 and 3 and of the thumb along with weakness of forearm pronation can point to a pure anterior interosseous nerve lesion in the forearm.

EMG/NCV

This test is upwards of 85% sensitive for carpal tunnel syndrome and more than 95% specific for it [2]. A basic understanding of the technique follows.

Motor nerves carry large myelinated fibers which conduct electrical impulses at 40–50 m/s. Sensory nerves carry large, medium, small and unmyelinated nerves which conduct electricity at anywhere from 50 m/s down to 2–3 m/s. Standard EMG nerve conduction study testing evaluates the large, fast conducting fibers of motor and sensory nerves. Electrical studies for entrapment neuropathy involve testing mixed motor and sensory nerves, isolated motor nerves, and isolated sensory nerves. The standard protocol for evaluating a patient with carpal tunnel syndrome is to place a recording electrode over the abductor policies brevis muscle (Fig. 1.3). A reference electrode is placed at a local, bony, non-electrically active reference area. A separate ground wire is applied to the skin for electrical safety. The median nerve is stimulated in the antecubital fossa and at the wrist with a handheld stimulation device. If one were to measure the distance between the stimulating and the recording electrode on the APB muscle, and divide that distance by the time it takes an electrical impulse generated from the stimulating electrode to the recording electrode, a falsely low velocity for motor nerve conduction would result. This is because one is measuring not only the conduction in nerve fibers, but also across the neuromuscular junction and across the muscle membrane, which conduct at extremely low velocities. Therefore the technique of measuring velocity in motor nerves involves stimulating the nerve at two separate points, recording at one particular point, and subtracting the distance from the distal stimulation point to the recording electrode, from that of the proximal stimulus point to the recording electrode, and dividing that by the difference in time it takes the impulse that is generated from the initial point of stimulation from the distal point of stimulation. This results in deriving a conduction velocity along

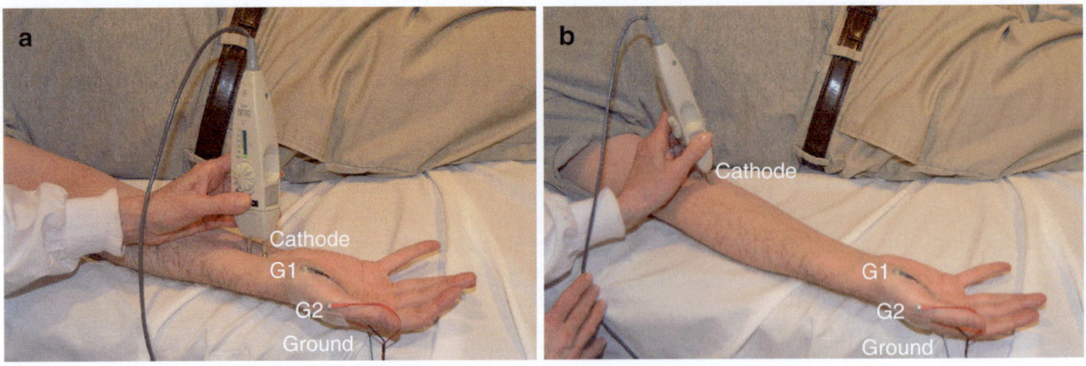

Fig. 1.3 Median motor study. (**a**) Distal stimulation site over median nerve at wrist, recording abductor pollicis brevis. (**b**) Proximal stimulation site at antecubital fossa

the forearm segment of the median nerve itself, subtracting out the time it takes the impulse to go from the distal stimulating point to the recording electrode, which is adulterated by neuromuscular junction and muscle membrane influences. This results in an accurate conduction velocity in the median motor nerve itself. This concept is also applied to stimulating all other motor nerves such as the ulnar nerve and other motor nerves in the body. Sensory nerve conduction velocities are a more simple practice. Since the nerve impulse does not traverse a neuromuscular junction or muscle membrane substance, simply stimulating a sensory nerve at one point, recording at another point, and dividing the distance between the two points by the time it takes the impulse to go from one point to the other results in measuring conduction velocity in the sensory nerve. The examiner must always be attentive to the effects of temperature on conduction velocities, and even on the amplitude of both sensory and motor responses. A surface skin temperature of 30 ° C generally reflects a normal body temperature which reflects the true parenchymal nerve temperature itself. A rule of thumb is that for every degree Celsius below body temperature measured for a nerve, there is a 2 m/s decrease in conduction velocity. Too many studies in general neurological practice reveal low conduction velocities which are due to low surface skin temperature and not to true pathology, frequently rendering a false positive diagnosis of peripheral neuropathy, resulting in inappropriate patient management.

In addition to velocities, the resulting waveform generated on the oscilloscope results in an amplitude measured from the baseline to the electrical peak of a biphasic waveform in units of microvolts, in the case of a motor nerve referred to as a compound motor action potential (CMAP), and in the case of a sensory nerve referred to as a sensory nerve action potential (SNAP). Each of these potentials is the algebraic sum of the number of either the number of sensory nerves recorded or muscle cells depolarized, measured within the nerve bundle itself or the muscle being tested. Any electromyography laboratory must have a reference set of normal values from which clinical test results are compared. It is impractical for each laboratory to determine its own normal values, which historically had been painstakingly measured. Historical normal values for amplitude and velocity in motor and sensory nerves can be applied as long as the EMG/NCV machine is set to the same filter settings, and the same type of electrodes and stimulators are used as were used to derive the original normative textbook values. One cannot overemphasize the importance of controlling skin temperature in providing accurate results, as mentioned above. A paradoxically slow conducting nerve with large amplitude should be a clue to that the test was done with inadequate temperature control. The study may then need to be repeated. Other than amplitude and velocities, the parameters measured in standard nerve conduction studies, include other data points - the "distal latency", and the "F response". Historically the F response, (which stands for "foot"), where the measure was first derived, is a method of stimulating motor nerves distally at a very high level of stimulus duration and amperage, and doing so repeatedly with recording over the muscle innervated by the nerve in question, and deriving approximately 10–20 responses which occur because of "back firing" of motor nerves near or in the anterior horn cell. The amplitude of these responses are very low normally, and appear much later on the oscilloscope than the CMAP, however when the latency of these responses is measured, it provides a general overview of the most myelinated nerves conducting along the proximal, middle, and distal segments of the motor nerve, and if very prolonged, can be a clinical sign of severe demyelination proximal to the point of stimulation. For entrapment neuropathies, this particular test has less use than the regular recording of amplitude, velocity and distal latency. Distal latency refers to the time it takes an electrical impulse from normal stimulation of a motor nerve at the point closest to its recording electrode to reach its innervated muscle. This value is usually on the order of less than 10 ms, and there are normative values for each motor nerve tested. Prolongation of distal latencies suggests distal demyelinating pathology in a nerve.

For sensory nerve action potentials, merely the recording of the amplitude of the SNAP and the velocity are adequate for the clinical report to the referring physician. Thus, an electrical study for any entrapment neuropathy or even for peripheral neuropathy, myopathy radiculopathy, or plexopathy should contain a data sheet which lists the amplitude and velocity of any sensory nerve tested as well as the amplitude, distal latency, F response latency and conduction velocity along any motor or sensory nerve measured.

The most sensitive indicator electrically of carpal says tunnel syndrome is a slowing in the conduction velocity and or decreased amplitude of the sensory nerve action potential of the median sensory branch to digits 1 or 2 [3]. Electrodes are placed at the distal end of digit two as well as at the wrist. Stimulation of the sensory nerve can be accomplished either at the finger, with recording at the wrist, or at the wrist with recording at the finger. Stimulating the nerve in its physiologically "correct" or orthodromic" direction or stimulating the mixed median nerve at the wrist with recording at the finger "antidromic" direction will result in a waveform representing the sensory nerves to the finger tested. The antidromic method may result in muscle artifact; however, it is a more sensitive method for recording sensory nerve action potentials. Either method is reasonable in practice as long as artifact is controlled for. The next most sensitive indicator of carpal tunnel syndrome is a prolonged distal latency when measuring the motor conduction as described above. Frequently, electrical studies will reveal some combination of sensory nerve slowing to digit 2 and a prolongation of the median motor distal latency. The normal median motor distal latency is <4.5 ms. The normal median sensory conduction is 50 m/s. Generally no median motor nerve conduction slowing is noted in the forearm in carpal tunnel syndrome, but it may occur as an artifact of an extremely prolonged distal latency (greater than 10 ms) as retrograde demyelination can occur from severe damage to the nerve within the carpal tunnel. In this case the sensory nerve action potential to digit 2 is usually found to be absent. In cases of extremely mild carpal tunnel syndrome the entire electrical study is normal- however, with the patient reporting typical carpal tunnel syndrome symptoms a more sensitive test that can be performed is to stimulate the median mixed motor and sensory nerve directly in the palm and recording over the median nerve at the wrist and determining the conduction velocity in that short segment of this median mixed motor/sensory nerve. If it is decreased, and all other data are normal, there is clear evidence of carpal tunnel syndrome. This portion of the study should be performed when the patient's symptoms are typical for carpal tunnel syndrome as mentioned, and the remainder of the test is normal. As part of a general electrical study for carpal tunnel syndrome, the ulnar motor nerve and ulnar sensory nerves should also be evaluated. When a generalized neuropathic process is not present, a normal ulnar motor and sensory nerve set of values serves as a nice control when median neuropathy at the wrist is electrically noted. This provides more confidence for the electromyographer to present to the surgeon of the lesion truly being at the carpal tunnel and not being part of a more generalized peripheral neuropathic process not requiring surgical intervention.

After the median and ulnar motor and sensory responses are recorded, needle EMG is then performed.

EMG or electromyography, is the process of inserting a needle electrode in a muscle and recording electrical impulses on an oscilloscope either at rest or while directing the patient to perform a muscle contraction. Normal muscle generally does not reveal unusual electrical potentials at rest. With activation of any muscle tested a number of motor units can be assessed to that muscle for any variance from normality. Motor unit action potentials (MUAPs), are representative of the algebraic sum of individual muscle cell action potentials representing the sum of all voltage changes from all muscle cells innervated by the nerve activated. No externally applied electrical shocks are required. The duration, amplitude and number of phases of the visualized potentials can determine whether a process resulting in weakness or spasm is on a neurogenic or a myogenic basis.

Individual muscles are innervated by a number of different motor nerves. The motor unit is defined as a motor nerve and all the muscle cells it innervates. If there is damage to a particular nerve, other nerves innervating other muscle cells within the muscle itself eventually will take over innervation of those muscle cells. The resulting motor unit action potential generated by a voluntary contraction will then appear larger than normal on the electromyography oscilloscope, since any individual surviving motor nerve will innervate more muscle cells than it usually does. Therefore, a chronic neurogenic process can be defined as an increased amplitude in motor unit potentials seen. In addition, the surviving motor neurons fire at a frequency which is faster than usual in order to maintain a specific force since other motor nerves are damaged and cannot do so. This denervation and reinnervation process is time-dependent, and a nerve conduction study performed immediately after nerve injury will not reflect this. Reinnervation of muscle cells which have been "abandoned" by their damaged motor nerves occurs approximately after 2 weeks for arm innervated muscles and 3 weeks for leg innervated muscles and 1 week for facial innervated muscles. This reflects the time it takes for reinnervation to occur as the axons of the reinnervating nerves must grow to innervate the muscle cells which have been denervated. Reinnervation may not be complete process. After mechanical trauma to the carpal tunnel, when weakness ensues, one may perform a baseline nerve conduction study near the time of trauma, however it is more important to perform a study more than 2 weeks after the trauma to determine what reinnervation has occurred. In addition, proper localization of the process to the carpal tunnel can only occur after such reinnervation occurs. In moderate to severe cases of carpal tunnel syndrome, the APB muscle will show changes of acute and/or chronic neurogenic change, such as increased amplitudes of the motor unit action potentials (MUAPs), and if the process is subacute to acute, spontaneous electrical discharges from denervated APB muscle cells will occur and are easily noted with the patient's muscle at rest (fibrillations and positive sharp waves) and the EMG electrode inserted into the APB muscle. All these changes require at least 2 week's delay in performing the electrical test after any particular acute inciting event thought to cause carpal tunnel syndrome has occurred. If the patient has had carpal tunnel symptoms for weeks, months, or years- then certainly the electrical study can be accomplished at any time.

Ulnar neuropathy most commonly occurs at the ulnar sulcus or at the cubital tunnel [4, 5]. When occurring at the ulnar sulcus historically the problem was referred to as the "tardy ulnar palsy", as it frequently was observed with some delay after some form of direct inciting trauma to the area had occurred [6]. Constant flexion and extension of the elbow is a clear risk factor for this process as well as the above-mentioned generalized peripheral neuropathic risk factors, distal humerus fracture, and olecranon fracture. The cubital tunnel is a virtual structure in the forearm through which the ulnar nerve passes after traversing the ulnar sulcus, piercing the aponeurosis between the two main heads of the flexor carpi ulnaris muscle. Compression of the nerve by these portions of the flexor carpi ulnaris muscle can result in the process referred to as the cubital tunnel syndrome. Although worth mentioning, but not the subject of this particular chapter, ulnar neuropathy may also occur at Guyon's canal at the wrist where the distal ulnar nerve enters the hand. Each of these processes is distinguishable, if not by clinical examination, then by nerve conduction study and electromyography.

The ulnar nerve is derived from the C8, T1 nerve roots and the lower trunk of the brachial plexus. The motor axons of the ulnar nerve to the flexor carpi ulnaris muscle generally branch from the main ulnar nerve trunk proximal to the cubital tunnel, and therefore in cases of cubital tunnel syndrome, examination via EMG of the flexor carpi ulnaris muscle is normal. Branches of the ulnar nerve to the flexor digitorum profundus muscles to digits four and five in the hand are generally not spared in cubital tunnel syndrome, and the finding of typical ulnar neuropathic symptoms with preserved flexor carpi ulnaris function via EMG and abnormal EMG examination of the FDP muscle and other distal muscles via EMG can help localize the process.

Stimulation of the ulnar nerve in the electromyography laboratory with recording over either the 1st dorsal interosseous muscle or the abductor digiti minimi muscle of the hand, generally is carried out recording at 3 points, above the elbow, below the elbow, and at the wrist. As described for the median nerve, the segmental velocities of the ulnar nerve in the above-elbow to below-elbow segment, and the below-elbow segment to wrist are derived via the method mentioned above to filter out the effects of muscle membrane and neuromuscular junction slowing, which adulterate calculated nerve velocity values. Both the above- elbow to below- elbow segment and the below- elbow to wrist segment should conduct at 50 m/s. When performing ulnar motor nerve conduction studies (Fig. 1.4) the forearm should be bent at a 45° angle, which more closely approximates its normal anatomic course. Performing ulnar motor nerve conduction studies with the elbow joint at 180° can result in "telescoping" of the nerve and its myelin upon itself, resulting in a falsely low conduction velocity being recorded. The ulnar nerve, in addition to innervating the flexor carpi ulnaris and flexor digitorum profundus muscles, innervates the abductor digiti minimi as well as a portion of the flexor pollicis brevis muscles and all the interosseous muscles of the hand. The sensory nerve action potential of the ulnar nerve is generally derived by either orthodromic stimulation of the digit 5 sensory nerve with recording over the ulnar nerve at the wrist, or antidromically as described for the median sensory nerve.

Ulnar neuropathy at the ulnar sulcus is readily demonstrated by revealing slowing in the ulnar motor nerve segment in the above- elbow to below- elbow segment, with relative preservation of the conduction velocity in the motor ulnar nerve in the below- elbow segment to wrist. In addition there is usually abnormality of the ulnar sensory nerve action potential from digit 5 noted. Usually an absent sensory

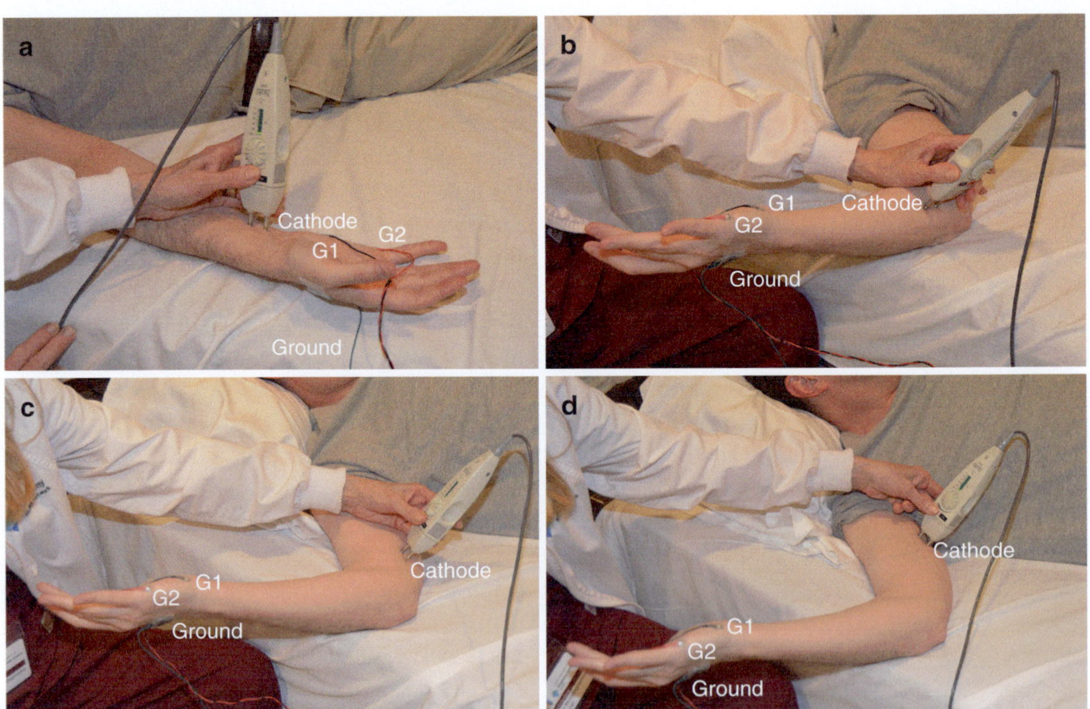

Fig. 1.4 Ulnar motor study. (**a**) Distal stimulation site over ulnar nerve at wrist. (**b**) Proximal stimulation site below elbow. (**c**) Proximal stimulation site above elbow. (**d**) Proximal stimulation site under upper arm

potential or low amplitude sensory potential accompanies ulnar neuropathy at the ulnar sulcus. In cubital tunnel syndrome, slowing in the ulnar motor nerve may not be readily perceptible. If ulnar neuropathy in general is suspected, then in addition to stimulating the ulnar motor nerve at the above elbow, below elbow and wrist segments, the ulnar nerve is serially stimulated at 1 cm intervals along the below-elbow to wrist segment in a separate graphical array available on any standard EMG nerve conduction study machine along perhaps 7–8 points. The conduction velocity along any of these 1 cm points can readily be derived, and a precise localization of pathology to a particular area in the below-segment to wrist may be identified, thus localizing in the process to the cubital tunnel. In addition, the ulnar sensory nerve action potential would be abnormal, and needle EMG of the flexor carpi ulnaris muscle (FCU) would be normal, with abnormalities seen in the needle examination via EMG of the flexor digitorum profundus muscle to digits 4 and 5, the abductor digiti minimi (ADM) muscle and the first dorsal interosseous (FDI) muscle. Thus, a combination of electromyography and ulnar nerve conduction studies, both motor and sensory, can be utilized to more precisely localize an ulnar nerve process.

One complicating factor in the electrophysiologic examination of patients with entrapment neuropathies is that there are fairly common variations in nerve innervation of voluntary muscle, particularly median and ulnar innervated muscles, by anomalous median to ulnar nerve connections in the forearm. In a study of cadavers, the anatomist Martin found anastomoses in 15% of patients, and another anatomist Gruber did as well. The former in 1763 and the latter in 1870. These common anastomoses of median to ulnar nerves, complicating, at times proper diagnosis of ulnar neuropathy and median neuropathy, have become to be known as the Martin-Gruber anastomoses. There are three main types. Upwards of 15–20% of patients with carpal tunnel syndrome may have this anastomosis, and approximately 20% of normal controls do as well. The anastomoses involve axons leaving the main trunk of the median nerve or anterior interosseous nerve and crossing through the forearm to join the main trunk of the ulnar nerve, ultimately innervating intrinsic hand muscles. Although a significant number of axons may participate in the anastomosis, all of the axons of the median nerve are not involved. The most common anastomosis is a median-to-ulnar anastomosis with innervation eventually of the 1st dorsal interosseous muscle. This is the type 2 Martin-Gruber anastomosis. It can be inherited as an autosomal dominant trait. In routine nerve conduction studies this most common Martin-Gruber anastomosis may not be found because the ADM muscle is usually the routine site of ulnar nerve recording. The type 1 Martin-Gruber anastomosis exists as the median crossing fibers to the ulnar nerve terminating in the abductor digiti minimi muscle. This can be noted on routine nerve conduction studies as a low ulnar CMAP amplitude with above-elbow stimulation and a larger CMAP with below-elbow and wrist stimulation, simulating an ulnar neuropathy at the ulnar sulcus. When this is noted on a routine nerve conduction study, the electromyographer should simply, as a general check for the crossover, stimulate the median nerve at the elbow and record over the abductor digiti minimi muscle. Without the anastomosis, there should be no CMAP found. If the anastomosis exists to the ADM muscle, then a small CMAP would be seen. This simple test can avoid over diagnosing ulnar neuropathy at the elbow potentially avoiding unnecessary surgery. The most common type of Martin-Gruber anastomosis of median nerve fibers crossing to the ulnar nerve, innervating the FDI muscle, will not present on routine nerve conduction studies. If one were to test specifically for a deep ulnar branch neuropathy which characteristically causes interosseous wasting and pain from palmar compression (i.e. often in cyclists from handlebar pressure) the recording electrode is purposely placed on the FDI muscle, this type of Martin-Gruber anastomosis will reveal itself as a larger CMAP from the FDI upon wrist stimulation than upon elbow stimulation. The least common type of Martin Gruber anastomosis (Type 3) may manifest on routine median motor conduction studies with the recording electrode on the APB muscle. It should be suspected when the CMAP of the thenar muscle is unusually larger after elbow stimulation than with wrist stimulation of the median nerve. In addition, if both carpal tunnel syndrome and this type of anastomosis co-exist, then not only will the median nerve stimulation at the elbow evoke a large CMAP with an unusual deflection pattern, but there would be and erroneously normal motor latency from the median nerve at the elbow with a prolongation of the distal motor latency and a factitiously high velocity noted in the forearm segment of the median nerve. The details of these anomalies can be left to the electromyographer, as well as the design of the study when such an anastomosis is present. These studies should be clearly explained in the summary portion of the electromyography report, not only for accurate documentation, but to avoid leading the surgeon down the path of over-diagnosing ulnar neuropathy at the ulnar sulcus and underdiagnosing median neuropathy at the wrist when the type 3 anastomosis occurs.

Conclusion

Electromyography and nerve conduction studies supplement the patient history, physical and neurological examination, and radiographic data to help the examining surgeon properly localize nerve entrapment processes, particularly when upper extremity median and ulnar nerve entrapments are suspected. These electrophysiological tests serve the patient and surgeon as well as to the correct place and timing of surgery in the management of these highly prevalent, uncomfortable, and often disabling conditions.

References

1. Padua L, Coraci D, Erra C, et al. Carpal tunnel syndrome: clinical features, diagnosis, and management. Lancet Neurol. 2016;15(12):1273–84.
2. Jablecki CK, Andary MT, Floeter MK, Miller RG, Quarterly CA, Vennix MJ, et al. Practice parameter: electrodiagnostic studies in carpal tunnel syndrome. Neurology. 2002;58:1589–92.
3. Buchtal F, Rosenfalck A, Trojaborg W. Electrophysiological findings in entrapment neuropathy of the median nerve at the wrist and elbow. J Neurol Neurosurg Psychiatry. 1974;37:340–63.
4. Brown WF, Yates SK. Cubital tunnel syndrome and ulnar neuropathy. Ann Neurol. 1980;7:289–90.
5. Ulnar neuropathy clinical presentation: history, physical examination, ulnar neuropathy at elbow. emedicine.medscape.com. 2016.
6. James GR, Grafton L. Diagnosis and treatment of tardy paralysis of the ulnar nerve: based on a study of 100 cases. J Bone Joint Surg. 1947;29:1087–97.

Ultrasound Anatomy of the Median and Ulnar Nerves

2

Antonios Kerasnoudis, Min-Suk Yoon, Georgios Barmpalios, and Aaron I. Venouziou

Introduction

Neuromuscular ultrasound is a well established, imaging method of the peripheral nervous system. It offers a holistic approach to peripheral nerve disease, adding valuable, diagnostic information to physical examination, nerve conduction studies and magnetic resonance imaging.

High frequency resolution ultrasound is commonly used in everyday practice to detect structural, peripheral nerve changes, especially in cases of entrapment, autoimmune, traumatic and neoplastic neuropathies [1–3]. The main advantages of nerve ultrasound are the non-invasive technique of examination, the good tolerance from the patients' point of view and the relative low cost.

The aim of this chapter is to present the basic topographic, ultrasound anatomy of the median and ulnar nerves and to describe the examination technique, following the example of the median and ulnar nerve, with a series of ultrasound images.

A. Kerasnoudis (✉)
Department of Neurology, St. Luke's Hospital, Panorama, Thessaloniki, Greece

M.-S. Yoon
Department of Neurology, EVK Hattingen, Hattingen, Germany

G. Barmpalios
Department of Radiology, Iatriki Diagnosi Private Imaging Centre, Serres, Greece

A. I. Venouziou
Division of Upper Extremity Surgery, Orthopaedic Department, St. Luke's Hospital, Panorama, Thessaloniki, Greece

Imaging Technique of Peripheral Nerves

General Requirements

The American Academy of Electrodiagnostic Medicine (AANEM) published in 2009 and updated, reapproved in 2014 a position statement, indicating the prerequisites for the performance and interpretation of neuromuscular ultrasound [4]. Among those requirements, the most significant are: the knowledge of the peripheral nerve and muscle anatomy, the distribution patterns of myopathic and neurological diseases and the risks and benefits of surgical and medical treatment of nerve and muscle diseases. In addition, the ability to correlate ultrasound imaging with clinical findings, including genetic, serological, histopathologic, radiographic, and electrodiagnostic tests, to understand and recommend appropriate correlative studies or to modify the examination based on real time findings are also required. Last but not least, a deep knowledge of the ultrasound equipment, ultrasound physics, technique and common artifacts are the key points for proficiency in neuromuscular ultrasound.

D. G. Sotereanos, L. K. Papatheodorou (eds.), *Compressive Neuropathies of the Upper Extremity*,
https://doi.org/10.1007/978-3-030-37289-7_2

Optimization of Sonographic Imaging

The ultrasound beam originates from mechanical oscillations of numerous crystals in a transducer, which is excited by electrical pulses (piezoelectric effect). The transducer converts one type of energy into another (electrical ↔ mechanical/sound). The resonance frequency is the one frequency at which the piezoelectric transducer is most efficient in converting electrical energy to acoustic energy and vice versa and it is determined by the thickness of the piezoelectric element.

The ultrasound waves (pulses of sound) are sent from the transducer, propagate through different tissues, and then return to the transducer as reflected echoes. The returned echoes are converted back into electrical impulses by the transducer crystals and are further processed to form the ultrasound image presented on the screen. Ultrasound waves are reflected at the surfaces between different density tissues and the reflection is proportional to the difference in impedance. If the difference in density is increased then the proportion of reflected sound is also increased, and the proportion of transmitted sound is respectively decreased.

If the difference in tissue density is very dissimilar, then the sound is completely reflected, resulting in total acoustic shadowing. Acoustic shadowing is present behind bones, calculi (stones in kidneys, gallbladder, etc.) and air (intestinal gas). Echoes are not produced if there is no density alteration in a tissue or between tissues. Homogenous fluids like blood, bile, urine, contents of simple cysts, ascites and pleural effusion are seen as echo-free structures.

The optimal visualization of peripheral nerves requires the use of a high frequency (>12 MHz) linear transducer. Modern linear transducers are designed to generate more than one frequency (broad band width), so that the examiner has the opportunity to adjust the frequency of the probe for optimal visualization of the area of interest.

Imaging of superficial structures (for example superficial sensory branch of the radial nerve) requires the application of high frequency transducers (>12 MHz), taking always into consideration, that the depth of penetration is often limited to 2–3 cm below the skin surface. On the other hand, visualization of deeper structures (for example brachial plexus in the infraclavicular region) demands the use of lower frequency transducers (<8 MHz), because they offer ultrasound penetration of 4–5 cm or more below the skin surface. However, the image resolution is often inferior to that obtained with a higher frequency transducer [5].

Additionally, the application of newest technology, such as tissue harmoning imaging or speckle reduction, improves significantly the visualization of the peripheral nerves. Another important aspect, is the evaluation of the vascularity of the nerves and their surroundings tissues, usually using color coded sonography (color Doppler or power Doppler). Color coded sonography is also helpful in localizing nerves that are often accompanied by vessels (e.g. sural nerve accompanied by lesser saphenous vein). For color Doppler, a small-flow-setting of the ultrasound device is recommended (pulse repetition frequency 500 Hz, band-pass filter 50 Hz) [5].

Imaging of Healthy Peripheral Nerves

A peripheral nerve is composed of multiple nerve fibers and connective tissue. The endoneurium is a layer of delicate connective tissue around the myelin sheath of each myelinated nerve fiber. The role of endoneurium is to supply blood capillaries to each nerve fiber. Multiple nerve fibers, targeting the same anatomical location, are bundled together and form a fascicle, which is wrapped in a fibrous perineurium. Several fascicles may be in turn bundled together with a blood supply and fatty tissue within yet another sheath, the epineurium. This grouping structure is analogous to the muscular organization system of epimysium, perimysium and endomysium.

In view of the fact that the basic unit of the peripheral nerve (neuron) is too thin to reflect an ultrasound beam, only groups of nerve fibers may be pictured with this imaging technique. On the other hand, the fibrous perineurium contains collagen, fibroblasts, blood and lymphatic vessels, and thus forms a layer, sufficiently thick to reflect ultrasound beam (hyperechogenic). The group of nerve fascicles are surrounded by the epineurium, that can be also easily seen clearly in ultrasound as a hyperechogenic layer.

The examiner evaluates peripheral nerves using two different planes, the transverse and longitudinal. In the longitudinal plane, the peripheral nerve is seen as several parallel hyperechogenic lines – representing the perineurium – between two more prominent and also hyperechogenic layers of the epineurium ("electric cable" pattern) (Fig. 2.1a). On the other hand, in the transverse plane, the nerve is seen as multiple hypoechogenic areas (nerve fascicles) with hyperechogenic rims of the epineurium ("honeycomb" pattern) (Fig. 2.1b).

In everyday practice, usually the examiner visualizes the peripheral nerve applying the transverse plane and using the so-called "elevator technique". The "elevator technique" consists of finding the nerve of interest at a characteristic anatomic point and "tracking it" either proximally or distally. In this way it is possible to evaluate at the same time multiple characteristics of the nerve, such as diameter, cross sectional area, vascularity, shape, echogenicity and its anatomic relation to the surrounding tissues. In cases of entrapment, sometimes additional longitudinal images are taken, in order to document in detail the exact anatomic point of interest.

A second important aspect is the change of echogenicity of a peripheral nerve, when moving from more proximal to distal segments. In concrete terms, the echogenicity of the nerve changes from hypo- to hyperechogenic, when followed more peripherally distally, due to the continously, increasing amount of connective tissue between the nerve bundles. In addition, the echoes received from musculoskeletal structures depend on the angle of insonation (anisotropy), therefore structures with highly fribrillar echostructure, such as tendons and ligaments, are more sensitive to transducer manipulation, than peripheral nerves. However, the property of anisotropy is seen in cases of nerves with large cross-sections [6] (Fig. 2.1c, d).

Median Nerve (C6–T1)

Introduction

The median nerve is one of the five terminal divisions of the brachial plexus. It provides motor innervation, not only to the flexors of the forearm and hand, but also to the flexion, abduction, extension and opposition of the thumb. In addition, its sensory innervation includes the dorsal aspect (nail bed) of the distal first two digits of the hand, the volar aspect of the thumb, index, middle, and half of the ring finger and the palm.

Innervation

The median nerve gives off no muscular branches until it reaches the elbow. In the anatomical space between the two heads of the pronator teres muscle, it innervates the following muscles

1. Pronator Teres (C6–C7): forearm pronator.
2. Flexor carpi radialis (C6–C7): radial flexor of the hand.
3. Palmaris longus (C7–T1): flexor of the wrist.
4. Flexor digitorum superficialis (C7–T1): flexor of the middle phalanges of the second, thirs, fourth and fifth fingers.

After it passes through the pronator teres, it gives off the anerior interosseous nerve, which innervates the following muscles:

1. Flexor pollicis longus (C7–C8): flexor of the terminal phalanx of the thumb.
2. Flexor digitorum profundus I and II (C7–C8): flexor of the terminal phalanges of the second and third fingers.
3. Pronator quadratus (C7–C8): forearm pronator.

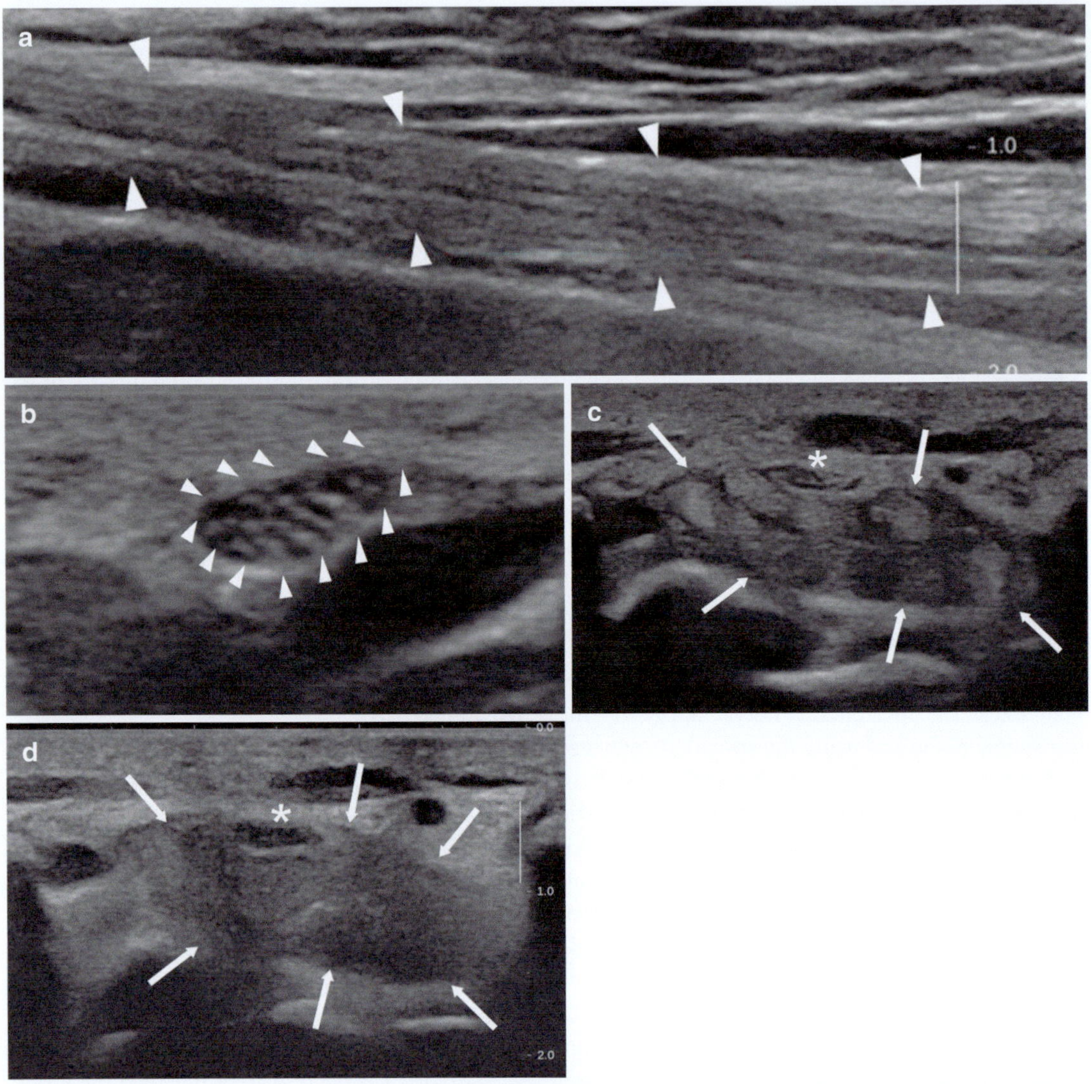

Fig. 2.1 Overview of the echogenicity of a peripheral nerve. (**a**) Longitudinal image of the median nerve showing several, parallel, hyperechogenic lines (perineurium), between two more prominent and also hyperechogenic layers of the epineurium (arrows), forming the so called "electric cable" pattern. (**b**) Transverse plane of the median nerve, showing multiple, hypoechogenic areas (nerve fascicles), with hyperechogenic rims of the epineurium (arrows), forming the so called "honeycomb" pattern. (**c**) Transverse image of the median nerve and flexor tendons in the carpal tunnel. The echoes received from musculoskeletal structures depend on the angle of insonation (anisotropy), therefore structures with highly fribrillar echostructure, such as tendons, are more sensitive to transducer manipulation, than peripheral nerves. In this image tendons are visualized hyperechoic, when compared to the median nerve (star). (**d**) Same transverse image of the median nerve and flexor tendons in the carpal tunnel, after changing the angle of insonation. Now tendons (arrows) are visualized hypoechoic, when compared to the median nerve (star)

At the distal end of the carpal tunnel the median nerve divides into its terminal branches, innervating thenar and lumbrical muscles:

1. Abductor pollicis brevis (C8–T1): abductor of the metacarpal of the thumb.
2. Opponens pollicis (C8–T1): a muscle that brings the metacarpal of the thumb into opposition.
3. Superficial head of the flexor pollicis brevis (C8–T1): flexor of the proximal phalanx of the thumb.
4. Lumbricals I and II (C8–T1): flexors of the proximal and extensors of the two distal phalanges of the second and third finger.

Topographic Ultrasound Anatomy

The median nerve is formed in the axilla, arising from the lateral (spinal segments C6–C7) and the medial cord (spinal segments C8–T1) of the brachial plexus. These roots joined in a form of letter 'Y' and embrace the third part of axillary artery [7]. Then, the nerve enters the axilla laterally to the brachial artery and crosses over to the medial side of the same vessel, descending medially to the coracobrachialis muscle down to the cubital fossa (Fig. 2.2a). Just proximally to the nerve fossa, the nerve is located posterior to the bicipital aponeurosis and anterior to the brachialis muscle (Fig. 2.2b).

The entrance of the nerve to the forearm is located between the humeral and the ulnar head of the pronator teres muscle. Exactly at this height the median nerve provides its first branch, the anterior interosseous nerve (AIN) (Fig. 2.2c). It then travels to the distal forearm, lying posterior and adherent to the flexor digitorum superficialis and anterior to the flexor digitorum profundus muscle (Fig. 2.2d). In the majority of individuals, about 5 cm proximal to the flexor retinaculum, it emerges behind the lateral margin of the flexor digitorum superficialis and becomes superficial just proximal to the wrist, lying between the tendons of flexor digitorum superficialis and flexor carpi radialis [7]. Just before passing deep to the flexor retinaculum at the wrist, it gives off the palmar cutaneous branch (Fig. 2.2e). It then passes through the carpal tunnel lying underneath the flexor retinaculum and above the flexor tendons of the digits (Fig. 2.2f). Distally to carpal tunnel it divides to its terminal branches for the thenar muscles and to the palmar digital nerves, which innervate the skin of the palmar aspect of the thumb, the second, the third and half of the fourth finger, the palm overlying the corresponding metacarpophalangeal joints and the posterior middle and distal phalanges of the second, third and half of the fourth finger.

Carpal Tunnel Syndrome

Fornage and Rifkin described for the first time the pathological ultrasound findings of CTS, opening the way for an innovative diagnostic approach to peripheral nerve disease. The most common pathological findings seen in symptomatic CTS patients are: (1) enlarged CSA of the median nerve proximal to the edge of the flexor retinaculum, (2) increased wrist to forearm swelling ratio (3) hypoechogenity and disturbed fascicular echostructure, (4) reduced slippage of the nerve and (5) increased vascularity (Fig. 2.3a–d).

Nerve conduction studies are traditionally used as the confirmatory test for the diagnosis of CTS; however, ultrasound has increasingly gained interest as an alternative diagnostic test for CTS. The diagnostic sensitivity and specificity of nerve ultrasound in the diagnosis of CTS varies among literature reports (sensitivity 77.6–91%, specificity 86.8–93%) [8–10], mainly depending on the reference standard used for the diagnosis. The cross-sectional area of the median nerve at the inlet of the carpal tunnel (at the level of the pisiform) is the most sensitive and specific ultrasound finding in patients with CTS [11]. While ultrasound will not replace electrodiagnostic testing in the diagnosis of CTS, especially in complicated or unclear cases, ultrasonography seems to provide significant improvement in the diagnostic accuracy according to a recently published evidence based guideline [12–14]. On the other hand, both the CSA enlargement and the hypervascularity detected with the Doppler technique seem to correlate with the clinical and electrophysiological severity of CTS [15].

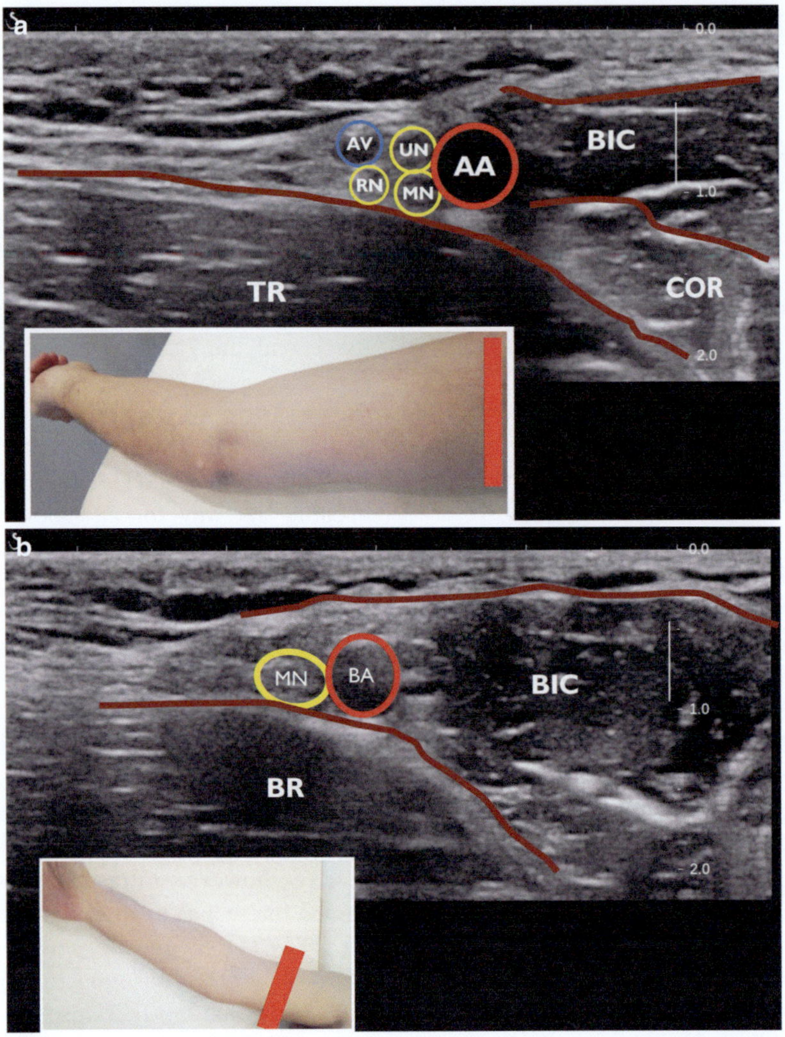

Fig. 2.2 Transverse ultrasound images of the median nerve in the axilla and upperarm. (**a**) Transverse image of the median nerve in the axilla. The median nerve (MN) is located between the axilary artery (AA) and axillary vein (AV), together with the radial (RN) and ulnar nerves (UN). The median nerve is descending medially to the coracobrachialis muscle (CB) down to the cubital fossa. BIC = biceps brachi muscle, TR = triceps brachi muscle. (**b**) Transverse image of the median nerve (MN) at the upperarm. Just proximally to the nerve fossa, the nerve is located next to the brachial artery (BA), posterior to the bicipital aponeurosis (BIC) and anterior to the brachialis muscle (BR). (**c**) Transverse image of the median nerve (MN) at the proximal forearm. The entrance of the nerve to the forearm is located between the humeral and the ulnar head of the pronator teres muscle (PT). The nerve is accompanied by the anterior, interosseous vessels (AIV). Exactly at this height the median nerve provides its first branch, the anterior interosseous nerve (AIN). RAD = radius, ULN = ulna, BRD = brachioradialis muscle, BR = brachialis muscle. (**d**) Transverse image of the median nerve (MN) at the mid-forearm. Here the nerve lies posterior and adherent to the flexor digitorum superficialis (FDS) and anterior to the flexor digitorum profundus muscle (FDP). RAD = radius, RA = radial artery, FCR = flexor carpi radialis muscle. (**e**) Transverse image of the median nerve (MN) at the distal forearm. Just before passing deep to the flexor retinaculum at the wrist, it gives off the palmar cutaneous branch (PCB). At this height the median nerve lies also posterior and adherent to the flexor digitorum superficialis (FDS) and anterior to the flexor digitorum profundus muscle (FDP). RAD = radius, RA = radial artery, FCRT = flexor carpi radialis tendon, FCUT = flexor carpi ulnaris tendon, UA = ulnar artery, UN = ulnar nerve, SC = scaphoid, LN = lunateTransverse image of the carpal tunnel. (**f**) Transverse image of the median nerve (MN) in the carpal tunnel. The nerve lies underneath the flexor retinaculum (RFL) and above the flexor tendons of the digits (FDST, FDPT). FDST = flexor digitorum superficialis tendon, FDPT = flexor digitorum profundus tendon, FCRT = flexor carpi radialis tendon, FPLT = flexor pollicis longus tendon, UA = ulnar artery, TRAP = trapezoid, CAP = capitatum, HAM = hamate

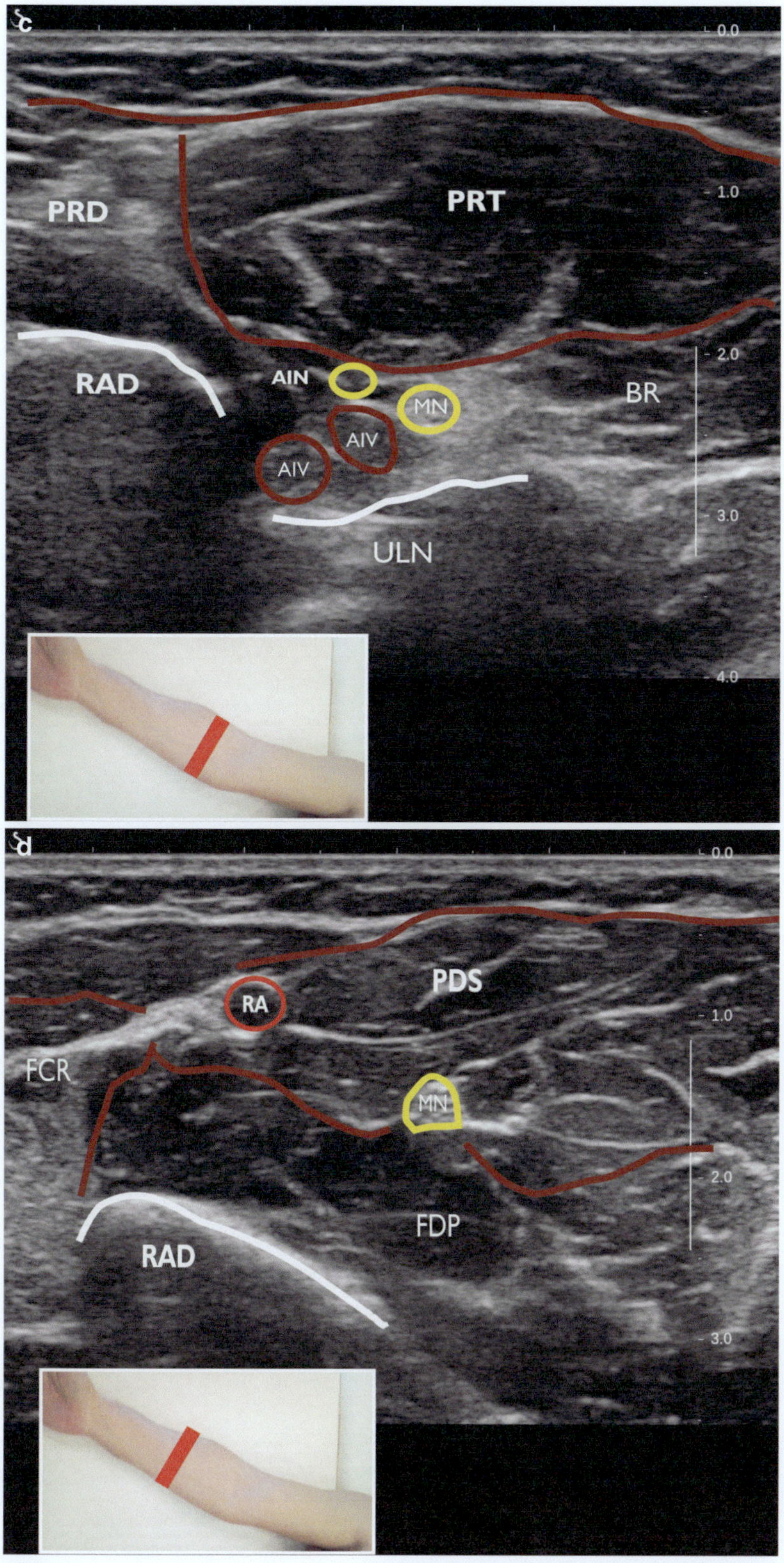

Fig. 2.2 (continued)

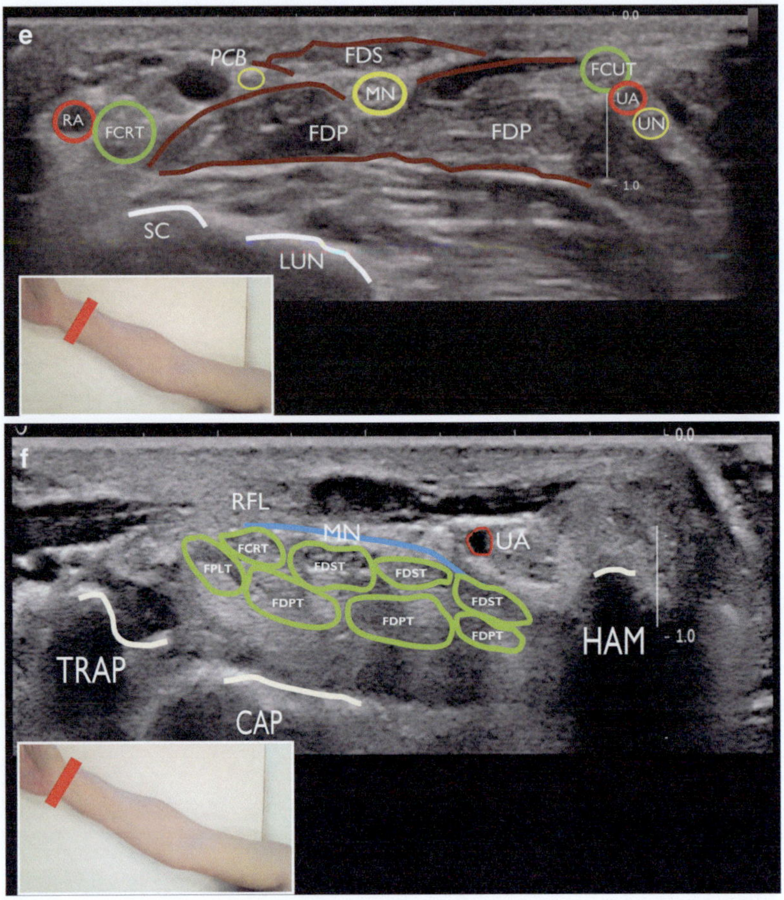

Fig. 2.2 (continued)

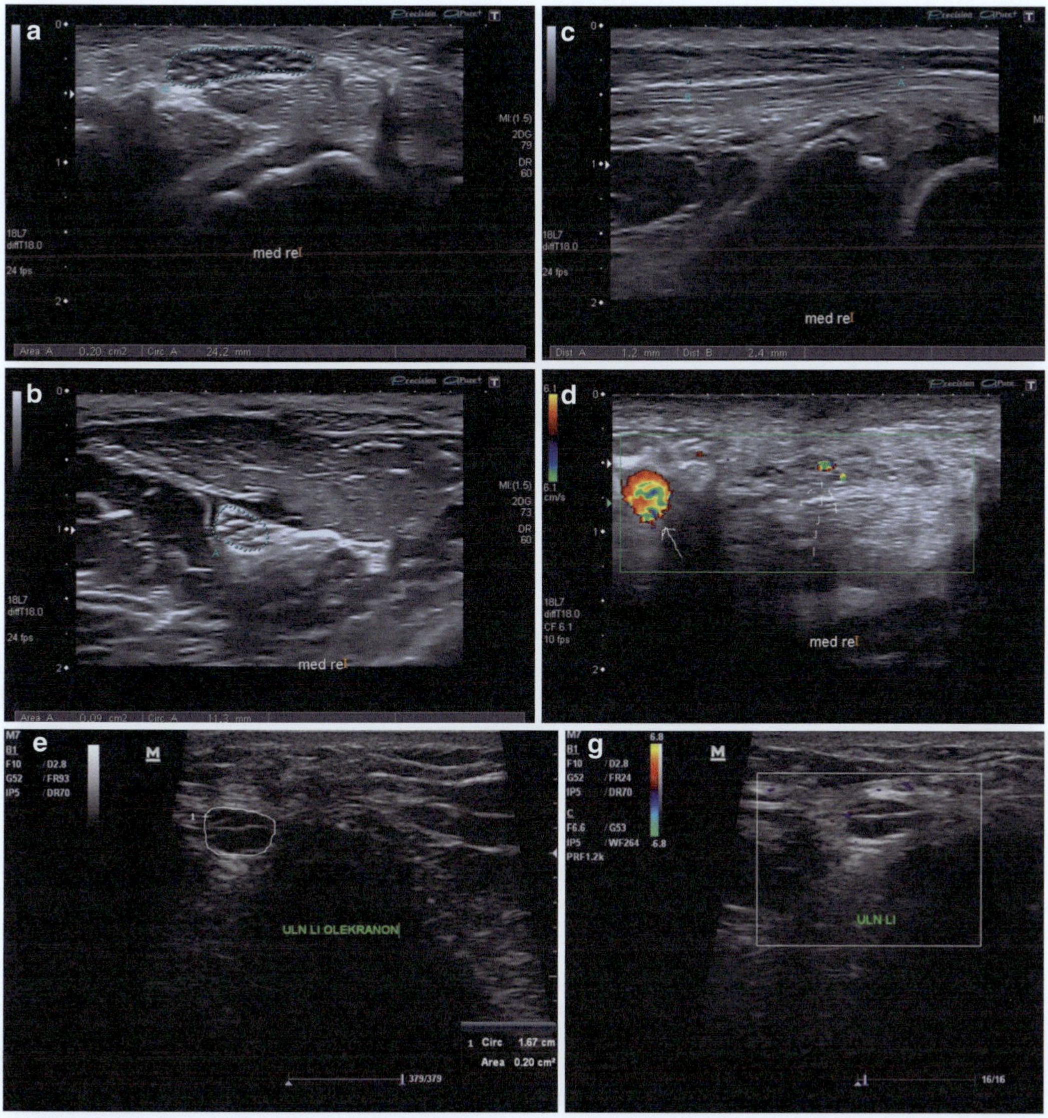

Fig. 2.3 Overview of the ultrasound findings in a patient with carpal (CTS) and cubital tunnel syndrome (CUTS). (**a**) Axial scan of the median nerve just proximal to the carpal tunnel, showing a pathological cross sectional area enlargement (CSA = 0.20 cm^2, normal values ≤0.11 cm^2) with relatively preserved fascicular echostructure, (**b**) axial scan of the median nerve in the middle forearm (between the flexor digitorum superficialus and profundus), showing the pathological wrist to forearm ratio = 0.20/0.09 = 2.22 (normal values <1.4), (**c**) longitudinal scan of the median nerve just proximal to carpal tunnel showing the site of entrapment, (**d**) colour duplex mode showing the hyervascularity of the median nerve in the carpal tunnel (dotted arrow) and the ulnar artery located near the nerve (continuous arrow), (**e**) Axial scan of the ulnar nerve in the cubital tunnel, showing a pathological cross sectional area enlargement (CSA = 0.20 cm^2, normal values ≤0.11 cm^2). The disturbed fascicular echostructure and the increase of the echogenicity of the epineurium, as sign of possible luxation are also noteworthy (**f**) longitudinal scan of the ulnar nerve in the cubital tunnel showing the pathological enlargement and the increase of the echogenicity of the epineurium, as sign of possible luxation, (**g**) axial, colour dupplex assessment of the ulnar nerve, showing absent signs of increased vascularity (**h**) longitudinal scan of the ulnar nerve in the cubital tunnel, showing the exact point of entrapment

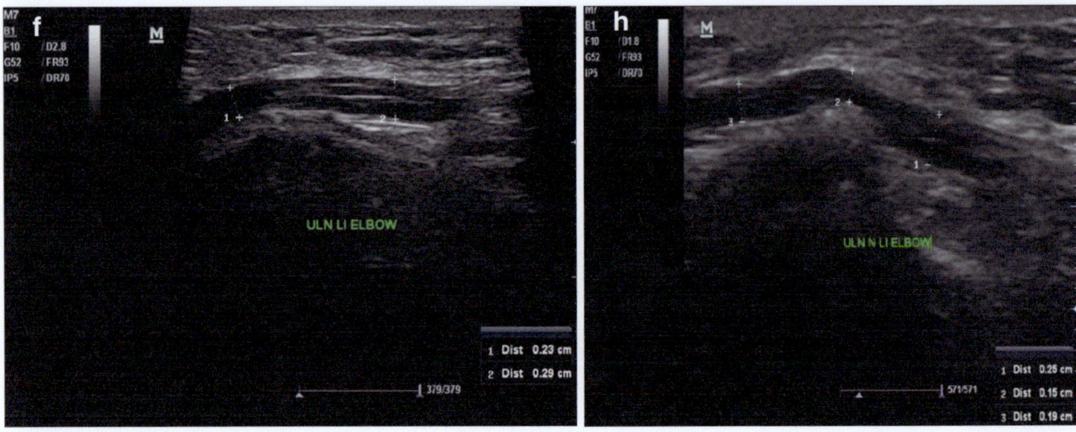

Fig. 2.3 (continued)

Ulnar Nerve (C7–T1)

Introduction

The ulnar nerve is an extension of the medial cord of the brachial plexus. It is a mixed nerve, that supplies innervation to forearm and hand muscles, but also provides sensation over the medial half of the fourth digit and the entire fifth digit (the ulnar aspect of the palm) and the ulnar portion of the posterior aspect of the hand (dorsal ulnar cutaneous distribution).

Topographic Ultrasound Anatomy

The ulnar nerve is the terminal branch of the medial cord, from the nerve roots of C8–T1 and sometimes C7. The nerve enters the axilla and descends along the medial aspect of the arm, being located medial to biceps brachii and anterior to brachialis muscles (Fig. 2.4a). Directly at the height of the coracobrachialis muscle, the ulnar nerve pierces the medial intermuscular septum and enters the posterior compartment of the arm. Here, the nerve lies on the anterior aspect of the medial head of the triceps, together with the superior ulnar collateral artery (Fig. 2.4b). The medial intermuscular septum extends from the coracobrachialis proximally, where it is a thin and weak structure, to the medial humeral epicondyle, where it is a thick, distinct structure [16].

In the majority of individuals the ulnar nerve passes under the arcade of Struthers. At this point, it must be clarified, that the Struthers' ligament and the arcade of Struthers are two different anatomical structures, that are often confused. The Struthers' ligament was first described by the anatomist John Struthersin 1854 [17]. It is a fibrous band, which is found in 1% of the population and extends from the supracondylar process and to the medial humeral epicondyle. From an anatomical point of view, it usually passes over the median nerve and the brachial artery, sometimes causing entrapment of these structures. It may be observed even in the absence of the supracondylar process; even when present, it may not cause the compression of these structures [17]. On the other hand, the arcade of Struthers was first described in 1973 by Kane et al. [18]. This arcade normally derives from the brachial fascia, but in rare cases it can appear as an aponeurotic or musculoaponeurotic structure extending from the medial intermuscular septa to the medial head of the triceps brachii muscle, at a variable distance above the medial humeral epicondyle [19] (Fig. 2.4c). This area is not usually a site for constriction of the nerve, however it can become so if an anterior transposition of the nerve is performed, in

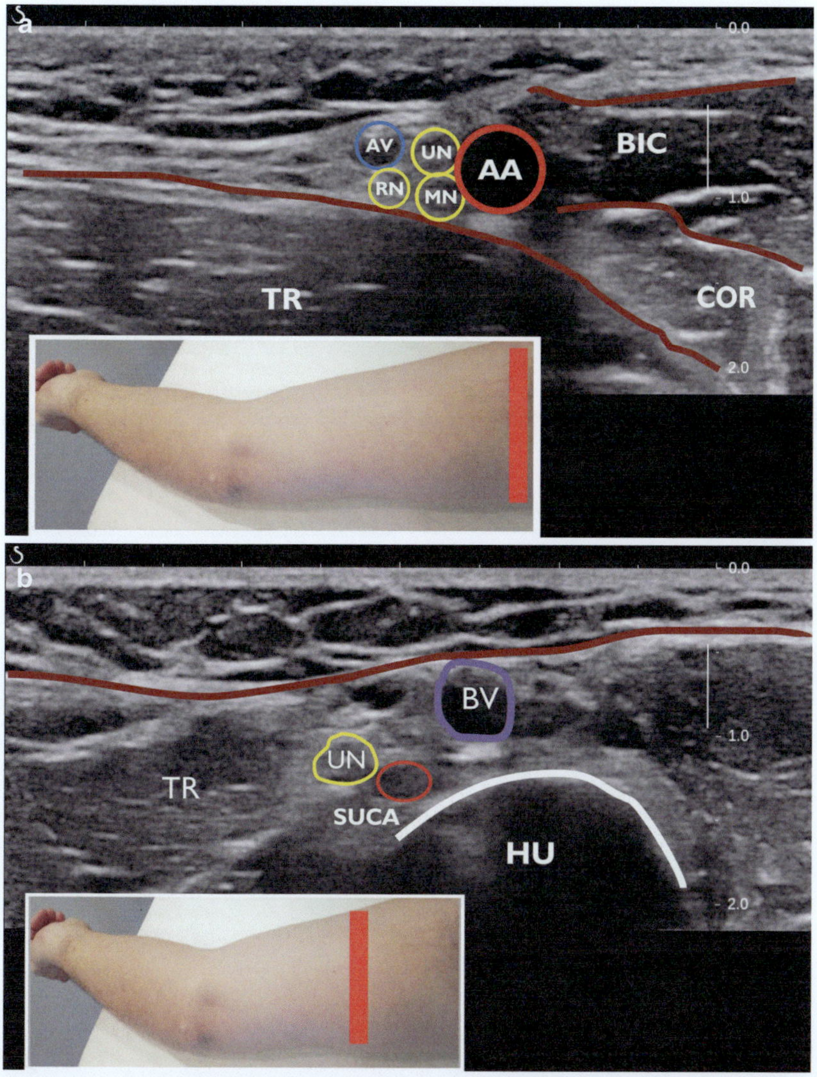

Fig. 2.4 Transverse ultrasound images of the ulnar nerve in the axilla and upperarm. (**a**) Transverse image of the ulnar nerve in the axilla. The nerve enters the axilla and descends along the medial aspect of the arm, being located medial to biceps brachii (BIC) and anterior to brachialis muscles (BR). Directly at the height of the coracobrachialis muscle (CB), the ulnar nerve pierces the medial intermuscular septum and enters the posterior compartment of the arm. AA = Axilary artery, AV = axillary vein, RN = radial nerve, MN = median nerve (M), TR = triceps brachi muscle. (**b**) Transverse image of the ulnar nerve (UN) in the posterior compartment of the upper arm. Here, the nerve lies on the anterior aspect of the medial head of the triceps (TR), together with the superior ulnar collateral artery (SUCA). HUM = Humerus, BV = basilar vein. (**c**) Transverse image of the ulnar nerve (UN) in the arcade of Struthers (SA). The arcade of Struthers normally derives from the brachial fascia, but in rare cases it can appear as an aponeurotic or musculoaponeurotic structure extending from the medial intermuscular septa (MIS) to the medial head of the triceps brachii muscle (TR). HU = Humerus. (**d**) Transverse image of the ulnar nerve (UN) in the cubital tunnel. The deep forearm investing fascia of the flexor carpi ulnaris and the arcuate ligament of Osborne (arrows), also known as the cubital tunnel retinaculum, form the roof of the cubital tunnel. EM = medial epicondyle, ON = olecranon. (**e**) Transverse image of the ulnar nerve (UN) in the proximal forearm. The ulnar nerve enters the forearm in the anatomical space between the two heads of flexor carpi ulnaris (FCU) and crosses the oblique ulnar collateral ligament. The ligament of Spinner (LS) is an additional aponeurosis between the flexor digitorum superficialis (FDS) of the ring finger and the humeral head of the flexor carpi ulnaris. FDP = flexor digitorum profundus, UA = ulnar artery

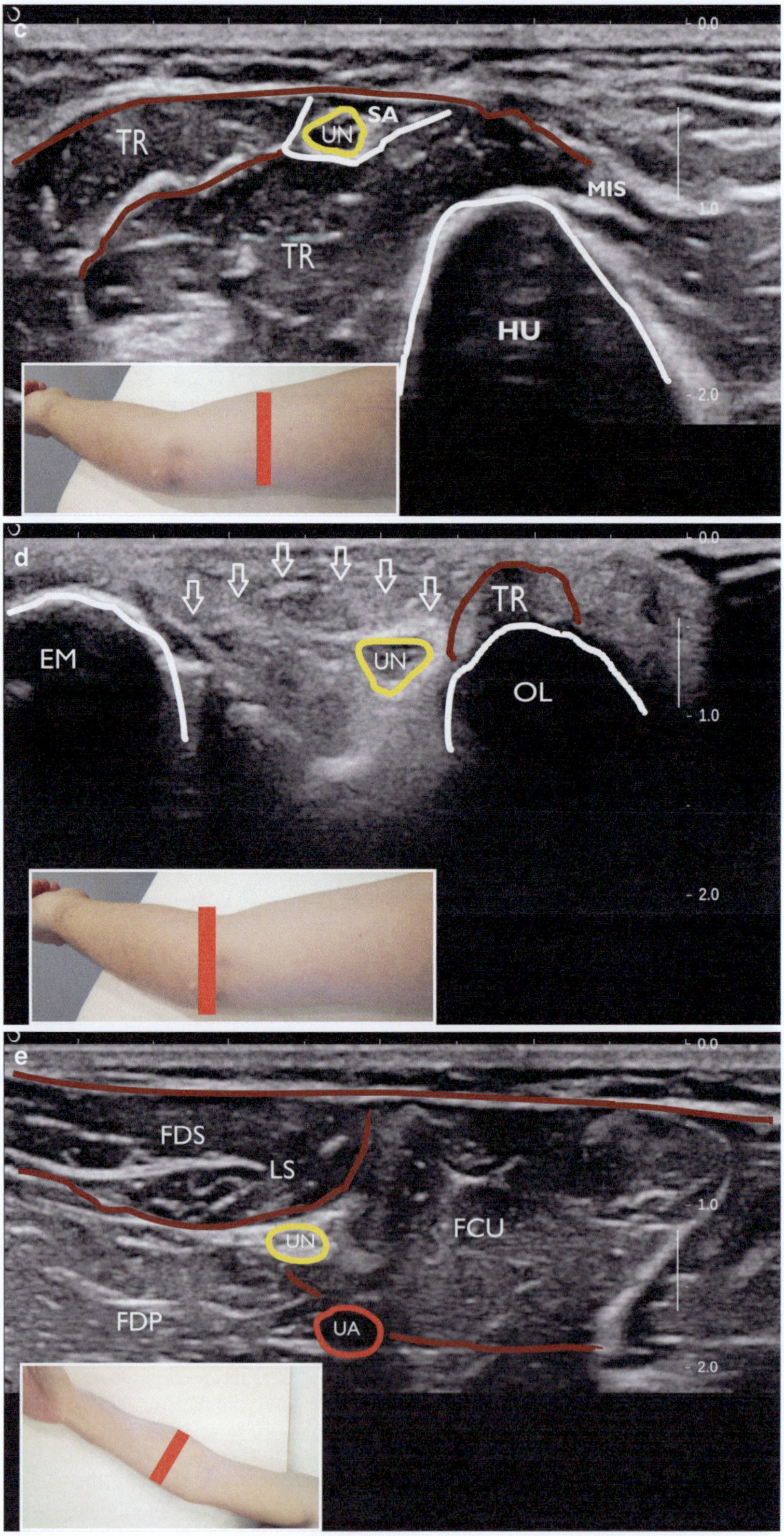

Fig. 2.4 (continued)

which case the surgeon should release the arcade if it appears under tension.

Then, the ulnar nerve enters the cubital tunnel, an anatomical space consisting of the following: the medial epicondyle (medial border), the olecranon (lateral border), the elbow capsule at the posterior aspect of the ulnar collateral ligament (floor), the Osborne ligament (roof). In the majority of the cases, both the deep forearm investing fascia of the flexor carpi ulnaris and the arcuate ligament of Osborne, also known as the cubital tunnel retinaculum, form the roof of the cubital tunnel. In addition, in 9% of the people undergoing cubital tunnel surgery an aberrant muscle, called anconeus epitrochlearis, may be found [17]. During elbow flexion, this muscle may insert on the olecranon, causing narrowing of the cubital tunnel and therefore entrapment of the ulnar nerve (Fig. 2.4d).

The ulnar nerve enters the forearm in the anatomical space between the two heads of flexor carpi ulnaris and crosses the oblique ulnar collateral ligament (Fig. 2.4e). It gives articular branches to elbow joint and passes through the cubital tunnel bordered by the medial epicondyle of the humerus, the olecranon process of ulna and tendinous arch joining the two heads of flexor carpi ulnaris. The ligament of Spinner is an additional aponeurosis between the flexor digitorum superficialis of the ring finger and the humeral head of the flexor carpi ulnaris. This septum is independent of the other aponeuroses and attaches directly to the medial epicondyle and the medial surface of the coronoid process of the ulna. With anterior transposition of the ulnar nerve, it is important to recognize and to release this structure to prevent kinking.

In the forearm, the ulnar nerve gives motor branches to the flexor carpi ulnaris and the flexor digitorum profundus of the ring and small fingers (Fig. 2.5a). The ulnar nerve may give as many as 4 branches to the flexor carpi ulnaris, ranging from 4 cm above to 10 cm below the medial epicondyle. Proximal dissection of the first motor branch to the flexor carpi ulnaris from the ulnar nerve may be performed up to 6.7 cm proximal to the medial epicondyle, facilitating anterior transposition of the nerve.

Posterior branches of the medial antebrachial cutaneous nerves cross the ulnar nerve anywhere from 6 cm proximal to 4 cm distal to the medial epicondyle. These branches are often injured during cubital tunnel release, creating an area of dysesthesia or resulting in neuroma formation.

As the ulnar nerve courses down the forearm toward the wrist, the dorsal ulnar cutaneous nerve arises from the main branch (Fig. 2.5b). A little further down, the palmar cutaneous branch takes off. Neither of these two branches go through the Guyon's canal. The remainder branch of the ulnar nerve enters the canal at the proximal portion of the wrist. This is bounded proximally and distally by the pisiform and the hook of the hamate (Fig. 2.5b). It is covered by the volar carpal ligament and the palmaris brevis.

The deep terminal branches innervate the vast majority of intrinsic hand muscles. These include all the interossei (3 palmar and 4 dorsal), the medial two lumbricals, and adductor pollicis. Hence, when considering the ulnar and median nerve, they should be considered a pair, with the median nerve doing the majority of the innervation in the forearm, and the ulnar nerve doing the majority of the innervation in the hand.

The superficial branch of the ulnar nerve supplies the palmar aspect of the little finger and the ulnar half of the ring finger and medial palmar skin. The dorsal cutaneous branch supplies the medial half of the dorsal surface and one and a half ulnar fingers dorsally. The palmar sensation is provided by the palmar cutaneous branch, which also supplies palmar aponeurosis.

Cubital Tunnel Syndrome

Cubital tunnel syndrome (CUTS) remains the second most common entrapment neuropathy after CTS. Although nerve conduction studies offer a 78% diagnostic sensitivity in cases with CUTS, the addition of nerve ultrasound may increase this to 98% [20]. The main ultrasound findings of CUTS are: (1) increased CSA of the ulnar nerve between olecranon and medial epicondyle and (2) increased elbow-to upper arm swelling ratio, showing a sensitivity of 80% [20, 21] (Fig. 2.3e–h). In addition, nerve ultrasound has been shown to make the diagnosis of CUTS

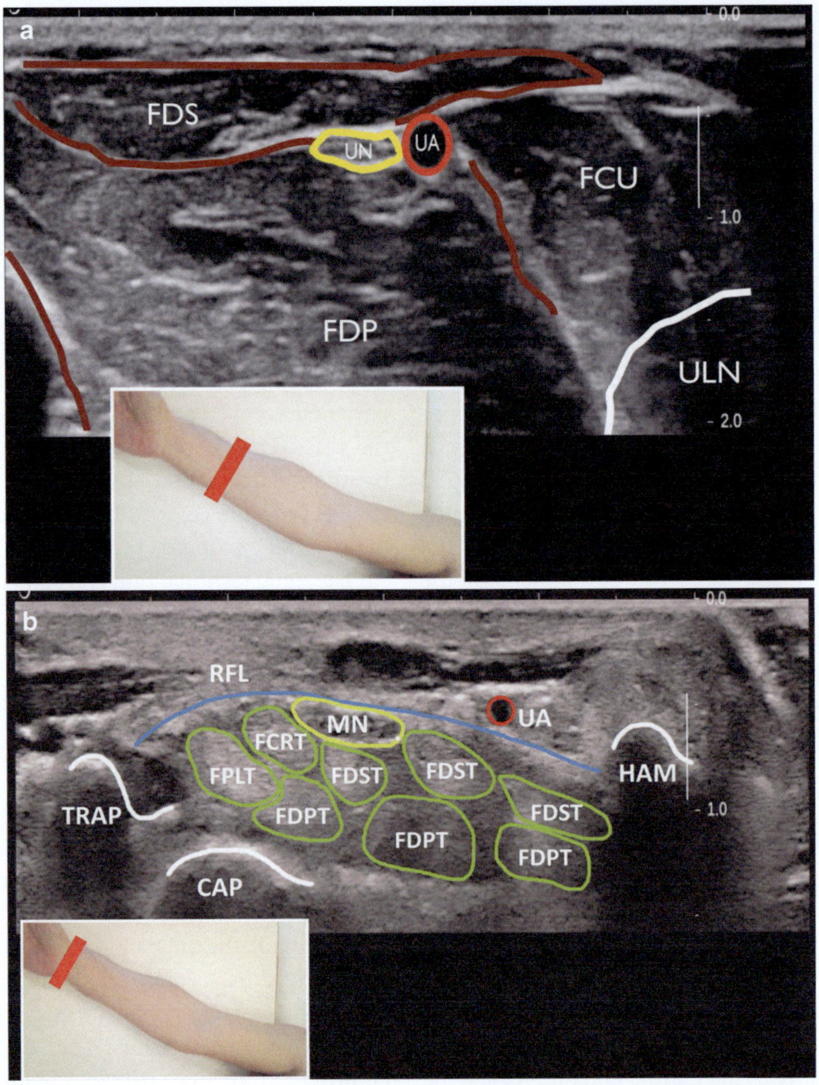

Fig. 2.5 Transverse ultrasound images of the ulnar nerve at the forearm and Guyon's canal. (**a**) Transverse image of the ulnar nerve (UN) at the proximal forearm. The nerve lies just next to the ulnar artery (UA), between the flexor carpi ulnaris (FCU) and the flexor digitorum profundus (FDP) of the ring and small fingers muscles. FDS = flexor digitorum superficialis muscle. (**b**) Transverse image of the ulnar nerve (UN) in Guyon's canal. The ulnar nerve enters the Guyon's canal at the proximal portion of the wrist, lying next to the ulnar artery (UA). This is bounded proximally and distally by the pisiform (PIS) and the hook of the hamate. It is covered by the volar carpal ligament (small blue line) and the palmaris brevis. MN = median nerve, FDST = flexor digitorum superficialis tendon, FDPT = flexor digitorum profundus tendon, FCRT = flexor carpi radialis tendon, FPLT = flexor pollicis longus tendon, SC = scaphoid, CAP = capitatum, RA = radial artery

possible in cases with typical clinical signs, but normal electrodiagnostic findings [22]. Considering the classification of severity, CSA seems to correlate significantly with the severity of CUTS, as defined via nerve conduction studies [23, 24]. According to a recent study from Simon et al, ulnar nerve CSA and hypoechoic fraction were significantly increased in patients with CUTS immediately distal and proximal to the medial epicondyle [25] The authors highlighted also, that CSA and hypoechoic fraction of individual segments did not correlate with corresponding latencies on inching studies. In view of these findings, the authors concluded, that ultrasound abnormalities may not be maximal at the site of electrophysiological nerve dysfunction and may reflect secondary pathophysiological changes in segments adjacent to regions of nerve compression [25].

Furthermore, neuromuscular ultrasound often highlights the underlying cause of ulnar neuropathy, such as structural abnormalities, ganglia or osteophytes [20], while increased intraneural vascularity has been reported in 15% of patients with CUTS [26]. The incidence of luxation/subluxation seems not to differ among patients with CUTS and normal subjects and therefore no etiological association between these two entities is documented yet [27].

Conclusion

New challenges continuously arise on how to obtain the best static and dynamic imaging of the pertinent nerve structures in different types of immune-mediated and entrapment nerve disorders, aiming to provide a complementary and holistic approach to nerve impairment. A detailed knowledge of the normal, ultrasound findings in the median and ulnar nerves, is a prerequisite for understanding peripheral nerve disorders of the upper extremity. This chapter describes in detail the basics to understand the topology and the basic principles of ultrasound neuroimaging in healthy individuals.

References

1. Kerasnoudis A, Tsivgoulis G. Nerve ultrasound in peripheral neuropathies: a review. J Neuroimaging. 2015;25(4):528–38.
2. Fisse AL, Pitarokoili K, Trampe N, Motte J, Kerasnoudis A, Gold R, Yoon MS. Clinical, sonographic, and electrophysiologic longitudinal features of chronic inflammatory demyelinating polyneuropathy. J Neuroimaging. 2019;29(2):223–32. https://doi.org/10.1111/jon.12579.
3. Walker FO, Cartwright MS, Alter KE, Visser LH, Hobson-Webb LD, Padua L, Strakowski JA, Preston DC, Boon AJ, Axer H, van Alfen N, Tawfik EA, Wilder-Smith E, Yoon JS, Kim BJ, Breiner A, Bland JDP, Grimm A, Zaidman CM. Indications for neuromuscular ultrasound: expert opinion and review of the literature. Clin Neurophysiol. 2018;129(12):2658–79.
4. Walker FO, Alter KE, Boon AJ, Cartwright MS, Flores VH, Hobson-Webb LD, Hunt CH, Primack SJ, Shook SJ. Qualifications for practitioners of neuromuscular ultrasound: position statement of the American Association of Neuromuscular and Electrodiagnostic Medicine. Muscle Nerve. 2010;42(3):442–4.
5. Kele H. Ultrasonography of the peripheral nervous system. In: Bartels E, Bartels S, Poppert H, editors. New trends in neurosonology and cerebral hemodynamics – an update, vol. 1. Munich: Elsevier; 2012. p. 417–21.
6. Kowalska B, Sudoł-Szopińska I. Normal and sonographic anatomy of selected peripheral nerves. Part I: sonohistology and general principles of examination, following the example of the median nerve. J Ultrason. 2012;12(49):120–30.
7. Arquez HF, Hurtado DKA. An anatomical study of formation of the median nerve. J Chem Pharm Res. 2016;8(5):22–6.
8. Fu T, Cao M, Liu F, et al. Carpal tunnel syndrome assessment with ultrasonography: value of inlet-to-outlet median nerve area ratio in patients versus healthy volunteers. PLoS One. 2015;10(1):e0116777.
9. Paliwal PR, Therimadasamy AK, Chan YC, Wilder-Smith EP. Does measuring the median nerve at the carpal tunnel outlet improve ultrasound CTS diagnosis? J Neurol Sci. 2014;339(1–2):47–51.
10. Tai TW, Wu CY, Su FC, Chern TC, Jou IM. Ultrasonography for diagnosing carpal tunnel syndrome: a meta-analysis of diagnostic test accuracy. Ultrasound Med Biol. 2012;38(7):1121–8.
11. Fowler JR, Gaughan JP, Ilyas AM. The sensitivity and specificity of ultrasound for the diagnosis of carpal tunnel syndrome: a meta-analysis. Clin Orthop Relat Res. 2011;469(4):1089–94.
12. Azami A, Maleki N, Anari H, Iranparvar Alamdari M, Kalantarhormozi M, Tavosi Z. The diagnostic value of ultrasound compared with nerve conduction velocity in carpal tunnel syndrome. Int J Rheum Dis. 2014;17(6):612–20.
13. Cartwright MS, Hobson-Webb LD, Boon AJ, American Association of Neuromuscular and Electrodiagnostic Medicine, et al. Evidence-based guideline: neuromuscular ultrasound for the diagnosis of carpal tunnel syndrome. Muscle Nerve. 2012;46(2):287–93.
14. Mhoon JT, Juel VC, Hobson-Webb LD. Median nerve ultrasound as a screening tool in carpal tunnel syndrome: correlation of cross-sectional area measures with electrodiagnostic abnormality. Muscle Nerve. 2012;46(6):871–8.
15. Kim JM, Kim MW, Ko YJ. Correlating ultrasound findings of carpal tunnel syndrome with nerve conduction studies. Muscle Nerve. 2013;48(6):905–10.
16. Struthers J. On some points in the abnormal anatomy of the arm. Br Foreign Med Chir Rev. 1854;14:170–9.
17. Caetano EB, Sabongi Neto JJ, Vieira LA, Caetano MF. The arcade of Struthers: an anatomical

study and clinical implications. Rev Bras Ortop. 2017;52(3):331–6.
18. Kane E, Kaplan EB, Spinner M. Observations on the course of the ulnar nerve in the arm. Ann Chir. 1973;27:487–96.
19. Spinner M, Kaplan EB. The relationship of the ulnar nerve to the medial intermuscular septum in the arm and its clinical significance. Hand. 1976;8:239–42.
20. Beekman R, Van Der Plas JP, Uitdehaag BM, et al. Clinical, electrodiagnostic, and sonographic studies in ulnar neuropathy at the elbow. Muscle Nerve. 2004;30:202–8.
21. Beekman R, Schoemaker MC, Van Der Plas JP, et al. Diagnostic value of high-resolution sonography in ulnar neuropathy at the elbow. Neurology. 2004;62(5):767–73.
22. Yoon JS, Walker FO, Cartwright MS. Ulnar neuropathy with normal electrodiagnosis and abnormal nerve ultrasound. Arch Phys Med Rehabil. 2010;91(2):318–20.
23. Bayrak AO, Bayrak IK, Turker H, et al. Ultrasonography in patients with ulnar neuropathy at the elbow: comparison of cross-sectional area and swelling ratio with electrophysiological severity. Muscle Nerve. 2010;41:661–6.
24. Mondelli M, Filippou G, Frediani B, Aretini A. Ultrasonography in ulnar neuropathy at the elbow: relationships to clinical and electrophysiological findings. Neurophysiol Clin. 2008;38:217–26.
25. Simon NG, Ralph JW, Poncelet AN, et al. A comparison of ultrasonographic and electrophysiologic 'inching' in ulnar neuropathy at the elbow. Clin Neurophysiol. 2015;126(2):391–8.
26. Frijlink DW, Brekelmans GJ, Visser LH. Increased nerve vascularization detected by color Doppler sonography in patients with ulnar neuropathy at the elbow indicates axonal damage. Muscle Nerve. 2013;47(2):188–93.
27. Van Den Berg PJ, Pompe SM, Beekman R, Visser LH. Sonographic incidence of ulnar nerve (sub) luxation and its associated clinical and electrodiagnostic characteristics. Muscle Nerve. 2013; 47(6):849–55.

3 Diagnosis and Clinical Presentation of Carpal Tunnel Syndrome

John R. Fowler

Introduction

Carpal tunnel syndrome (CTS) is the most common entrapment neuropathy with a bimodal age distribution of 50–54 and 75–84 years of age [1, 2] The majority of cases are idiopathic and genetic predisposition has been found to be the strongest predictor for development of carpal tunnel syndrome [3].

Carpal tunnel syndrome, by definition, is a constellation of signs and symptoms. However, it is unclear how many or what combination of signs and/or symptoms a patient must have in order to make the diagnosis. Expert physicians may reasonably disagree on the presence or absence of CTS in some cases. The lack of a clear reference standard makes research on the diagnosis and outcomes of carpal tunnel syndrome more difficult.

Symptoms may include paresthesia and/or anesthesia of the radial three and a half fingers, weakness of the thenar muscles, and nocturnal symptoms. Signs may include a Tinel sign, Phalen test, compression test, increased two-point discrimination, increased Semmes-Weinstein monofilament testing, atrophy and/or weakness of the thenar musculature, and many other physical examination findings. It is important to recognize that any one sign or symptom, in isolation, has a low sensitivity and specificity for diagnosis of carpal tunnel syndrome [4]. Multiple studies have demonstrated that additional diagnostic testing in cases of "classic" carpal tunnel syndrome adds little additional value [5, 6].

The purpose of this chapter is to review the clinical presentation of carpal tunnel syndrome and to review the clinical and diagnostic tests that are commonly utilized to make the diagnosis of carpal tunnel syndrome.

Clinical Presentation

The classic presentation of carpal tunnel syndrome is numbness and paresthesias in the radial three and a half fingers. The symptoms are often exacerbated at night and with activities that require wrist flexion such as driving, knitting, etc. As the syndrome becomes more advanced, patients may experience weakness of the thenar muscles and clumsiness of the hand. Pain is not typically considered to be part of classic carpal tunnel syndrome, although the "pins and needles" sensation can certainly be interpreted as painful. In addition, in patients where the main driver of nerve compression is flexor tendonitis/tenosynovitis, these patients may complain of radiating pain into the forearm and/or hand.

J. R. Fowler (✉)
Department of Orthopaedics, University of Pittsburgh Medical Center, Pittsburgh, PA, USA
e-mail: fowlerjr@upmc.edu

D. G. Sotereanos, L. K. Papatheodorou (eds.), *Compressive Neuropathies of the Upper Extremity*,
https://doi.org/10.1007/978-3-030-37289-7_3

Compression of the median nerve within the carpal tunnel results in decreased epineural blood flow, edema, and changes in nerve conduction [7, 8]. The majority of cases are idiopathic, meaning there is not an identifiable systemic, anatomic, or traumatic etiology [7]. Systemic conditions with known associations with carpal tunnel syndrome include amyloidosis, renal failure, diabetes, hypothyroidism, congestive heart failure, obesity, rheumatologic conditions (rheumatoid arthritis, lupus, scleroderma), vitamin deficiencies, and alcoholism [7, 9]. Anatomic causes can include space occupying lesions such as ganglions, lipomas, neurofibromas, schwannomas and other rare tumors. Anomalous muscles may be present in the carpal tunnel and include the palmaris profundus, extra slips of the flexor pollicis longus, and a more proximal origin of the lumbricals. A persistent median artery is also described as a potential anatomic variation that can result in carpal tunnel syndrome. Traumatic etiologies include median nerve contusion from a distal radius fracture and/or perilunate dislocation, distal radius malunion, and post-traumatic arthritic changes [7].

Certain activities have been postulated as contributing to carpal tunnel syndrome. Typing is probably the most widely cited in the lay press, however, several large studies have failed to find a difference in the rates of carpal tunnel syndrome in patients who type and those who do not [10, 11]. Occupations with vibrational exposure and those which require a high volume of repeated heavy grasp appear to have more clear associations with carpal tunnel syndrome [10, 11].

Physical Examination

The physical examination shoulder should start with inspection. The entire arm should be inspected for signs of atrophy, color changes, and differences in skin moisture. The cervical spine is evaluated for range of motion, tenderness to palpation, and a Spurling's maneuver is performed to determine if cervical radiculopathy is present. Examination for thoracic outlet syndrome should also be considered. This may include shoulder abduction, external rotation, and asking the patient to inhale deeply (Wright's test) and having the patient extend his/her neck, look toward the affected side, and take a deep breath (Adson's test). A positive test would be reproduction of the patient's symptoms with the maneuver.

Sensation in the digits is evaluated using Semmes-Weinstein monofilament testing and 2-point discrimination. Semmes-Weinstein is a threshold sensory test and has been shown to have a sensitivity of 91% and specificity of 80% for CTS [12, 13]. Numerous provocative maneuvers have been described for carpal tunnel syndrome. It is important to note that, individually, the provocative maneuvers have low specificity and sensitivity for CTS [4]. Percussion of the median nerve resulting in radiating paresthesias to the median nerve distribution represents a positive Tinel's sign. Flexion of the wrist for 60 seconds that results in paresthesias in the median nerve distribution represents a positive Phalen's test. Durkan's compression test involves compression of the median nerve within the carpal tunnel for 30 seconds. A positive test is reproduction of paresthesias in the median nerve distribution. MacKinnon described the scratch collapse test, where the examiner asks the patient to bilaterally externally rotate the shoulder with the shoulder abducted, elbow flexed to 90°, wrist in neutral, and shoulder in neutral rotation while the examiner applies an internal rotation force. The examiner then scratches over the carpal tunnel on the affected side and repeats the internal rotation force against patient resistance [14]. In patients with carpal tunnel syndrome, the patient "collapses" against the internal rotation force on the affected side, but not the unaffected side. Follow-up studies have questioned the diagnostic ability of this test [15].

Clinical Diagnostic Tools

In an effort to standardize the physical examination and to determine which combination of history and physical examination findings were most predictive of carpal tunnel syndrome, a number of diagnostic tools have been developed. The Katz hand diagram was one of the first attempts to standardize findings from the history and physical examination and to compare the constellation of these findings to the results of EMG/NCS [16]. Subjects were provided with a hand diagram and asked to mark the areas on the diagram corresponding to their symptoms. Subjects also underwent moving 2-point discrimination testing, assessment for thenar atrophy, thumb abduction strength testing, Phalen test, Tinel sign, and EMG/NCS. After multivariate regression, only the Tinel sign and hand diagram were significant predictors in the model. The authors found that subjects older than 55 with a positive Tinel sign had a positive EMG/NCS in 89% of cases while subjects young than 40 with a positive Tinel sign had a positive EMG/NCS in 71% of cases [16]. Levine et al. developed a self-administered questionnaire, now known as the Levine-Katz or Boston Carpal Tunnel Questionnaire [17]. This questionnaire assesses both functional and symptom severity. The questionnaire has been shown to be reproducible, internally consistent, and sensitive to change after treatment [17].

The CTS-6 was developed by Graham and colleagues to determine the probability of carpal tunnel syndrome based on the presence or absence of 6 criteria (Table 3.1). The authors started with 57 signs and symptoms associated with carpal tunnel syndrome and an expert panel ranked them in order of importance. The top 8 criteria were then used to create 256 unique case presentations. An expert panel made a binary decision as to whether each case represented carpal tunnel syndrome. A logistic regression model was created and it was determined that only 6 of the criteria contributed to the model. A CTS-6 score of 12 represents an 80% probability for a diagnosis of carpal tunnel syndrome. The CTS-6 was found to have a higher sensitivity and specificity than EMG/NCS using latent class analysis [18] and has been used as the reference standard in a prospective study comparing EMG/NCS and ultrasound for diagnosis of carpal tunnel syndrome [19].

Table 3.1 CTS-6

Finding	Points
Numbness predominately or exclusively in median nerve territory	3.5
Nocturnal numbness	4
Thenar atrophy and/or weakness	5
Positive Phalen test	5
Loss of 2-point discrimination	4.5
Positive Tinel sign	4

Several other clinical diagnostic tools have been developed. Lo et al. developed a clinical prediction rule which included the following components: gender, duration of symptoms, nocturnal symptoms, neck pain, wrist pain, median nerve sensory symptoms, abductor pollicis brevis (APB) weakness, thenar atrophy, and pinprick sensation [20]. Point values were assigned to each component, some with negative points (neck pain, wrist pan, and female gender), and a higher total point score was found to have a higher probability of having a positive electromyogram (EMG)/nerve conduction study (NCS). Wainner and colleagues developed a clinical prediction rule which included five variables: hand shaking improves symptoms, a wrist-ratio >0.67 (calculated by dividing the anteroposterior diameter of the wrist by the mediolateral diameter of the wrist), a symptom severity score (from Levine-Katz Carpal Tunnel Questionnaire) >1.9, diminished sensation in the thumb, and age >45 years [21]. The authors found that when all five variables were present, EMG/NCS was positive in 90% of cases. When at least four out of five variables were present, EMG/NCS was positive in 70% of cases [21]. Kamath et al. used a nine question assessment based on patient symptoms and found that a score of 5 or more on the assessment would allow it to replace EMG/NCS as a screening tool [22].

EMG/NCS

Electrodiagnostic testing, a combination of NCS and EMG, has historically been the most widely utilized diagnostic test for carpal tunnel syndrome. NCS involves placing electrodes along the path of the nerve being tested. The proximal electrode sends an electrical impulse along the nerve and the more distal electrode measures the result. NCS evaluation of a pure motor nerve produces a motor nerve action potential (MNAP) and evaluation of a pure sensory nerve produces a sensory nerve action potential (SNAP). Evaluation of a mixed nerve results in a compound nerve action potential (CNAP). Latencies and nerve conduction velocity (NCV) are calculated using the distance between the electrodes. Factors such as age, height, and weight can affect the latencies and NCV [23].

Large, myelinated fibers are most affected in chronic compressive neuropathies such as carpal tunnel syndrome [24]. As the myelin is damaged (demyelination), the electrical impulse is able to "leak" into surrounding tissues, resulting in increased latency [25]. As compression becomes more chronic, axonal degeneration occurs. Sensory fibers are more sensitive to compression and therefore SNAP values typically decrease before MNAP/CNAP values [25].

EMG evaluates the muscle contraction through either surface or intramuscular electrodes. There has been much interest in using surface electrodes to reduce patient pain and discomfort, however, intramuscular needle EMG remains the reference standard. When stimulated with a needle, normal muscle exhibits brief activity and then quickly returns to electrical silence. This is called insertional activity. If the tip of the EMG needle approaches a motor end plate, miniature endplate potentials (MEPPs) may be recorded. Voluntary muscle contraction is also recorded and termed the muscle unit action potential (MUAP) [26]. Muscle denervation leads to membrane instability, spontaneous depolarization, and cyclical activation of muscle fibers. If these depolarizations occur due to needle movement, they are called fasciculations. Positive sharp waves are similar to fasiculations, but are monophonic waveforms of larger amplitude [27].

The American Association of Neuromuscular and Electrodiagnostic Medicine (AANEM) practice parameters for electrodiagnostic studies reports a high sensitivity (>85%) and high specificity (>95%) for the diagnosis of carpal tunnel syndrome [28, 29]. Sensitivity and specificity are highly dependent on the cut-off values used for diagnosis and one often sacrifices sensitivity to increase specificity and vice versa. There has been an anecdotal trend to lower the absolute cut-off values for distal motor latency and distal sensory latency and to include other comparisons such as relative sensory latencies and the combined sensory index [30]. The effect of these changes has been to increase the sensitivity of nerve conduction studies by detecting "early" or "very mild" cases of CTS, but it also likely leads to an increase in the number of false positive EMG/NCS tests in patients without clinical signs and symptoms of CTS [31]. A recent systematic review of EMG/NCS for diagnosis of carpal tunnel syndrome found only three studies that met criteria for inclusion in the review and those studies found cut-off values of 3.3 ms for peak sensory latency and 4.5 ms for distal motor latency [32]. These values are much higher than those used by my local EMG/NCS laboratory and have the effect of lowering the specificity of the test.

The use of EMG/NCS for diagnosis of carpal tunnel syndrome has several potential benefits, including grading the severity of carpal tunnel syndrome, identification of additional or unexpected causes of nerve compression (cervical radiculopathy, pronator syndrome, polyneuropathy), and documenting recovery of the nerve after intervention [6, 18, 33, 34]. Several different grading schemes have been proposed. The simplest scales classify CTS as mild, moderate or severe using absolute cut-off values for distal motor and sensory latencies [35–37]. Bland developed a 7-point scale ranging from "no abnormality" to "no recordable sensory or motor potential" [38]. There is conflicting evidence regarding whether or not EMG/NCS is a predictor of outcome after carpal tunnel release. Bland et al. found that EMG/NCS was the best predictor of successful outcome after CTR [35, 39]. In contrast, Braun et al. and Grundberg found no correlation between EMG/NCS and outcome after CTR [40, 41]. These studies are hampered by arbitrarily chosen delineations between groups and confounding factors such as age and gender.

Recent studies have questioned the benefit of EMG/NCS in the diagnostic workup when compared to other commonly used diagnostic tests and/or clinical diagnostic tools [5, 18, 19, 34, 39]. Glowacki and colleagues found no differences in outcomes between patients who underwent carpal tunnel release with pre-operative EMG/NCS and those who had the diagnosis based on the history and physical examination alone [6]. In addition, several studies document and high rate of false positives and false negatives for EMG/NCS [42, 43]. Atroshi et al. noted that 18% of patients in their series had a positive EMG/NCS despite no clinical signs and symptoms of CTS and 30% of patients had negative nerve tests despite "clinically certain" CTS based on clinical signs and symptoms [42]. Buch-Jaeger and Foucher found EMG/NCS was positive in only 61% of patients with clinical signs and symptoms of CTS [44]. Additionally, most studies have found a poor correlation between patient reported symptoms and function and the results of nerve conduction studies. Levine et al. reported a correlation coefficient of 0.11 between median nerve sensory latency and symptom severity and a correlation coefficient of 0.12 between median nerve sensory latency and functional severity [17].

Ultrasound

Ultrasound has emerged as a viable alternative to NCS for diagnosis of CTS. Median nerve compression within the carpal tunnel results in nerve swelling proximal and distal to the location of the compression. Nerve swelling is likely multifactorial; however, compression of the nerve leads to changes in the permeability of the blood-nerve barrier. Based on animal models, the epineurium is the first layer to experience changes and the result is isolated swelling in this layer. The endoneurium than becomes involved, resulting in changes in nerve conduction. Chronic nerve compression may lead to fibrosis of the intrafascicular tissues [25–27, 45–47]. Nerve swelling results in an increased in the cross-sectional area (CSA) of the nerve. If the CSA exceeds a pre-defined cut-off, then the diagnosis of carpal tunnel syndrome is confirmed (Figs. 3.1 and 3.2).

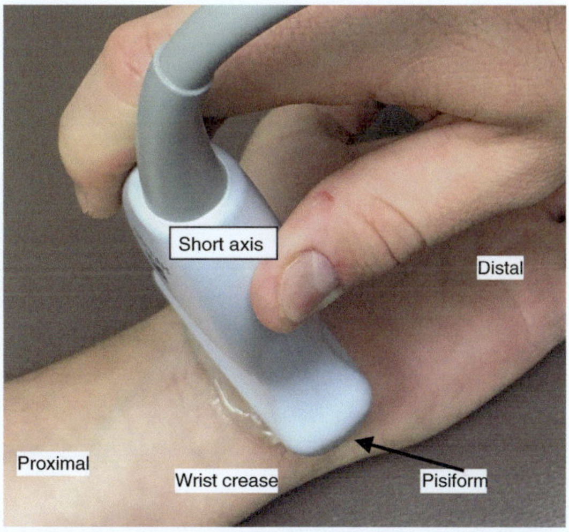

Fig. 3.1 Photograph demonstrating the technique and location for the short axis measurement of the cross-sectional area of the median nerve at the level of the pisiform

While MRI is widely considered the most accurate diagnostic modality to evaluate and measure soft-tissue structures such as nerve, obtaining an MRI to evaluate patients with CTS is not a cost-effective strategy. Musculoskeletal ultrasound was proposed as a lower cost modality and Buchberger et al. demonstrated that ultrasound measurements of the median nerve were comparable to MRI measurements [48]. Nakamichi et al. compared CSA measurements in the distal forearm, carpal tunnel inlet (level of pisiform), middle of carpal tunnel, and carpal tunnel outlet (level of hook of hamate [49]. The authors found that the most sensitive and specific level to measure the CSA was at the carpal tunnel inlet/level of the pisiform [49]. Various cut-off values have been utilized in the literature for a positive diagnosis of carpal tunnel syndrome, ranging from 10 to 14 mm^2 [19, 50–53]. Fowler and colleagues used a cut-off of 10 mm^2 and demonstrated that US had a similar sensitivity and greater specificity that EMG/NCS in patients with a clinical diagnosis of carpal tunnel syndrome [19]. However, Cartwright et al. has suggested an upper limit of 14.6 mm^2 as being 2 standard deviations above

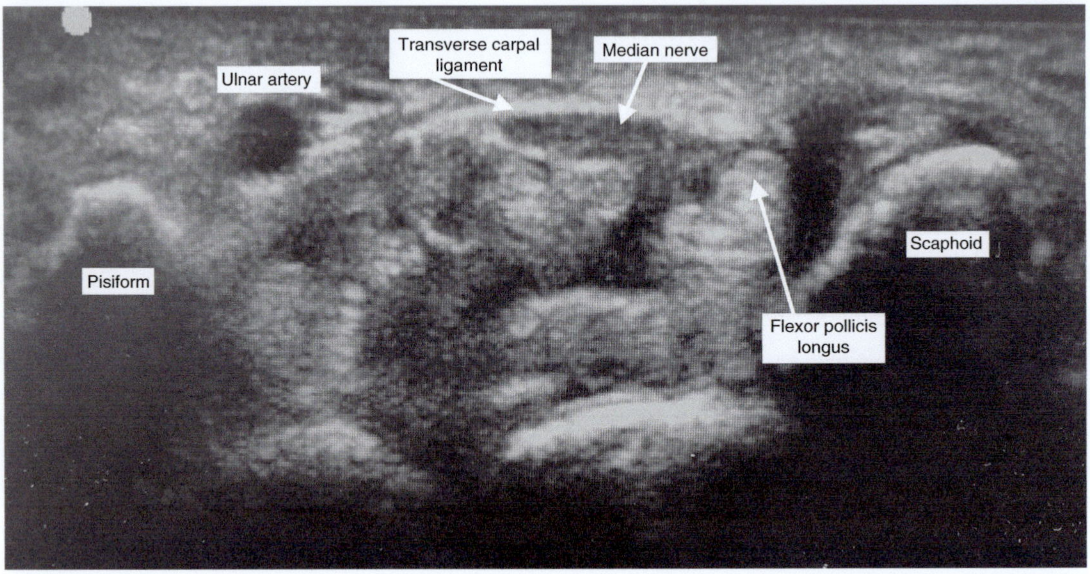

Fig. 3.2 Ultrasound image demonstrating the view obtained from Fig. 3.1

the mean in their study of 100 arms [54]. Age, gender and ethnicity may play a role in the baseline values used for cross-sectional area.

Numerous studies have been performed in an attempt to compare the sensitivity and specificity of EMG/NCS and US for diagnosis of carpal tunnel syndrome. A systematic review of these studies demonstrated similar sensitivity and specificity between US and EMG/NCS when clinical diagnosis was used as the reference standard [55]. Ziswilier and colleagues found a 98% probability of CTS in a prospective study of 110 wrists using a cut-off CSA of 12 mm^2 [56]. A meta-analysis of high quality studies concluded that US "as accurate as" EMG/NCS with respect to sensitivity, specificity, and accuracy for diagnosis of CTS [57].

Some authors have criticized the use of absolute CSA values when using US for diagnosis of CTS and have proposed the use of ratios to account for differences in nerve size and morphology. Hobson-Webb and colleagues [58] described the wrist-to-forearm ratio (WFR), a ratio between the CSA of the median nerve at the wrist crease and CSA of the median nerve 12 cm proximal to the wrist crease. In this series, if the WFR was ≥ 1.4, there was 100% sensitivity for CTS. Buchberger et al. described bowing of the flexor retinaculum, calculated by drawing a line on the short axis ultrasound from the trapezium to the hamate and then measuring from that line to the most volar part of the transverse carpal ligament. The authors noted the amount of palmar displacement of the transverse carpal ligament in normal controls was 2.1 mm, compared to 3.7 mm in patients with carpal tunnel syndrome [48]. The flattening ratio of the median nerve is determined on the short axis ultrasound by dividing the nerve's medial-lateral diameter by the anterior-posterior diameter. The flattening ratio is typically greatest at the level of the hamate in patients with carpal tunnel syndrome [48].

Ultrasound may be a useful adjunct in patients with normal nerve conduction studies despite signs and symptoms consistent with carpal tunnel syndrome. Al-Hashel and colleagues found that nearly 50% of the patients in their series with normal nerve conduction studies but clinically certain carpal tunnel syndrome had an elevated CSA of the median nerve at the level of the pisiform [59]. Aseem et al. found 92% of wrists with clinical evidence of CTS and normal NCS had an increased CSA and 100% had an elevated WFR [60]. At a minimum, ultrasound should be considered an alternative test to EMG/NCS in the correct clinical scenario. Fowler and colleagues demonstrated that ultrasound as a first line test is a cost-effective strategy for diagnosis of carpal tunnel syndrome [61].

References

1. Blumenthal S, Herskovitz S, Verghese J. Carpal tunnel syndrome in older adults. Muscle Nerve. 2006;34(1):78–83. https://doi.org/10.1002/mus.20559.
2. Bland JD. Carpal tunnel syndrome. BMJ. 2007;335(7615):343–6. https://doi.org/10.1136/bmj.39282.623553.AD.
3. Hakim AJ, Cherkas L, Zayat El S, MacGregor AJ, Spector TD. The genetic contribution to carpal tunnel syndrome in women: a twin study. Arthritis Rheum. 2002;47(3):275–9. https://doi.org/10.1002/art.10395.
4. American Academy of Orthopaedic Surgeons. Management of carpal tunnel syndrome evidence-based clinical practice guideline. Feb 2016. www.aaos.org/ctsguideline.
5. Graham B. The value added by electrodiagnostic testing in the diagnosis of carpal tunnel syndrome. J Bone Joint Surg Am. 2008;90(12):2587–93. https://doi.org/10.2106/JBJS.G.01362.
6. Glowacki KA, Breen CJ, Sachar K, Weiss AP. Electrodiagnostic testing and carpal tunnel release outcome. J Hand Surg Am. 1996;21(1):117–21. https://doi.org/10.1016/S0363-5023(96)80164-X.
7. Cranford CS, Ho JY, Kalainov DM, Hartigan BJ. Carpal tunnel syndrome. J Am Acad Orthop Surg. 2007;15(9):537–48.
8. Gelberman RH, Hergenroeder PT, Hargens AR, Lundborg GN, Akeson WH. The carpal tunnel syndrome. A study of carpal canal pressures. J Bone Joint Surg Am. 1981;63(3):380–3.
9. Michelsen H, Posner MA. Medical history of carpal tunnel syndrome. Hand Clin. 2002;18(2):257–68.
10. Jenkins PJ, Srikantharajah D, Duckworth AD, Watts AC, McEachan JE. Carpal tunnel syndrome: the association with occupation at a population level. J Hand Surg Eur Vol. 2013;38(1):67–72. https://doi.org/10.1177/1753193412455790.
11. Nathan PA, Keniston RC, Myers LD, Meadows KD. Longitudinal study of median nerve sensory conduction in industry: relationship to age, gender, hand dominance, occupational hand use, and clinical diagnosis. J Hand Surg Am. 1992;17(5):850–7.
12. Gelberman RH, Szabo RM, Williamson RV, Dimick MP. Sensibility testing in peripheral-nerve compression syndromes. An experimental study in humans. J Bone Joint Surg Am. 1983;65(5):632–8.
13. Szabo RM, Gelberman RH, Dimick MP. Sensibility testing in patients with carpal tunnel syndrome. J Bone Joint Surg Am. 1984;66(1):60–4.
14. Cheng CJ, Mackinnon-Patterson B, Beck JL, Mackinnon SE. Scratch collapse test for evaluation of carpal and cubital tunnel syndrome. J Hand Surg Am. 2008;33(9):1518–24. https://doi.org/10.1016/j.jhsa.2008.05.022.
15. Simon J, Lutsky K, Maltenfort M, Beredjiklian PK. The accuracy of the scratch collapse test performed by blinded examiners on patients with suspected carpal tunnel syndrome assessed by electrodiagnostic studies. J Hand Surg Am. 2017;42(5):386.e1–5. https://doi.org/10.1016/j.jhsa.2017.01.031.
16. Katz JN, Larson MG, Sabra A, et al. The carpal tunnel syndrome: diagnostic utility of the history and physical examination findings. Ann Intern Med. 1990;112(5):321–7.
17. Levine DW, Simmons BP, Koris MJ, et al. A self-administered questionnaire for the assessment of severity of symptoms and functional status in carpal tunnel syndrome. J Bone Joint Surg Am. 1993;75(11):1585–92.
18. Fowler JR, Cipolli W, Hanson T. A comparison of three diagnostic tests for carpal tunnel syndrome using latent class analysis. J Bone Joint Surg Am. 2015;97(23):1958–61. https://doi.org/10.2106/JBJS.O.00476.
19. Fowler JR, Munsch M, Tosti R, Hagberg WC, Imbriglia JE. Comparison of ultrasound and electrodiagnostic testing for diagnosis of carpal tunnel syndrome: study using a validated clinical tool as the reference standard. J Bone Joint Surg Am. 2014;96(17):e148. https://doi.org/10.2106/JBJS.M.01250.
20. Lo JK, Finestone HM, Gilbert K. Prospective evaluation of the clinical prediction of electrodiagnostic results in carpal tunnel syndrome. PM R. 2009;1(7):612–9. https://doi.org/10.1016/j.pmrj.2009.05.004.
21. Wainner RS, Fritz JM, Irrgang JJ, Delitto A, Allison S, Boninger ML. Development of a clinical prediction rule for the diagnosis of carpal tunnel syndrome. Arch Phys Med Rehabil. 2005;86(4):609–18. https://doi.org/10.1016/j.apmr.2004.11.008.
22. Kamath V, Stothard J. A clinical questionnaire for the diagnosis of carpal tunnel syndrome. J Hand Surg. 2003;28(5):455–9.
23. Slutsky DJ. Use of nerve conduction studies and the pressure-specified sensory device in the diagnosis of carpal tunnel syndrome. J Hand Surg Eur Vol. 2009;34(1):60–5. https://doi.org/10.1177/1753193408094921.
24. Dahlin LB, Shyu BC, Danielsen N, Andersson SA. Effects of nerve compression or ischaemia on conduction properties of myelinated and non-myelinated nerve fibres. An experimental study in the rabbit common peroneal nerve. Acta Physiol Scand. 1989;136(1):97–105. https://doi.org/10.1111/j.1748-1716.1989.tb08634.x.
25. Tapadia M, Mozaffar T, Gupta R. Compressive neuropathies of the upper extremity: update on pathophysiology, classification, and electrodiagnostic findings. J Hand Surg Am. 2010;35(4):668–77. https://doi.org/10.1016/j.jhsa.2010.01.007.

26. Slutsky DJ. Electromyography in hand surgery. J Am Soc Surg Hand. 2004;4(3):176–88. https://doi.org/10.1016/j.jassh.2004.06.008.
27. Sonoo M, Menkes DL, Bland JDP, Burke D. Nerve conduction studies and EMG in carpal tunnel syndrome: do they add value? Clin Neurophysiol Pract. 2018;3:78–88. https://doi.org/10.1016/j.cnp.2018.02.005.
28. Jablecki CK, Andary MT, Floeter MK, et al. Practice parameter: electrodiagnostic studies in carpal tunnel syndrome. Report of the American Association of Electrodiagnostic Medicine, American Academy of Neurology, and the American Academy of Physical Medicine and Rehabilitation. Neurology. 2002;58(11):1589–92.
29. American Association of Electrodiagnostic Medicine, American Academy of Neurology, American Academy of Physical Medicine and Rehabilitation. Practice parameter for electrodiagnostic studies in carpal tunnel syndrome: summary statement. Muscle Nerve. 2002;25(6):918–22. https://doi.org/10.1002/mus.10185.
30. Lew HL, Wang L, Robinson LR. Test-retest reliability of combined sensory index: implications for diagnosing carpal tunnel syndrome. Muscle Nerve. 2000;23(8):1261–4.
31. Redmond MD, Rivner MH. False positive electrodiagnostic tests in carpal tunnel syndrome. Muscle Nerve. 1988;11(5):511–8. https://doi.org/10.1002/mus.880110515.
32. Chen S, Andary M, Buschbacher R, et al. Electrodiagnostic reference values for upper and lower limb nerve conduction studies in adult populations. Muscle Nerve. 2016;54(3):371–7. https://doi.org/10.1002/mus.25203.
33. Szabo RM, Slater RRJ, Farver TB, Stanton DB, Sharman WK. The value of diagnostic testing in carpal tunnel syndrome. J Hand Surg Am. 1999;24(4):704–14.
34. Wang WL, Buterbaugh K, Kadow TR, Goitz RJ, Fowler JR. A prospective comparison of diagnostic tools for the diagnosis of carpal tunnel syndrome. J Hand Surg Am. 2018;43(9):833–836.e2. https://doi.org/10.1016/j.jhsa.2018.05.022.
35. Fowler JR, Munsch M, Huang Y, Hagberg WC, Imbriglia JE. Pre-operative electrodiagnostic testing predicts time to resolution of symptoms after carpal tunnel release. J Hand Surg Eur Vol. 2016;41(2):137–42. https://doi.org/10.1177/1753193415576248.
36. Beck JD, Wingert NC, Rutter MR, Irgit KS, Tang X, Klena JC. Clinical outcomes of endoscopic carpal tunnel release in patients 65 and over. J Hand Surg Am. 2013;38(8):1524–9. https://doi.org/10.1016/j.jhsa.2013.05.016.
37. Chang M-H, Wei S-J, Chiang H-L, Wang H-M, Hsieh PF, Huang S-Y. Forearm mixed nerve conduction velocity: questionable role in the evaluation of retrograde axonal atrophy in carpal tunnel syndrome. J Clin Neurophysiol. 2003;20(3):196–200.
38. Bland JD. A neurophysiological grading scale for carpal tunnel syndrome. Muscle Nerve. 2000 Aug;23(8):1280-3.
39. Bland JD. Do nerve conduction studies predict the outcome of carpal tunnel decompression? Muscle Nerve. 2001;24(7):935–40.
40. Grundberg AB. Carpal tunnel decompression in spite of normal electromyography. J Hand Surg Am. 1983;8(3):348–9.
41. Braun RM, Jackson WJ. Electrical studies as a prognostic factor in the surgical treatment of carpal tunnel syndrome. J Hand Surg Am. 1994;19(6):893–900. https://doi.org/10.1016/0363-5023(94)90086-8.
42. Atroshi I, Gummesson C, Johnsson R, Ornstein E, Ranstam J, Rosen I. Prevalence of carpal tunnel syndrome in a general population. JAMA. 1999;282(2):153–8.
43. Witt JC, Hentz JG, Stevens JC. Carpal tunnel syndrome with normal nerve conduction studies. Muscle Nerve. 2004;29(4):515–22. https://doi.org/10.1002/mus.20019.
44. Buch-Jaeger N, Foucher G. Correlation of clinical signs with nerve conduction tests in the diagnosis of carpal tunnel syndrome. J Hand Surg. 1994;19(6):720–4.
45. Rydevik B, Lundborg G. Permeability of intraneural microvessels and perineurium following acute, graded experimental nerve compression. Scand J Plast Reconstr Surg. 1977;11(3):179–87.
46. Yoshii Y, Nishiura Y, Terui N, Hara Y, Saijilafu, Ochiai N. The effects of repetitive compression on nerve conduction and blood flow in the rabbit sciatic nerve. J Hand Surg Eur Vol. 2010;35(4):269–78. https://doi.org/10.1177/1753193408090107.
47. Mackinnon SE, Dellon AL, Hudson AR, Hunter DA. Chronic nerve compression--an experimental model in the rat. Ann Plast Surg. 1984;13(2):112–20.
48. Buchberger W, Judmaier W, Birbamer G, Lener M, Schmidauer C. Carpal tunnel syndrome: diagnosis with high-resolution sonography. AJR Am J Roentgenol. 1992;159(4):793–8. https://doi.org/10.2214/ajr.159.4.1529845.
49. Nakamichi K, Tachibana S. Ultrasonographic measurement of median nerve cross-sectional area in idiopathic carpal tunnel syndrome: diagnostic accuracy. Muscle Nerve. 2002;26(6):798–803. https://doi.org/10.1002/mus.10276.
50. Wong SM, Griffith JF, Hui AC, Lo SK, Fu M, Wong KS. Carpal tunnel syndrome: diagnostic usefulness of sonography. Radiology. 2004;232(1):93–9. https://doi.org/10.1148/radiol.2321030071.
51. Kaymak B, Ozcakar L, Cetin A, Candan Cetin M, Akinci A, Hascelik Z. A comparison of the benefits of sonography and electrophysiologic measurements as predictors of symptom severity and functional status in patients with carpal tunnel syndrome. Arch Phys Med Rehabil. 2008;89(4):743–8. https://doi.org/10.1016/j.apmr.2007.09.041.

52. Nakamichi KI, Tachibana S. Enlarged median nerve in idiopathic carpal tunnel syndrome. Muscle Nerve. 2000;23(11):1713–8.
53. Kele H, Verheggen R, Bittermann HJ, Reimers CD. The potential value of ultrasonography in the evaluation of carpal tunnel syndrome. Neurology. 2003;61(3):389–91.
54. Cartwright MS, Shin HW, Passmore LV, Walker FO. Ultrasonographic reference values for assessing the normal median nerve in adults. J Neuroimaging. 2009;19(1):47–51. https://doi.org/10.1111/j.1552-6569.2008.00256.x.
55. Fowler JR, Gaughan JP, Ilyas AM. The sensitivity and specificity of ultrasound for the diagnosis of carpal tunnel syndrome: a meta-analysis. Clin Orthop Relat Res. 2011;469(4):1089–94. https://doi.org/10.1007/s11999-010-1637-5.
56. Ziswiler HR, Reichenbach S, Vogelin E, Bachmann LM, Villiger PM, Juni P. Diagnostic value of sonography in patients with suspected carpal tunnel syndrome: a prospective study. Arthritis Rheum. 2005;52(1):304–11. https://doi.org/10.1002/art.20723.
57. Cartwright MS, Hobson-Webb LD, Boon AJ, et al. Evidence-based guideline: neuromuscular ultrasound for the diagnosis of carpal tunnel syndrome. Muscle Nerve. 2012;46(2):287–93. https://doi.org/10.1002/mus.23389.
58. Hobson-Webb LD, Massey JM, Juel VC, Sanders DB. The ultrasonographic wrist-to-forearm median nerve area ratio in carpal tunnel syndrome. Clin Neurophysiol. 2008;119(6):1353–7. https://doi.org/10.1016/j.clinph.2008.01.101.
59. Al-Hashel JY, Rashad HM, Nouh MR, et al. Sonography in carpal tunnel syndrome with normal nerve conduction studies. Muscle Nerve. 2015;51(4):592–7. https://doi.org/10.1002/mus.24425.
60. Aseem F, Williams JW, Walker FO, Cartwright MS. Neuromuscular ultrasound in patients with carpal tunnel syndrome and normal nerve conduction studies. Muscle Nerve. 2017;55(6):913–5. https://doi.org/10.1002/mus.25462.
61. Fowler JR, Maltenfort MG, Ilyas AM. Ultrasound as a first-line test in the diagnosis of carpal tunnel syndrome: a cost-effectiveness analysis. Clin Orthop Relat Res. 2013;471(3):932–7. https://doi.org/10.1007/s11999-012-2662-3.

Standard Open Carpal Tunnel Release

4

Hannah H. Lee and Robert J. Goitz

Open Carpal Tunnel Release

Currently the most common open approach is performed through a longitudinal incision directly over the transverse carpal ligament (TCL), just distal to the wrist crease. It allows good visualization of the carpal tunnel contents. Variations in the anatomy of the palmar cutaneous and recurrent motor nerves can be visualized and avoided. Taleisnik recommended an incision ulnar to the axis of the flexed ring finger for this purpose [1].

Technique

A local anesthetic including a median nerve block at the wrist with or without sedation is used. Either an upper arm or forearm tourniquet is inflated to 250 mmHg. The skin incision is marked, and approximately 3-cm longitudinal incision is made in line with the third webspace (Fig. 4.1). A longer incision may be necessary for large hands or obese patients. With self-retaining retractor in place, dissection is carried out through the soft tissue (Fig. 4.2). The palmar fascia is visualized and incised longitudinally. Retractors

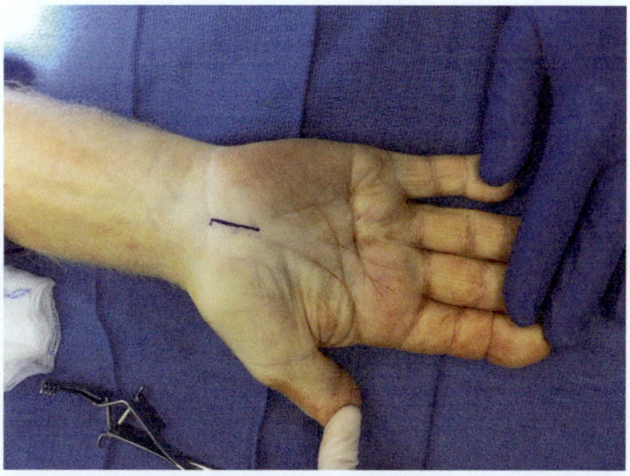

Fig. 4.1 An approximately 3-cm longitudinal skin incision is marked along the third webspace distal to the wrist crease in line with the third web space

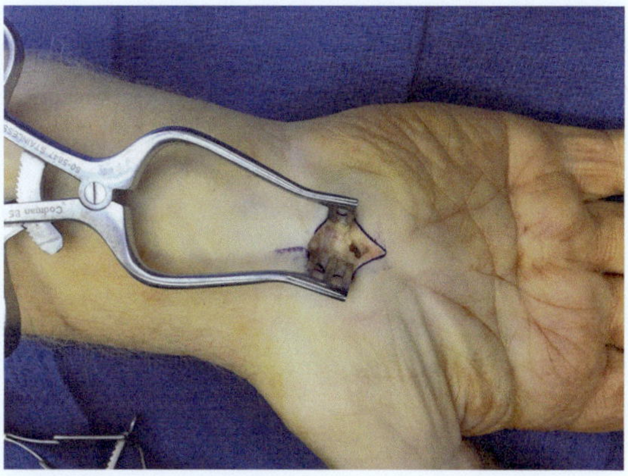

Fig. 4.2 Soft tissue dissection is carried out with a self-retaining retractor in place to visualize and release the palmar fascia

H. H. Lee · R. J. Goitz (✉)
Department of Orthopaedic Surgery, University of Pittsburgh Medical Center, Pittsburgh, PA, USA
e-mail: goitzrj@upmc.edu

D. G. Sotereanos, L. K. Papatheodorou (eds.), *Compressive Neuropathies of the Upper Extremity*,
https://doi.org/10.1007/978-3-030-37289-7_4

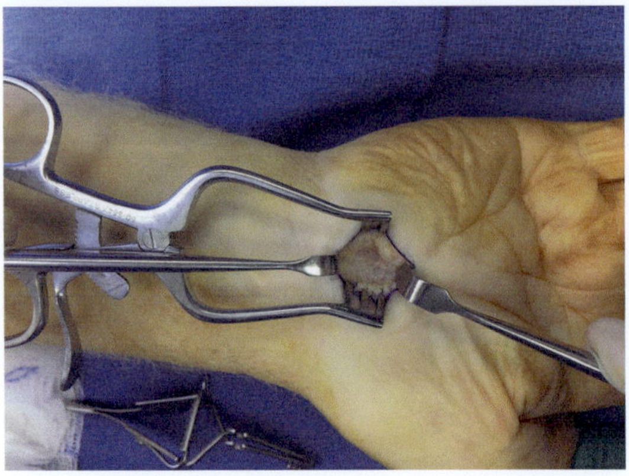

Fig. 4.3 The distal portion of the antebrachial fascia and the proximal portion of the flexor retinaculum, as well as the central TCL are visualized

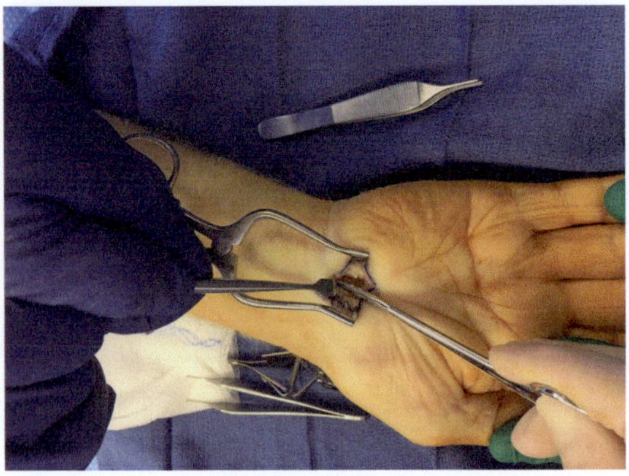

Fig. 4.4 Transverse carpal ligament is cut using a No. 15 blade, and scissors are used to cut the proximal forearm fascia under direct vision with proximal retraction

are used distally and proximally to retract and expose the proximal portion of the flexor retinaculum and the distal portion of the antebrachial fascia, respectively (Fig. 4.3). A No. 15 blade is then used to cut the TCL (Fig. 4.4). Proximally the antebrachial fascia should be well visualized and cut with scissors. Bipolar cautery is used for hemostasis, the incision is closed, and a bulky dressing is applied, prior to deflating the tourniquet. The patient is instructed to follow up in office in 10–14 days for suture removal.

Open Carpal Tunnel Release with Tenosynovectomy

The indication for tenosynovectomy is the presence of inflammatory tenosynovium within the carpal tunnel that can act as a space-occupying lesion [2]. The hypertrophic tenosynovium can increase the carpal tunnel pressure and compress the median nerve, thus playing a significant role in the development of carpal tunnel syndrome. When swelling on the volar aspect of the forearm proximal to the TCL and/or diminished grip or finger flexion strength are/is observed, one can anticipate the need for tenosynovectomy [3]. If it is indicated, the traditional open carpal tunnel release incision can be extended up the volar aspect of the forearm.

Technique

The incision for standard open carpal tunnel release is extended approximately 2–3 cm into the distal volar forearm in a curved fashion crossing the wrist crease at 45° angle to limit scar contracture across the wrist (Fig. 4.5). After the transverse carpal ligament is divided, the tenosynovium is sharply dissected away from the median nerve and the flexor tendons (Figs. 4.6, 4.7, 4.8, and 4.9). The closure and postoperative care are the same as that of traditional open carpal tunnel release procedures.

Carpal Tunnel Release Using Indiana Tome

The mini-open technique through a small palmar incision utilizing the Indiana Tome was first reported by Lee and Strickland in 1998 [4]. This technique further reduces soft tissue dissection with the goal to minimize pillar pain. More recent studies have confirmed the efficacy and safety of this technique, with most patients able to return to their pre-operative activities, with nonmanual laborers resuming regular job tasks in 2 days to 3 weeks [5]. The scar and pillar tenderness, and grip, key pinch, and three-point pinch strength

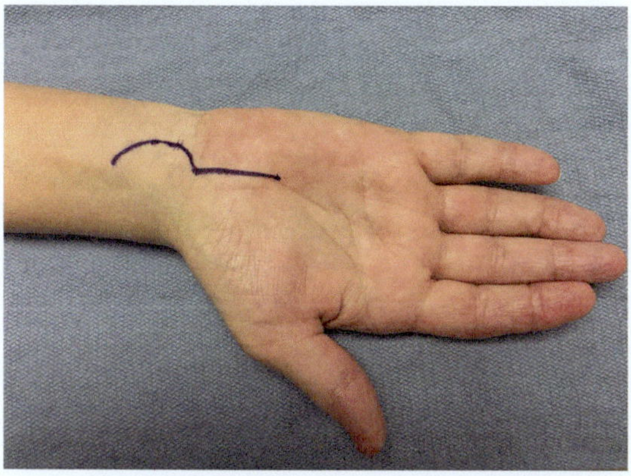

Fig. 4.5 The skin marking for traditional open carpal tunnel release is extended approximately 2–3 cm into the distal volar forearm in a curved fashion

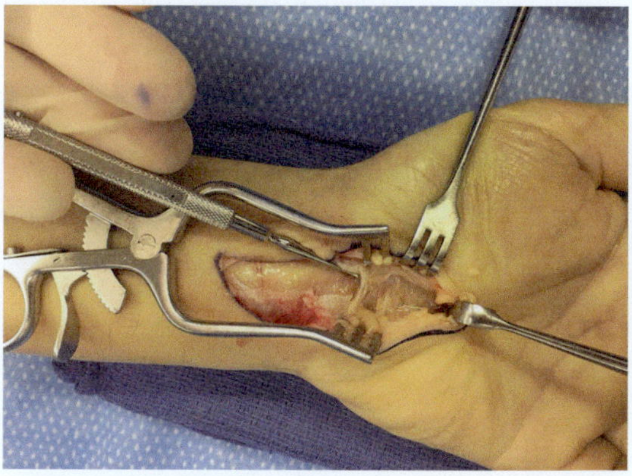

Fig. 4.6 TCL is exposed and cut after release of the forearm fascia

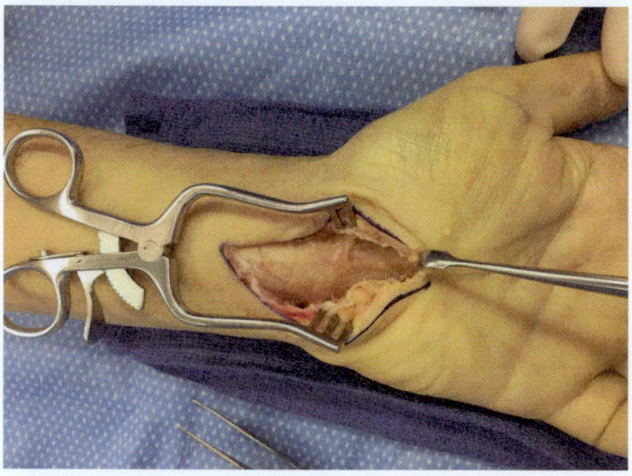

Fig. 4.7 After TCL is divided, the contents of the carpal tunnel with hypertrophic tenosynovium are exposed

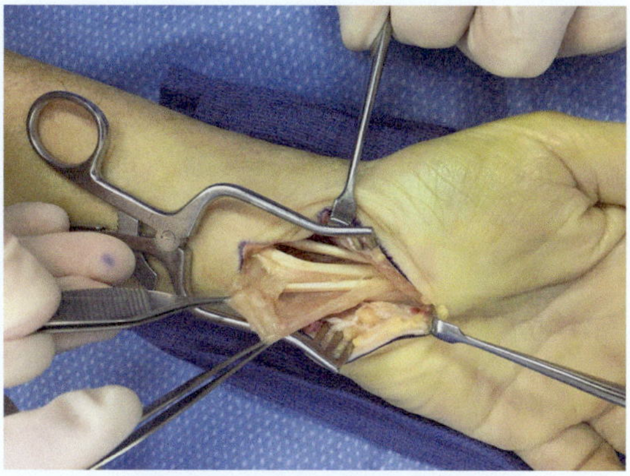

Fig. 4.8 The tenosynovium is sequentially removed from each of the 9 flexors tendons in the carpal tunnel

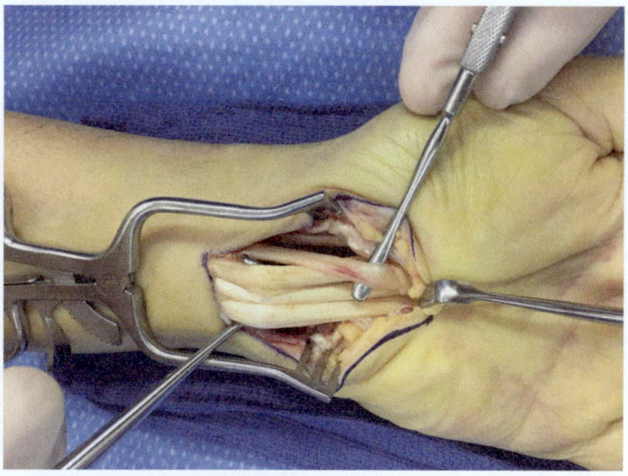

Fig. 4.9 After the tenosynovium is removed, note the perineural blush of the median nerve due to compression at the level of the released TCL

values were similar to those reported in studies utilizing endoscopic release techniques [4]. The authors noted that the key to reducing complications with the minimally invasive technique is to have a low threshold to convert to a standard open approach whenever the anatomy appears unclear or the technique does not proceed easily.

Technique

The procedure is performed under local anesthesia with or without sedation, with an upper arm tourniquet inflated to 250 mmHg. A median nerve block is provided. The skin incision utilized is a 1–1.5 cm longitudinal incision along the third web space

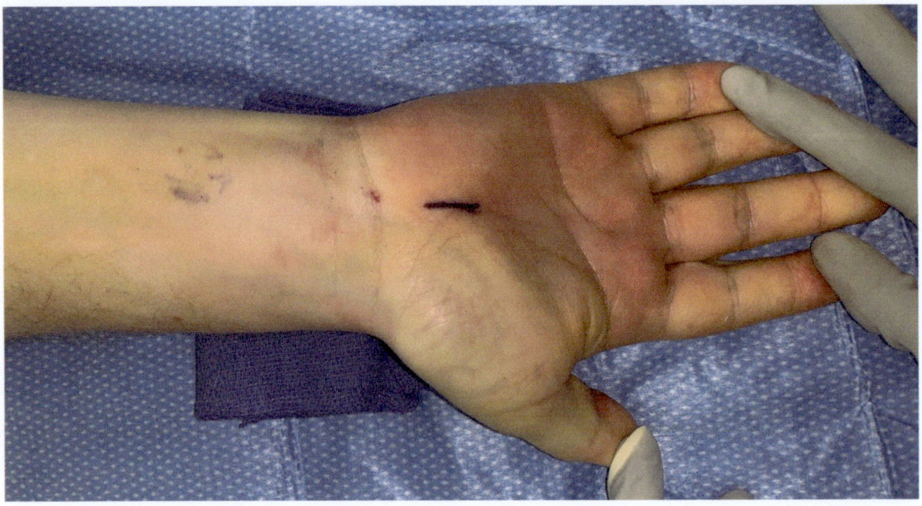

Fig. 4.10 The skin incision is marked – a 1–1.5 cm longitudinal incision along the third web space, centered over the distal edge of the TCL but proximal to Kaplan's line

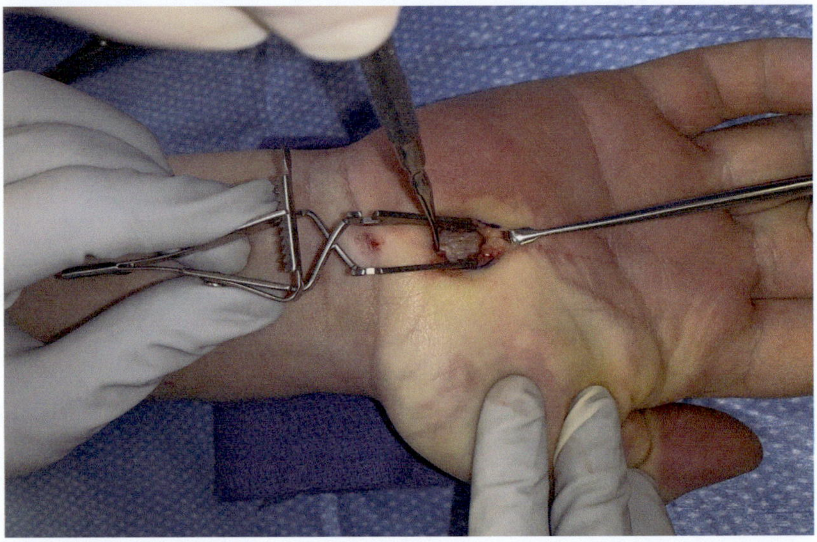

Fig. 4.11 Five-mm of the distal edge of TCL is divided using a No. 15 blade under direct visualization, allowing access to the carpal tunnel

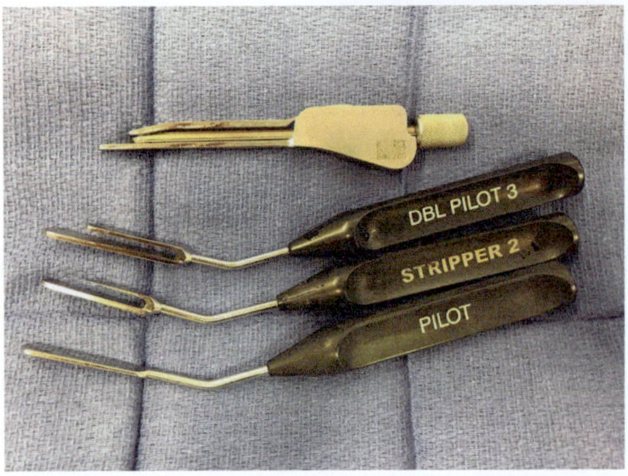

Fig. 4.12 Three dilators and a "safety clip" are shown this this photo that are sequentially used to isolate the TCL

centered over the distal edge of the TCL (Fig. 4.10). A self-retaining retractor is inserted and palmar fascia released. Deep inspection is performed for any anomalous structures that would preclude this procedure and convert to larger exposure. Using a No. 15 blade under direct visualization, 5-mm of the distal edge of transverse carpal ligament is divided, allowing access to the carpal tunnel (Fig. 4.11). A series of dilators is then used to separate the TCL from surrounding structures followed by a "safety clip" to isolate the TCL (Figs. 4.12 and 4.13). With the wrist positioned in mild extension, the first dilator or pilot is inserted underneath the transverse carpal ligament, displacing the contents

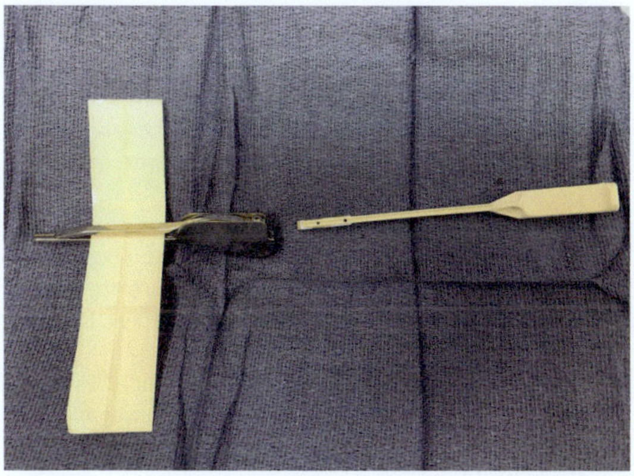

Fig. 4.13 Safety clip in this photograph is placed around paper similar to how it is used to isolate the TCL

of the carpal tunnel dorsally (Fig. 4.14). Two dilators are placed to further isolate the TCL and the safety clip is then placed around the TCL. The carpal tunnel knife or tome is placed through the safety clip that has isolated the TCL. The Indiana Tome is then engaged against the distal undivided edge of the TCL and advanced to divide the remaining ligament and distal antebrachial fascia through the safety clip (Fig. 4.15). The contents of the carpal tunnel can be seen between the separated radial and ulnar edges of the divided TCL. The skin incision is closed with 2–3 sutures, and a soft dressing is applied to the palm and wrist. Patients are encouraged to move the digits and return to office in 10–14 days suture removal.

Fig. 4.14 Here the first of three dilators is placed under the TCL

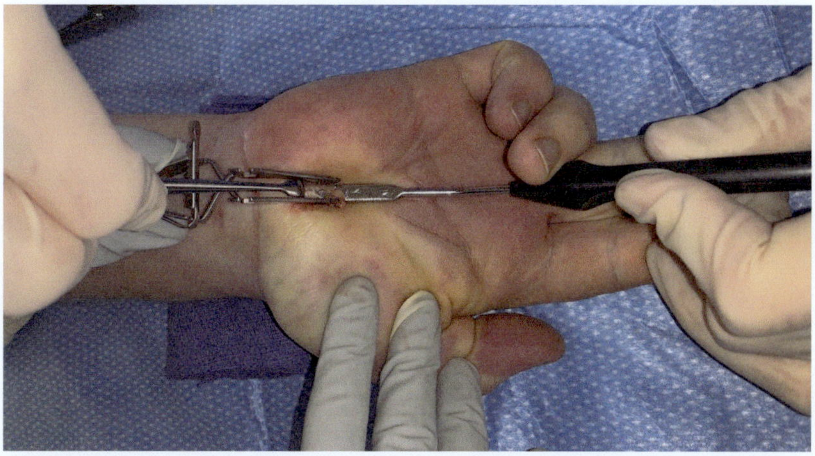

Fig. 4.15 The carpal tunnel knife or tome is placed through the safety clip that has isolated the TCL

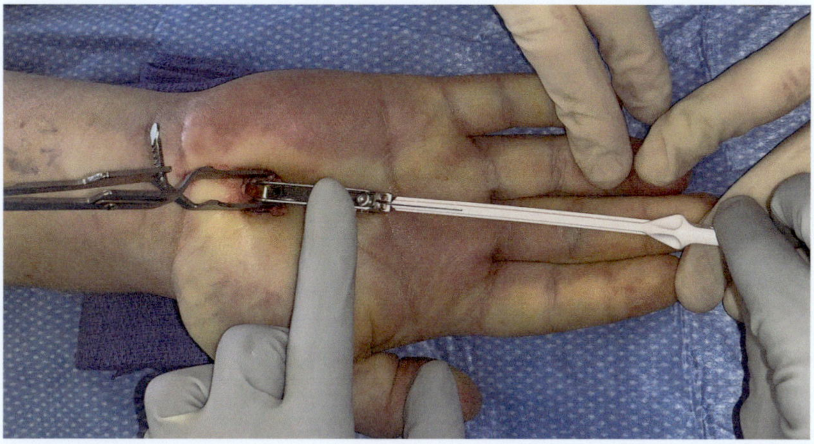

Conclusion

Numerous techniques exist to release the transverse carpal ligament to relieve the symptoms of carpal tunnel syndrome. Traditional open carpal tunnel release has been the standard procedure for many years, whereas more extensile exposure allows for concomitant tenosynovectomy but recovery is longer related to scar sensitivity and weakness. Limited exposure methods can be utilized to allow for faster return to activities with similar long-term outcomes. All three procedures provide similar outcomes and the procedure should be chosen based on experience and comfort with the approach.

References

1. Taleisnik J. The palmar cutaneous branch of the median nerve and the approach to the carpal tunnel. An anatomical study. J Bone Joint Surg Am. 1973;55(6):1212–7.
2. Ketchum LD. A comparison of flexor tenosynovectomy, open carpal tunnel release, and open carpal tunnel release with flexor tenosynovectomy in the treatment of carpal tunnel syndrome. Plast Reconstr Surg. 2004;113(7):2020–9.
3. Phalen GS. The carpal-tunnel syndrome. Seventeen years' experience in diagnosis and treatment of six hundred fifty-four hands. J Bone Joint Surg Am. 1966;48(2):211–28.
4. Lee WP, Strickland JW. Safe carpal tunnel release via a limited palmar incision. Plast Reconstr Surg. 1998;101(2):418–24; discussion 425–6.
5. Lee WP, Schipper BM, Goitz RJ. 13-year experience of carpal tunnel release using the Indiana Tome technique. J Hand Surg Am. 2008;33(7):1052–6.

Carpal Tunnel Release with Two Small Cross-Aligned Incisions

5

Konstantinos N. Malizos, Antonios Koutalos, Fotis Papageorgiou, Anna Ziogou, and Marianthi Papanagiotou

Carpal Tunnel Syndrome: Demographics and Historical Data

Median nerve compression neuropathy at the wrist level, widely known as carpal tunnel syndrome (CTS), is the most common peripheral nerve entrapment syndrome affecting 3.8% in the general population, mainly middle-aged females either as an acute or chronic CTS [1]. Acute CTS is relatively uncommon, caused by any acute injury increasing the pressure into the carpal tunnel. Chronic CTS is the commonest type, associated with a variety of etiologies ranging from local (such as tumors or anatomic abnormalities) to systematic (hypothyreoidism, sarcoidosis, diabetes mellitus) and several occupations that rising the pressure within the carpal tunnel [2].

The earliest symptoms of the CTS initially appear as sensory function deficit with paresthesia, numbness and pain variably involving the thumb, the index, the median and the radial half of the ring finger [2]. Patients are commonly complaining for nocturnal awakening pain and numbness in the early stage, followed by muscular weakness and loss of grip and pinch strength in the more advanced stage. In more severe and neglected cases, the patients may develop thenar muscles atrophy due to involvement of the motor brunch of the median nerve. Pain radiating to the forearm and the shoulder is often mentioned by the patient without clinical evidence of apparent neuropathy or compression proximal to the wrist.

There are several clinical tests to assist to the diagnosis of the CTS. Tinel's and Phalen's sign, are the most common in use [2–4]. The diagnosis is confirmed with the use of nerve conduction and complete electro-physiology studies, which in a number of patients may not turn positive.

Historically, the median nerve compression neuropathy at the wrist level (carpal tunnel syndrome-CTS) was described in 1854 by Sir James Paget, in a patient suffering from pain and impaired sensation of the hand after a distal radius fracture [5]. Almost 30 years later in 1880 Putnam presented a series of 37 patients with sensibility disturbances in the median nerve distribution area of the hand [6]. The pathology of CTS and the role of the transverse carpal ligament (TCL) on the median nerve compression were further elucidated in 1913 by Marie and Foix [7]. Twenty years later, in 1933, Learmonth described the first TCL release as a

K. N. Malizos (✉)
Hand Unit – Department of Orthopaedics & Musculoskeletal Trauma, University of Thessaly Medical School, Larissa, Greece
e-mail: kmalizos@otenet.gr

A. Koutalos · F. Papageorgiou · A. Ziogou
M. Papanagiotou
Department of Orthopaedics & MusculoSkeletal Trauma, University of Thessaly, Larissa, Greece

D. G. Sotereanos, L. K. Papatheodorou (eds.), *Compressive Neuropathies of the Upper Extremity*,
https://doi.org/10.1007/978-3-030-37289-7_5

surgical treatment to medial nerve entrapment neuropathy at the wrist [8]. Since then several techniques have been reported in the literature each one of them expressing both benefits and pitfalls.

Anatomy of the Carpal Tunnel and the Variations of the Median Nerve

The carpal tunnel is dorsally defined by the proximal carpal row (floor), the hook of the hamate and the pisiform at the ulnar side, the scaphoid tubercle and the trapezium on the radial side and the TCL at the volar side.

Ten anatomical structures pass through the carpal tunnel, including the nine flexor tendons of the fingers and the median nerve. The median nerve after exiting the carpal tunnel divides into the first and second common digital nerves, and the digital nerve for the radial side of the index which supply sensory innervation to lateral palm and through the digital cutaneous branches innervates the radial 3 1/2 digits (palmar) and can also supply the index, long, and ring fingers dorsally. The recurrent motor branch of the median nerve innervates the 1st and 2nd lumbricals, the opponens pollicis, the abductor pollicis brevis and the flexor pollicis brevis muscle. The take off of this recurrent motor branch presents several anatomical variations classified into three groups, by Lanz in 1977 [9]. The first variation occurs in the majority of cases (49%) with the origin of the recurrent motor branch from the median nerve radially, and distal to the transverse carpal ligament. In the second most common variation (30%) the branch is taking off within the carpal tunnel, while in the third less common type (20%) the recurrent motor brunch arises from the median nerve and tenets the transverse carpal ligament. Two more, rare variations have been also described, in the first of them the recurrent motor branch takes off from the ulnar and anterior area, bridging the median nerve as it approaches the thinner musculature [10], while in the other one, occurring in 9% of cases, the motor branch may have a course superficial to the transverse carpal ligament [11]. The identification of these variations is essential in order to avoid iatrogenic injury of the recurrent motor branch during the carpal tunnel release.

Surgical Techniques and Complains or Complications Following CTS Surgery

Since 1933, when Learmonth described the first surgical approach for the TCL release as a treatment to CTS [8], several surgical techniques have been described ranging from extended open to minimally invasive operations, to endoscopic techniques.

There are three basic techniques for treating CTS, Open Carpal Tunnel Release (OCTR), Minimal Incision Carpal Tunnel Release (MICTR), including mini distal incision release and double mini incision release and Endoscopic Carpal Tunnel Release (ECTR).

Open carpal tunnel release provides direct visualization of all anatomical structures, preventing iatrogenic complications such as palmar arch artery or median nerve injury. Although it is associated with a low intra-operative complication rate, a number of patients may be dissatisfied after open carpal tunnel release due to painful scar, loss of grip strength, reflex sympathetic dystrophy, bow stringing of flexor tendons and pillar pain [12, 13]. Pillar pain is the term used to describe pain and tenderness in the thenar or hypothenar area. The etiology is unclear but in some cases it is associated with disruption of the carpal arch structures during surgery, soft tissue edema, injury to the cutaneous branches of the palm or relaxation of the muscles of opposition and pinch following sectioning of TCL [12].

In order to avoid certain postoperative complications related to the OCTR, alternative minimally invasive techniques have been introduced, including a limited transverse incision of ≤2 cm technique at the same area as open release. Atik et al in 2001 [14] described a modification of the mini open technique but no difference in the long term results on patients undergoing open or mini open CTS release were demonstrated.

ECTR was first performed by Okutsu in 1987 [15] and since then several different endoscopic approaches were described. The most widely used are Agee's single-portal technique [16] and Chow's two-portal technique [17]. Although endoscopic techniques seemed promising there were no differences between them and the open techniques on the long term results, with the exception of the more aesthetically appealing scar, the reduced scar tenderness and increase in pinch grip and pinch strength at 12 weeks follow up.

The Mini Open Surgical Technique with Two Small Cross Aligned Incisions (TSCAI)

The patient is placed supine on the surgical table with an addition of arm support extension. Very few surgical instruments are needed to perform this surgical procedure (Fig. 5.1). A tourniquet is applied at the arm and the surgical field of the forearm and the hand is prepared with 4% chlorexidine scrub and solution. The local anaesthesia is applied prior to the tourniquet inflation in order to avoid excess of tourniquet time and also to achieve diffusion of its components during the bloodletting. A mixture of local anaesthetics including 2% lidocaine, 7.5% ropivacaine and normal saline 0.9% in a 5-3-2 ratio is prepared and injected slowly under the skin proximal to the palmar wrist creases (Fig. 5.2). Following this the needle is re-entered through the previously anaesthetised skin, now directed distally under the palmar skin between the thenar and hypothenar in the axis of the Taleisnik's line towards the distal surgical incision.

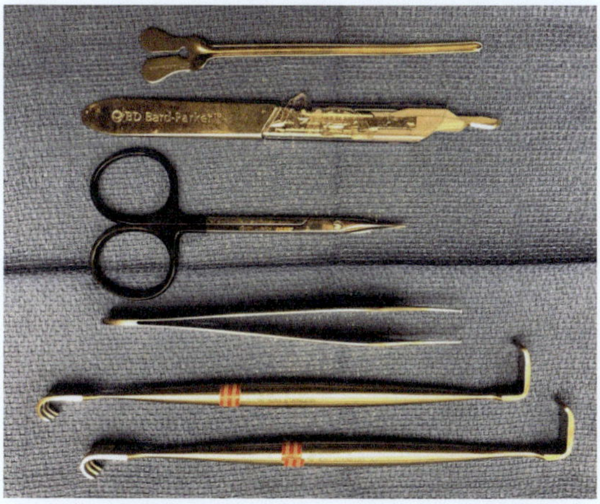

Fig. 5.1 The basic instruments that are needed to successfully release the TCL with the two small cross aligned incisions technique

The incisions are marked on the skin using the distal crease of the wrist as the proximal anatomical landmark and the intersection between Kaplan's line and Taleisnik's line as demonstrated as the distal landmark (Fig. 5.3). Then, the tourniquet is inflated, usually at 250 mmHg, and a 1.5 cm transverse skin incision is performed at the distal crease of the wrist, ulnarly to the flexor carpi radialis (FCR) tendon (Fig. 5.4a). The superficial dissection begins proximally to identify and incise the superficial forearm fascia. The Palmaris Longus (PL) tendon is identified when present and protected and then the deep forearm fascia is incised in a pointed way with the knife tip, with particular care to prevent damage to the median nerve running underneath. It is worth mentioning that in case of accidental damage of the PL tendon, there will not be any real functional deficit, as there is no proximal retraction due to its junction with the distal forearm fascia. Careful dissection is required to avoid injury of the palmar cutaneous branch of the median nerve. Through the small longitudinal incision of the fascia, a thin grooved knife guide with a blunt tip is inserted from distal to proximal direction. Then the distal forearm fascia is incised for approximately 2 cm with a #15 scalpel blade sliding within the guide from distal to proximal (Figs. 5.4b and 5.5). After the release of the distal forearm fascia, the median nerve comes in direct vision at its entrance into the proximal part of the carpal tunnel. Meticulous dissection under loop magnification prevents iatrogenic damage to the palmar cutaneous branch of the median nerve at its course on the distal forearm.

The second 10–12 mm distal skin incision is longitudinal at the level of the exit of the carpal tunnel following the "Taleisnik's line" (Fig. 5.6). This incision should always be placed into a palmar skin crease for an aesthetically more appealing scar. After the superficial dissection of the

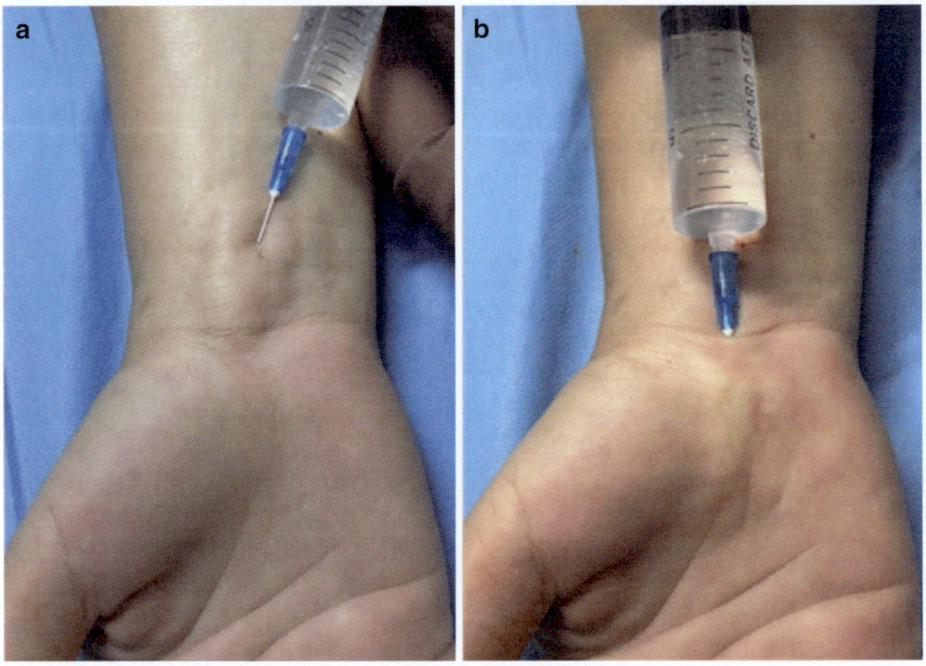

Fig. 5.2 The mixture of local anaesthetics is injected firstly under the skin proximal to the palmar wrist crease until a bump is created (**a**) and then under the skin from the wrist crease up to the distal incision (**b**). No anaesthetic is injected bellow the TCL in the carpal tunnel

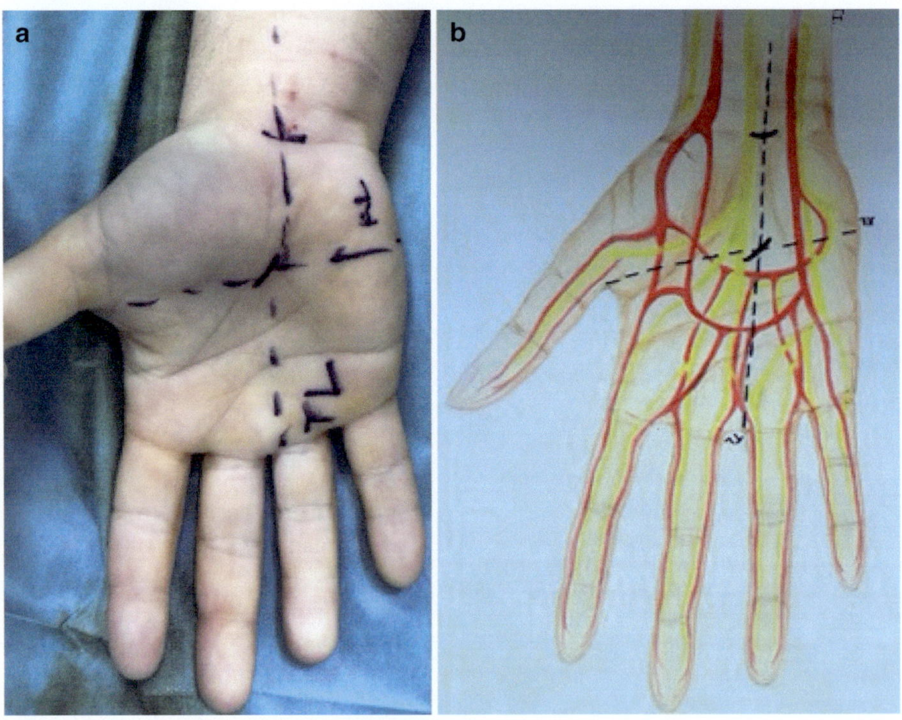

Fig. 5.3 (**a**) Pre-operative drawing of the two incisions. The proximal 1.5 cm incision is a transverse incision ulnar to flexor carpi radialis tendon in line with the Taleisnik's line (TL). The distal 1 cm incision is at the intersection of Taleisnik's and Kaplan's line (KL), with longitudinal or oblique direction to be more aesthetically appealing. (**b**) Schematic of the Taleisnik's and Kaplan's lines

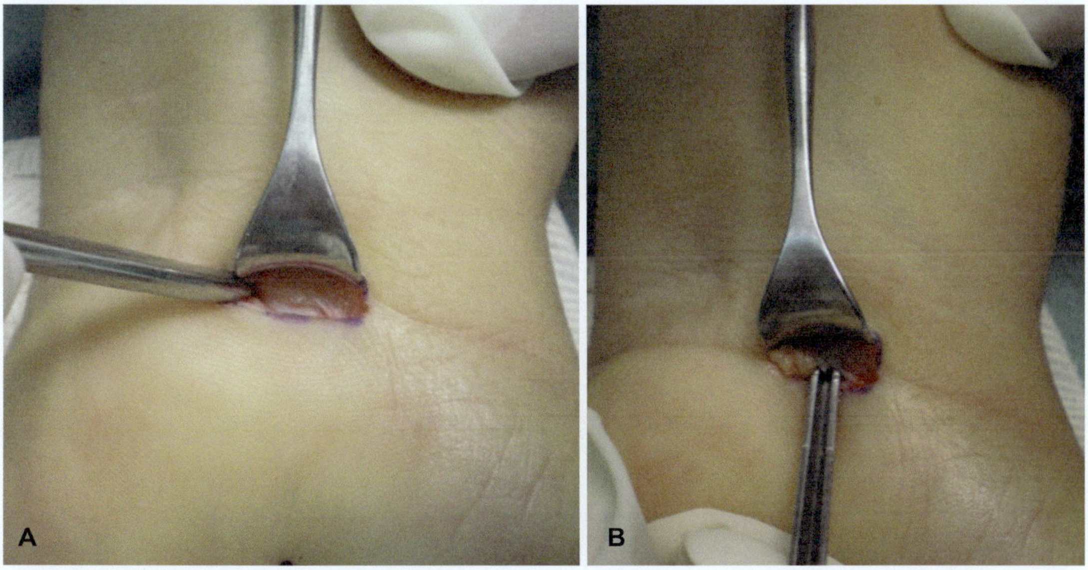

Fig. 5.4 (**a**) The palmaris longus is identified in the proximal incision and retracted radially. The forearm fascia is then incised proximally to reveal the median nerve. (**b**) Insertion of the grooved knife guide into the proximal incision from distal to proximal direction

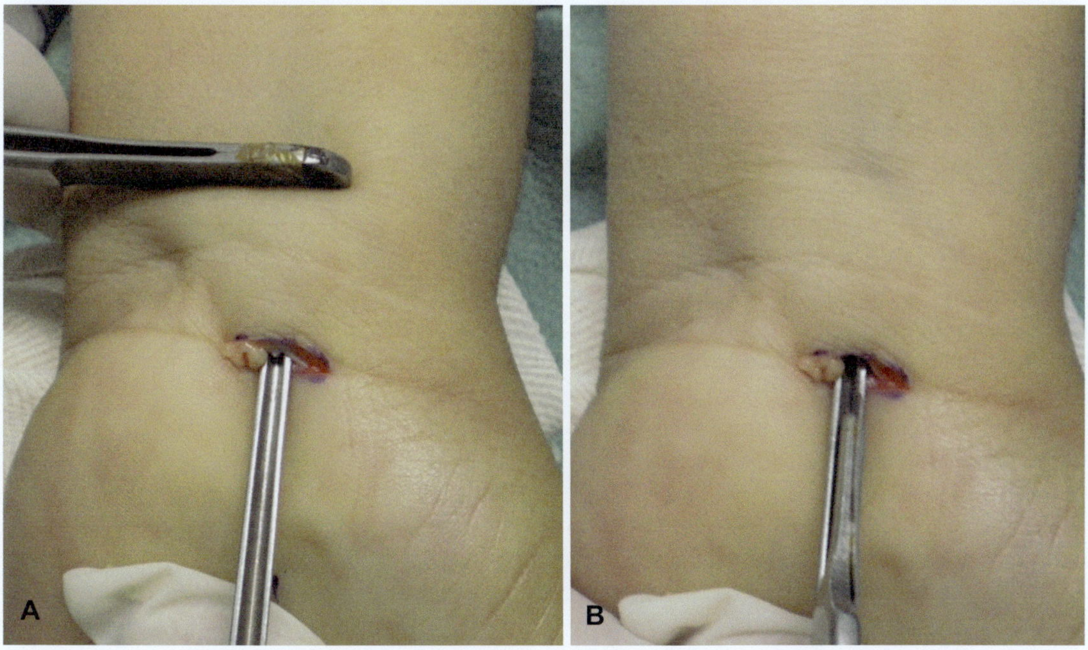

Fig. 5.5 (**a**) Insertion of the grooved knife guide into the proximal incision with distal to proximal direction. (**b**) Incision of the distal forearm fascia for approximately 2 cm with a knife sliding within the guide from distal to proximal

subcutaneous fat under the glabrous skin, opening the palmar aponeurosis the deeper "soft-substance" fat is recognized indicating the outlet of the carpal tunnel. Then, the slightly curved tip grooved knife guide is introduced from the proximal incision directed distally, in the same direction as the Talaisnik's line, and is gently passed distally through the distal incision

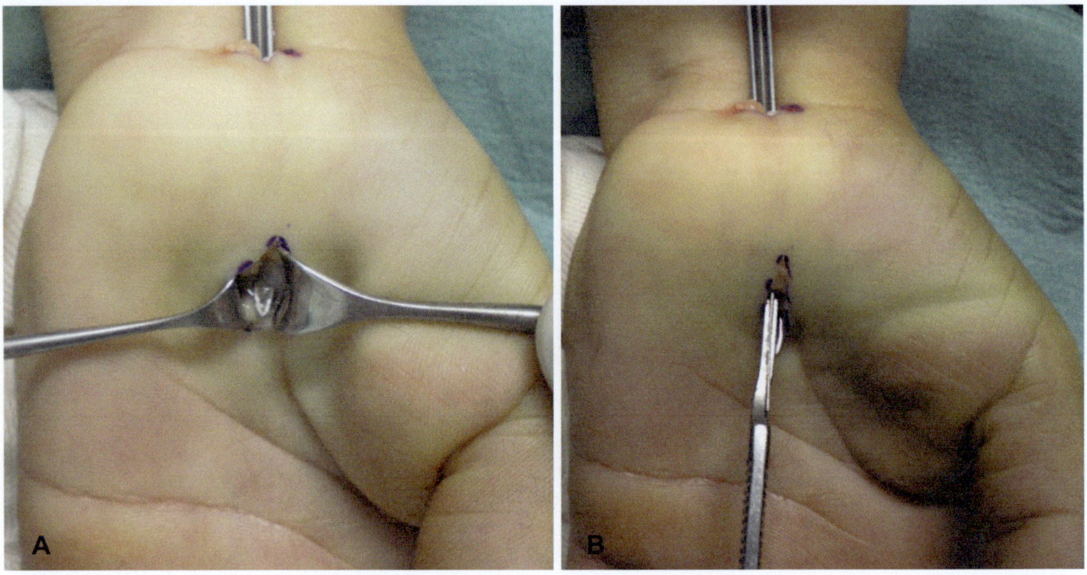

Fig. 5.6 (**a**) Insertion of the grooved knife guide from the proximal incision to the distal incision. (**b**) The knife, with the cutting edge of the scalpel facing upwards, is sliding within the guide from proximal to distal incising the transverse carpal ligament

(Fig. 5.6a). The knife guide turned slightly to an ulnar inclination of 20°, in order to avoid damaging possible trans-ligamentous course of the thenar motor branch of the median nerve. The knife, with the cutting edge of the scalpel facing upwards, is passed from distal to proximal (sliding within the guide) incising the transverse carpal ligament (Fig. 5.6b). At the end of the procedure the complete transection of the transverse carpal ligament is confirmed under direct vision through the proximal and distal incisions (Figs. 5.7 and 5.8) and by passing a broader blunt instrument (i.e. the needle holder tip) through the now widened carpal tunnel.

Neurolysis and excision of the synovium are not routinely performed, except in cases of hypothyroidism or possible inflammatory arthritis that may require a more extensile distal incision. The wound is irrigated with normal saline, and the skin is closed with absorbable sutures and covered by sterile gauzes and bandage.

Postoperative Care

The patient is instructed to elevate the arm and mobilize his fingers several times a day, with the wrist in extension to avoid irritation of the incised TCL by the finger flexor tendons. The long acting ropivacaine local anaesthetic is helping the patient to avoid discomfort for more than 12 hours. Paracetamol orally up to 3 g the first day, is usually enough for analgesia, but most of the patients do not need more than one tablet. The use of the hand is allowed as tolerance. The skin incisions are healed after the first week, and the patient is encouraged to gradually exercise and use the hand during the second week in order to regain the grip strength.

Results

The senior author has applied this technique since January 1995 and has operated on over eleven hundred hands. There were three patients in which the two-incision technique was intra-operatively abandoned and switched to open carpal tunnel release. This happened in manual labor workers with very thick palmar skin and dense subcutaneous fat, which didn't allowed adequate visualization of the carpal tunnel entrance and outlet through the two small incisions.

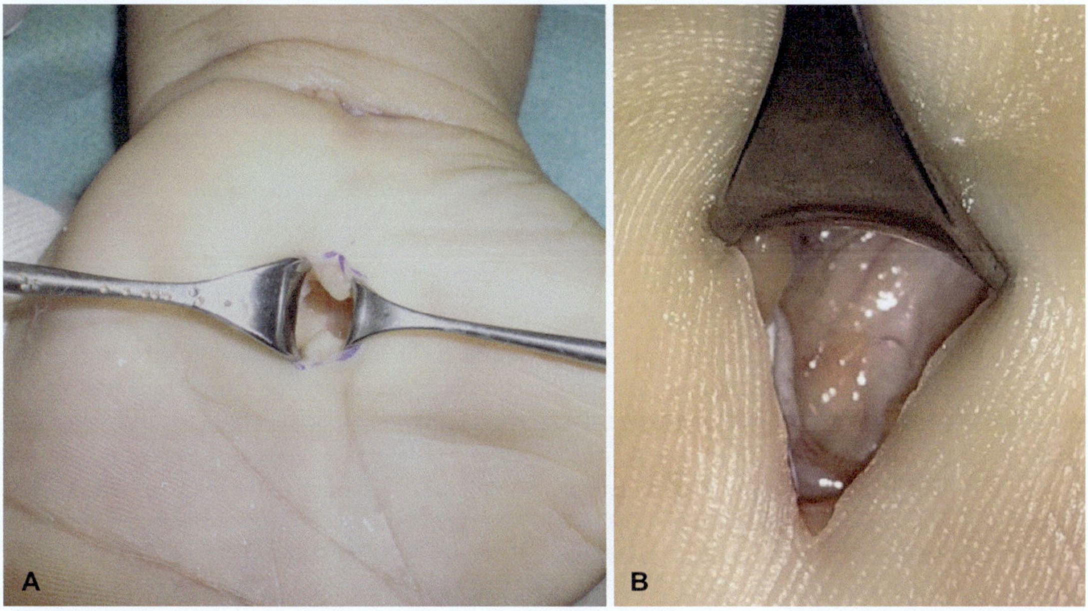

Fig. 5.7 (**a**, **b**) After the release of the transverse carpal ligament, direct inspection of the median nerve through the distal incision

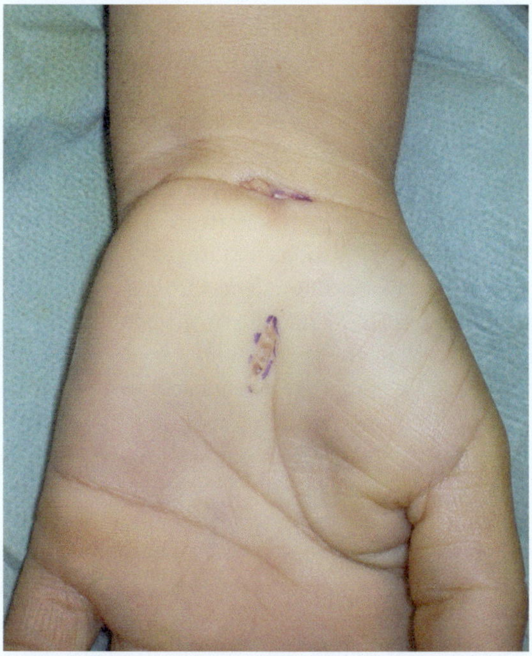

Fig. 5.8 Final appearance of the two cross aligned incisions before wound closure

The although rare but well recognized in the literature early complications are incomplete release of TCL, neuropraxia or injury to the median or ulnar nerve, inadvertent entry to Guyon's canal, injury to the palmar cutaneous or recurrent motor branch of the median nerve and injury to the superficial palmar arch or ulnar artery. The late complications are scar tenderness, loss of grip strength, pillar pain, and rarely the reflex sympathetic dystrophy or complex regional pain syndrome (CRPS), and bowstringing of flexor tendons. Pillar pain is a frequent complication of both open and endoscopic release procedures.

In a recent survey, we reviewed 189 patients with carpal tunnel syndrome who had treated with two-incision mini open technique and had a minimum follow up of 3 months. One of the current chapter authors (F.P.) has conducted all patients through a telephone questionnaire to evaluate the recurrence, painful scars, pillar pain and CRPS. None of the patients complained for neuroma formation, thenar atrophy, or insensate skin at the palm or distal forearm. These results were compared with the outcomes of 643 patients who were treated with the conventional open approach and 144 patients who were treated with minimally invasive surgery (MIS) using Knifelight technique. The findings of the comparison demonstrated no

Table 5.1 Results of comparison between open carpal tunnel release (OCTR), minimally invasive surgery (MIS) using Knifelight technique and two-incision mini open technique for carpal tunnel syndrome

	Group A OCTR	Group B MIS-Knifelight	Group C Two-incision
N (patients)	643 (65.8%)	144 (14.7%)	189 (19.3%)
Recurrence	6 (0.93%)	2 (1.4%)	0
Painful scars	12 (1.7%)	2 (1.4%)	0
Pillar pain	9 (1.4%)	0	0
Complex regional pain syndrome	8 (1.2%)	0	2 (1.0%)

recurrence and no painful scars for the two-incision technique, no pillar pain for both the mini open with the Knifelight and the two-incision decompression (Table 5.1). There was a trend from more CRPS in the open and two-incision techniques. Similarly, there were more patients with recurrences, painful scars in the open and the Knifelight decompressions (Table 5.1).

Discussion

OCTR is an operation easy to perform and in majority of patients it leads to relief from symptoms with a low complication rate. The overall success rate of OCTR is more than 95% with a complication rate of less than 3%. To minimize trauma and post-operative complications, several modifications to the length, location and shape of the incision in OCTR have been described. One of the modifications of classical OCTR is to make a limited transverse incision of ≤2 cm in the same location as classical OCTR. Another modification is a limited open release performed by Atik et al in 2001 [14]. Studies have found no difference between patients who undergo bilateral simultaneous OCTR with modified techniques when compared with classical in terms of the post-operative complication rate, hospital stay, time to return work and the overall cost.

The first ECTR was performed by Okutsu and his colleagues in Japan in 1987 [15]. Later several modifications of the endoscopic technique have been described in the literature, but the underlying principle is the same: to release transverse carpal ligament. ECTR techniques can be carried out either with single portal or with dual portal techniques depending on the number of ports used to access the carpal tunnel. The two most commonly used techniques are the single-portal technique described by Agee [16] and the two-portal technique described by Chow [17]. The reported success rates for surgical treatment range from 70% to 90%.

In an extensive review of all articles on ECTR covering six different types of techniques, Jimenez et al. found that the endoscopic release techniques offer similar success and complication rate as open techniques [18]. The overall success rate for ECTR was 96.52% with a complication rate of 2.67% and a failure rate of 2.61% [18]. The Cochrane database group reviewed all available evidence from randomized controlled trials comparing various surgical techniques in terms of efficacy in relieving symptoms, promoting early return to work and post operative complications and found no strong evidence to favour alternative surgical techniques compared to the standard open technique [19]. More specifically, the authors found conflicting evidence in support of endoscopic release in leading to an earlier return to work and/or activities of daily living when compared to open CTR [19]. These findings have been replicated by another meta-analysis study of randomized controlled trials comparing endoscopic and open carpal tunnel decompression, which also found no conclusive evidence favouring ECTR with regard to symptom relief and return to work [20]. However, they found that ECTR was associated with reduced scar tenderness and increase in pinch grip and pinch strength at 12 weeks follow up. The most common complications noted by the authors were paresthesia of the ulnar and median nerves, injury to superficial palmar arch, CRPS, flexor tendons lacerations and incomplete division of TCL.

As in other fields of surgery, less invasive techniques have been introduced into carpal tunnel surgery to facilitate earlier return to work and reduce post-operative pillar pain. The two small cross aligned incisions (TSCAI) surgical approach is causing minimal trauma and at the same time allows direct visualization of the median nerve. The transverse proximal incision always carried out under loop magnification allows protection of the superficial sensory branch for the palm, thus avoiding neuroma formation. The introduction of the thin grooved knife guide is safe when the patient is able to communicate and react in case of nerve encroachment. Directing upwards the cutting edge of the knife driven by the inserted guide, against the TCL with a slight ulnar inclination has been proven safe, as there has been no accidental injury of the thenar motor branch. The knife guide is a grooved metallic instrument of 4 mm in width and 2.5 mm in depth having a triangular cross section (Fig. 5.1). Its dimensions are considerably smaller compared to the bulk of the endoscopic guide. Thus entering the carpal tunnel is less irritable for the median nerve, and this might be one of the reasons of lower rates of CRPS with this technique.

In conclusion, the TSCAI technique with the use of few surgical instruments under local anaesthesia described above is a safe and reliable alternative treatment option for the release of the TCL to relieve the symptoms of the carpal tunnel syndrome.

Acknowledgement The authors want to thank our colleague physician Georgia Ioannou, for creating the Fig. 5.3b drawing.

References

1. Bai J, Kong L, Zhao H, Yu K, Zhang B, Zhang J, Tian D. Carpal tunnel release with a new mini-incision approach versus a conventional approach, a retrospective cohort study. Int J Surg. 2018;52:105–9.
2. Aroori S, Spence RA. Carpal tunnel syndrome. Ulster Med J. 2008;77(1):6–17.
3. Phalen GS. The carpal-tunnel syndrome. Seventeen years' experience in diagnosis and treatment of six hundred fifty-four hands. J Bone Joint Surg Am. 1966;48(2):211–28.
4. Hoffmann P, Buck-Gramcko D, Lubahn JD. The Hoffmann-Tinel sign. 1915. J Hand Surg Br. 1993;18(6):800–5.
5. Paget J. Lectures on surgical pathology. Philadelphia: Lindsay and Blakiston; 1854.
6. Putnam JJ. A series of cases of paraesthesia, mainly of the hand, of periodic occurence, and possibly of vaso-motor origin. Arch Med (NY). 1880;4:147–62.
7. Marie P, Foix C. Atrophie isolee de l'eminence thenar d'origine nevritique, role du legamente anulaire anterieur du carpe dans la pathogenie de la lesion Revue. Neurology. 1913;21:647.
8. Learmont JR. The principle of decompression in the treatment of certain diseases of peripheral nerves. Surg Clin North Am. 1933;13:905–13.
9. Lanz U. Anatomical variations of the median nerve in the carpal tunnel. J Hand Surg Am. 1977;2(1):44–53.
10. Henry BM, Zwinczewska H, Roy J, Vikse J, Ramakrishnan PK, Walocha JA, Tomaszewski KA. The prevalence of anatomical variations of the median nerve in the Carpal tunnel: a systematic review and meta-analysis. PLoS One. 2015;10(8):e0136477.
11. Hurwitz PJ. Variations in the course of the thenar motor branch of the median nerve. J Hand Surg Br. 1996;21(3):344–6.
12. Karl JW, Gancarczyk SM, Strauch RJ. Complications of carpal tunnel release. Orthop Clin North Am. 2016;47(2):425–33.
13. Hunt TR, Osterman AL. Complications of the treatment of carpal tunnel syndrome. Hand Clin. 1994;10(1):63–71.
14. Atik TL, Smith B, Baratz ME. Risk of neurovascular injury with limited-open carpal tunnel release: defining the "safe-zone". J Hand Surg Br. 2001;26(5):484–7.
15. Okutsu I, Ninomiya S, Takatori Y, Ugawa Y. Endoscopic management of carpal tunnel syndrome. Arthroscopy. 1989;5(1):11–8.
16. Agee JM, McCarroll HR, North ER. Endoscopic carpal tunnel release using the single proximal incision technique. Hand Clin. 1994;10(4):647–59.
17. Chow JC. Endoscopic carpal tunnel release. Clin Sports Med. 1996;15(4):769–84.
18. Jimenez DF, Gibbs SR, Clapper AT. Endoscopic treatment of carpal tunnel syndrome: a critical review. J Neurosurg. 1998;88(5):817–26.
19. Scholten RJ, Mink van der Molen A, Uitdehaag BM, Bouter LM, de Vet HCW. Surgical treatment options for carpal tunnel syndrome. Cochrane Database Syst Rev. 2007;(4):CD003905.
20. Zuo D, Zhou Z, Wang H, Liao Y, Zheng L, Hua Y, Cai Z. Endoscopic versus open carpal tunnel release for idiopathic carpal tunnel syndrome: a meta-analysis of randomized controlled trials. J Orthop Surg Res. 2015;10:12.

Endoscopic Carpal Tunnel Release

6

Aaron I. Venouziou and Antonios Kerasnoudis

Introduction

Carpal tunnel syndrome (CTS) is the most common compressive neuropathy of the upper extremity, with approximately 5% incidence in the general population [1]. Compression of the median nerve at the wrist level can cause hand pain, numbness, and tingling in the early stages of the syndrome and motor weakness of the hand in the late stages. CTS initially is addressed with non-operative measures such as rest, night splints, NSAIDs and corticosteroid injection. When non-operative treatment fails then surgical release of the transverse carpal ligament (TCL) is indicated.

The first carpal tunnel release (CTR) was performed by Learmonth in 1933 [2]. Since then, numerous surgical techniques have been described to release the TCL and decompress the underlying median nerve. The open CTR (OCTR) approach remains the gold standard and the most commonly used technique. Approximately 500,000 CTRs are performed every year in the US, with an annually cost of over two billion USD [3]. Based on 2009 US Department of Labour figures, a sick leave of at least 30 days per year is documented in about 45% of people with CTS, with a median of 28 days absent from work [4]. In the last three decades endoscopic carpal tunnel release (ECTR) techniques were introduced to reduce morbidity and to expedite recovery from surgery. ECTR offers the theoretical advantages of reduced postoperative pain, faster recovery of grip strength, earlier return to work and activities of daily living, and fewer wound-related complications [5]. Amongst the endoscopic techniques that have been developed the last decades, our preferred one is the single proximal portal approach described by Agee in 1992 [6]. This chapter describes in detail the single proximal portal ECTR technique.

Indication: Contraindications

Generally, the indications for ECTR are the same as for conventional OCTR. Most of the primary cases of CTS can be treated by endoscopic release. However, ECTR is absolutely contraindicated in cases where additional procedures must be performed in the carpal tunnel, such as exploration or dissection of the median nerve and/or the carpal tunnel contents, for e.g. space occupying lesions and prolific tenosynovitis that needs synovectomy. Severe median nerve neuropathy requiring extensive neurolysis is another relative

A. I. Venouziou (✉)
Division of Upper Extremity Surgery, Orthopaedic Department, St. Luke's Hospital, Panorama, Thessaloniki, Greece

A. Kerasnoudis
Department of Neurology, St. Luke's Hospital, Panorama, Thessaloniki, Greece

D. G. Sotereanos, L. K. Papatheodorou (eds.), *Compressive Neuropathies of the Upper Extremity*,
https://doi.org/10.1007/978-3-030-37289-7_6

contraindication for ECTR according to several authors [7]. Although, many surgeons advocate that ECTR should be avoided in patients with recurrent CTS, we agree with Trumble et al. that ECTR can be performed safely in selected cases, such as incomplete release of TCL which remains one of the leading causes for recurrence [8]. This can be successfully diagnosed preoperatively with an ultrasound examination of the wrist, by an experienced radiologist or neurologist on nerve and musculoskeletal sonography. For this reason, we routinely perform preoperative ultrasound of the wrist in every case of primary and recurrent CTS. If the ultrasound examination reveals incomplete sectioning of the TCL then ECTR can be safely performed. On the other hand, whenever scaring of the median nerve is demonstrated by the ultrasound then a revision open CTR should be executed.

Surgical Technique

Anatomy

On the dorsal side carpal tunnel has three walls that are formed by the volar arch of the carpal bones. On the palmar side, the roof of the carpal tunnel is the transverse carpal ligament. The TCL radially attaches to the scaphoid and the trapezium and ulnarly to the pisiform and the hook of the hamate. Proximally the TCL continues and blends with the antebrachial fascia. Before entering the carpal tunnel, the median nerve is superficial and lies beneath the antebrachial fascia, between the tendons of the flexor carpi radialis (FCR) and flexor digitorum superficialis (FDS) and deep to the palmaris longus, whenever the latter tendon is present. The median nerve enters the carpal tunnel in its palmar and radial quadrant, along with the nine digital flexor tendons. In an anatomic study, Rotman and Manske found that inserting the endoscope into the carpal tunnel in line with the ring finger axis is the safest approach because it maximizes the interval between the endoscope and the median nerve, and the distance from the superficial palmar arch, thus decreasing the risk of injury to these structures [9]. Concerning anatomical variations in the course of the thenar muscle branch (TMB) and the median nerve in the carpal tunnel we recommend an ulnar side approach along the axis of the fourth ray, to avoid iatrogenic damage to the TMB, as proposed in a recent meta-analysis [10].

Positioning

The patient is placed supine with the shoulder in 70–80° of abduction and the hand on a broad operating arm table. The surgical suite should be set up to offer the surgeon the best view of the video monitor. The surgeon should be able to easily shift his/her gaze upward from the surgical field to the video image. Surgeons who are ambidextrous using the endoscope generally take the axillary position when performing either a left or right carpal tunnel release (holding the instrument in their right hand for a right carpal tunnel and in their left hand for a left carpal tunnel). Those favouring right-handed use will usually prefer a position in the axilla for a right carpal tunnel release and cephalic position for a left release. The assistant is always positioned on the opposite side of the surgeon. The upper extremity is prepped and draped free and a non sterile pneumatic tourniquet is used, which is inflated to 250 mmHg to avoid bleeding.

Instrumentation

Special equipment is needed for the single proximal portal technique, first described by Agee in 1992 [6]. This technique utilizes a patented device (MicroAire Smart Release, Charlottesville, VA, USA) which is composed by a 2.7 mm/30° angle arthroscope, a camera, a fiber optic light source, and a pistol like handpiece with an attached disposable blade cartridge into which the endoscope is inserted. The sterile field should also include:

- 2 double-pronged skin hooks
- 2 Senn rake retractors
- 1 Adson tissue forceps with serrated tips

- 1 pair of tenotomy scissors
- 1 scalpel, #15 blade
- 1 Sterile skin marking pen
- 1 small hamate finder
- 1 standard hamate finder
- 1 Blade-shaped coequal hamate finder
- 1 synovium elevator

Anaesthesia

The operation may be performed, at the preference of the patient and surgeon, under general, regional, or local anaesthesia. In our practice we prefer local anaesthesia for ECTR. Injecting a large volume of local anesthetic may impair the view by fogging of the endoscope and poor visualization of the canal. For this reason, we infiltrate the distal wrist crease and proximal forearm fascia with 5 ml of a solution of 1% lidocaine with 1:100,000 epinephrine and 0.5% bupivacaine. The tourniquet is elevated and the solution is injected intracutaneously/subcutaneously in the wrist flexion crease, extending from the flexor carpi ulnaris to the flexor carpi radialis. It is very important to remember that only when the surgeon has gained experience with the surgical approach and instrumentation should the procedure be performed using local anesthesia.

Approach and Release of TCL

Before inflation of the tourniquet, it is recommended (especially for the first cases) to mark with a sterile skin marking pen the key anatomical landmarks on the patient's hand, such as the tendons of the flexor carpi ulnaris and flexor carpi radialis, pisiform bone and hook of the hamate (Fig. 6.1). The incision line at a wrist flexion crease should also be marked. Finally, the surgeon should draw a line from the middle of the wrist flexion crease to the base of the ring finger. This line should pass radial to the hook of hamate.

A 2 cm transverse incision between the tendons of the flexor carpi radialis and the flexor carpi ulnaris is used at the level of proximal wrist flexion crease (Fig. 6.2). The more proximal crease is technically easier to use because of less subcutaneous fat. Blunt, spreading longitudinal dissection is

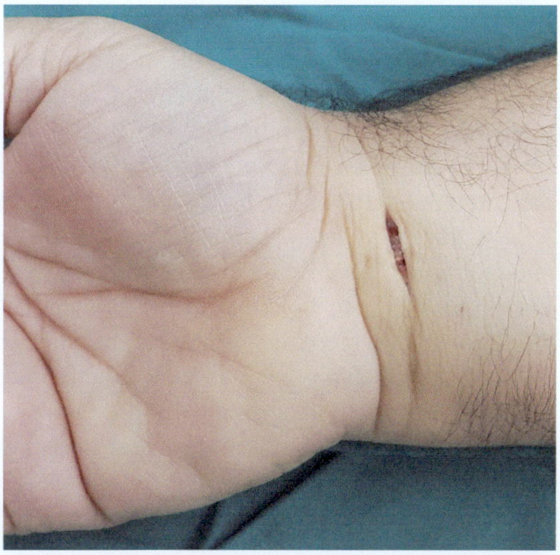

Fig. 6.2 The length of the incision is about 1.5–2 cm and located between PL and FCU

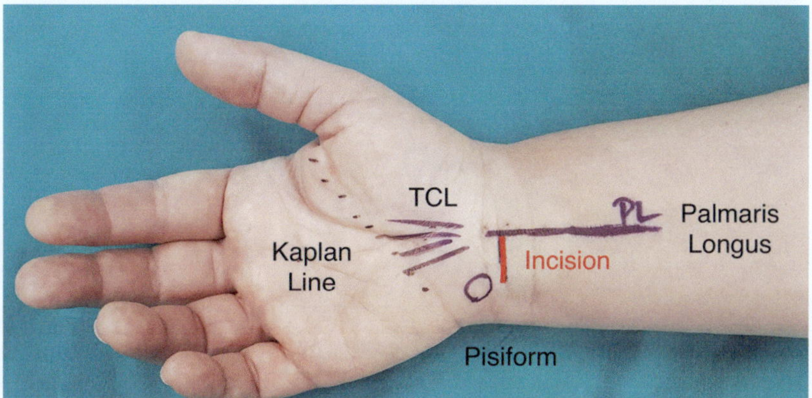

Fig. 6.1 Landmarks of endoscopic CTR. The incision is located between palmaris longus (PL), whenever is present, and the flexor carpi ulnaris (FCU). The distal edge of TCL is at the level of Kaplan's line

done in the subcutaneous layer, deep and ulnar to palmaris longus (thereby staying out of the territory of the palmar cutaneous branch of the median nerve which is located between palmaris and flexor carpi radialis), to expose and visualize the antebrachial fascia. Then a U-shaped incision is made in the forearm fascia, creating a rectangular flap distally based on the transverse carpal ligament. Elevating this flap from the underlying finger flexor synovium (ulnar bursa) allows the surgeon to create a plane between the synovium and the deep side of the transverse carpal ligament. The surgeon should always have in mind that the median nerve is immediately beneath this flap.

After elevating the forearm fascia flap from the underlying synovium the surgeon positions a synovium elevator in line with the base of the ring finger and radial to the hook of the hamate. Using the synovium elevator the surgeon feels the roughness ("washboard effect") of the TCL transverse fibers and continues distally until the tip of the elevator is palpable at the distal end of the carpal tunnel. Next, with the use of the small hamate finder a path is created for the blade assembly (Fig. 6.3). While aiming at the base of the ring finger and holding the wrist in slight extension, the surgeon gently passes the hamate finder distally down the ulnar side of the tunnel, hugging the hook of the hamate until the finder's curved tip can be palpated subcutaneously at the distal exit of the carpal tunnel. One or two passes is sufficient to create a path. In the case of a large hand the surgeon should use the standard or blade shaped hamate finder to create the path. While holding the patient's wrist in slight extension, the blade assembly is inserted into the carpal tunnel aiming at the base of the ring finger and hugging the hook of the hamate to assure an ulnar course (Fig. 6.4). When a clear view of the TCL is achieved, the distal edge of the TCL is identified *easily* (Fig. 6.5a). A fingertip pressed gently onto the palmar skin at the estimated point of the distal edge of the TCL can be helpful for confirmation of the endoscopic visualization of the distal TCL edge. Indentation and motion of the softer, yellowish subcutaneous fatty tissues will be seen through the endoscope just distal to the rigid distal edge of the TCL. The cutting blade of the device is deployed at the distal edge by pressing the trigger fully, and the device is then slowly withdrawn proximally to a point about one third to one half between the proximal and distal edges of the TCL (Fig. 6.5b). With the trigger released and the cutting blade retracted, the endoscope is advanced again distally and the incised portion of the TCL is inspected for any remaining superficial intact TCL fibers (Fig. 6.5c). Undivided fibers of the TCL can be incised with one or more additional distal-to-proximal passes with the endoscope in the distal half of the canal. Incising initially only the distal half of the TCL helps to avoid the visibility problem of fatty midpalm tissues hanging down between the cut edges of the TCL in the middle of the canal, and obscuring the

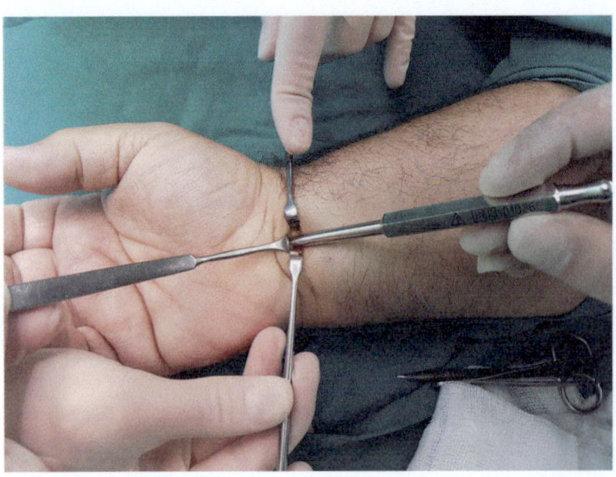

Fig. 6.3 The hamate finder is used to create a path for the blade assembly beneath the TCL

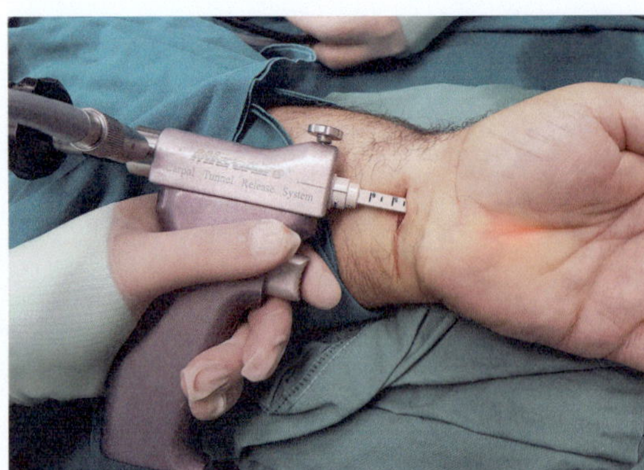

Fig. 6.4 The blade assembly is inserted into the carpal tunnel aiming at the base of the ring finger and hugging the hook of the hamate to assure an ulnar course

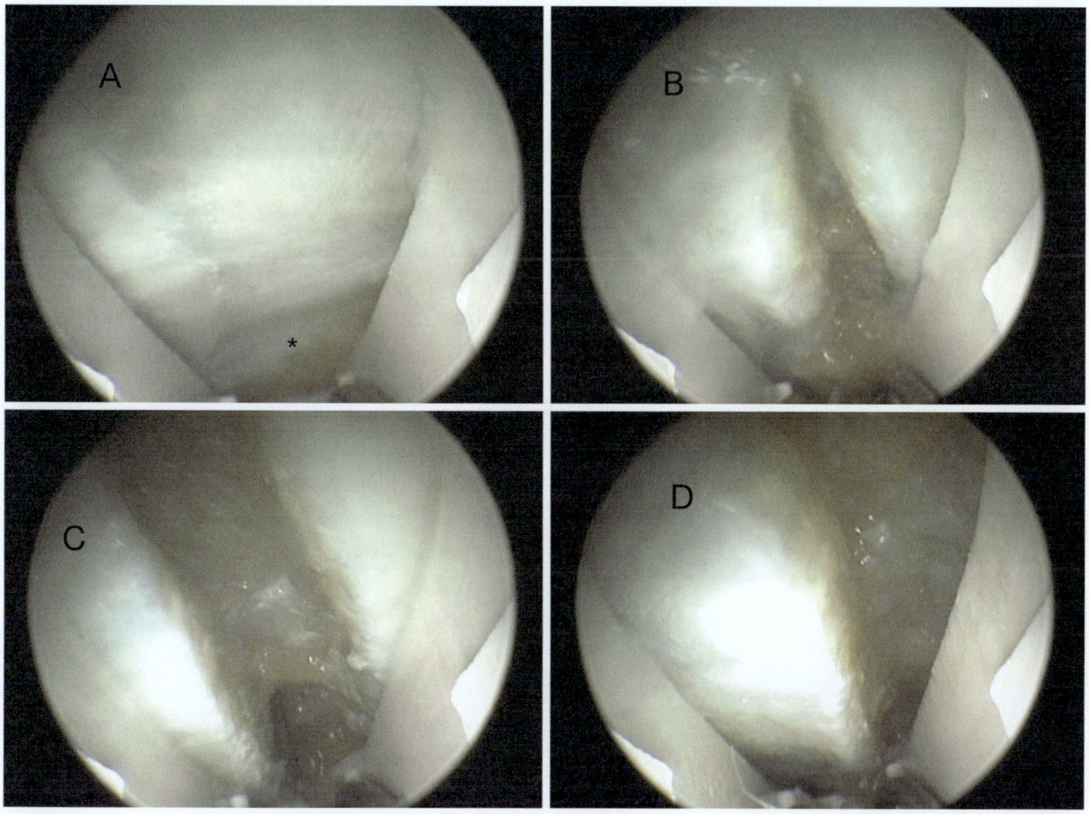

Fig. 6.5 (**a**) The distal edge of the TCL is identified easily by the presence of yellowish subcutaneous fat tissue (asterisk). (**b**) Initially the TCL is partially incised to a point about one third to one half between the proximal and distal edges of it. (**c**) The incised portion of the TCL is inspected for any remaining superficial intact TCL fibers. (**d**) Complete release is indicated by the retraction of the two halves of the ligament in radial and ulnar directions

view of the cut or uncut ligament through the endoscope. When division of the distal half of the TCL is complete, the endoscope is positioned distal to the most proximal portion of the cut ligament, the blade is deployed and the scope is withdrawn proximally to the proximal edge of TCL. With the blade retracted, the scope assembly is reinserted, the entire incised TCL is inspected, and any remaining intact fibers are divided. Complete release is indicated by the retraction of the two halves of the ligament in radial and ulnar directions. The canal will now be and feel much larger, and light transmission through palmar skin is increased. A small right-angled blunt retractor can be used after endoscope removal to inspect the proximal part of the carpal tunnel under direct vision, to confirm satisfactory wide separation of the cut edges of the TCL (Fig. 6.5d). After the completion of the TCL release, using a tenotomy scissors, the forearm fascia is released proximal to the skin incision, taking care to protect the median nerve. This prevents the forearm fascia from acting as a constricting band that could continue to compromise median nerve function.

Before closure the wound is copiously irrigated, the tourniquet is deflated and meticulous hemostasis is obtained. The skin is closed with a subcuticular running absorbable monofilament 4.0 suture and sterile strips (Fig. 6.6). A sterile dressing is then applied and the patient is discharged.

Follow-up Protocol

Active range of motion is encouraged immediately after discharge. We generally schedule the first postoperative follow up visit 3–5 days after

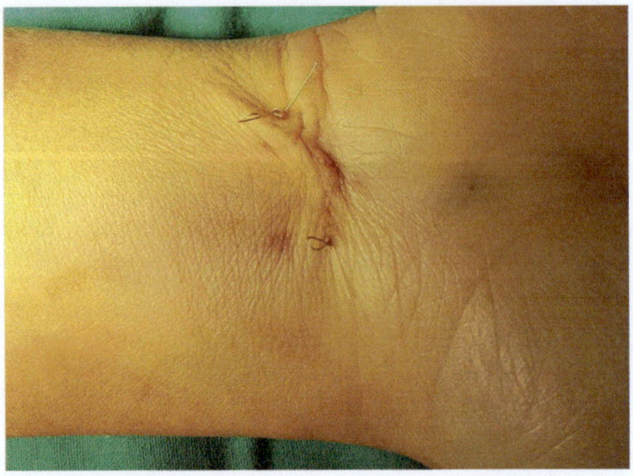

Fig. 6.6 The wound is closed with a running subcuticular 4.0 absorbable suture

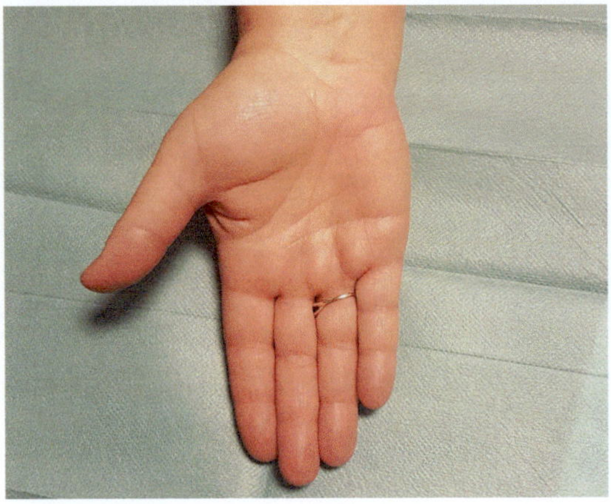

Fig. 6.7 At 3 months post surgery the cosmetic outcome is remarkable

surgery where we remove all the dressings and we apply to the incision a band-aid. At that point hand motion has fully recovered and light activities are resumed as per patient comfort. In general, heavy duties are resumed at about 4–6 weeks. Patients are seen by the physician at about 4 weeks post surgery and then followed as needed. At 3 months post surgery the cosmetic outcome of endoscopic release is remarkable (Fig. 6.7).

Complications

The reported complication rates of ECTR compare favorably with published series of open carpal tunnel release. Complications include incomplete ligament release, nerve injuries, palmar hematomas, adhesions between nerves and tendons, reflex sympathetic dystrophy, deep wound infections, scar tenderness, pillar pain, tendon lacerations and vascular injuries [11–17]. The damage to the surrounding anatomic structures that occurs during endoscopic carpal tunnel surgery usually requires a second surgical procedure to be repaired. For this reason, the surgeon should always inform the patients that he/she reserve the option of converting the endoscopic release to an open release if all of the conditions for a safe and effective, complete endoscopic-method release are not fulfilled intraoperatively. We never cut when we can not see everything that must be seen, at all times, and we should always remember that *when in doubt we get out*.

Outcomes

Controversy continues to dispute any method of ECTR. Advocates proclaim less postoperative pain, faster recovery of grip strength, and quicker return to work [18–20]. Criticizers cite the higher occurrence of incomplete release of the transverse carpal ligament, worrying reports of neurovascular injury, and a comparable rate of pillar pain [21–26].

Agee et al. carried out a 10-center randomized prospective multicenter study of endoscopic release using his technique. There were 122 patients in the study. Twenty-five had carpal tunnel surgery on both hands and 97 had surgery on one hand. Of the surgical procedures, 65 were in the control group and 82 were in the endoscopic group. For patients in the endoscopic group with one affected hand, the median time for return to work was 21.5 days less than that for the control group. Another benefit of the endoscopic method is the ability to perform simultaneous bilateral CTR without significantly increasing patient morbidity.

Another large multicenter prospective study of 192 cases demonstrated at least in the short term that the patients treated with the endoscopic method had significantly greater grip strength, pinch strength, and hand dexterity. The open technique resulted in greater scar tenderness during the first 3 months after surgery, as well as a longer time until the patients could return to work [27].

In a recent meta-analysis of 21 randomized control trials on open versus endoscopic carpal tunnel release, Sayegh and Strauch found that endoscopic release allows earlier return to work and improved strength during the early postoperative period. Results at 6 months or later are similar according to current data except that patients undergoing endoscopic release are at greater risk of nerve injury and lower risk of scar tenderness compared with open release [5].

Conclusions

The Agee ECTR technique represents a single-portal, minimally invasive procedure to treat patients with median nerve compression at the wrist who meet the criteria for surgery. General advantages of this technique over open CTR include less scar tenderness, decreased pillar pain, faster recovery of pinch and grip strength, and earlier return to work and daily activities. While endoscopic release may appeal to patients who require an early return to work and activities, surgeons should be cognizant of its elevated incidence of transient nerve injury among its similar overall efficacy to open carpal tunnel release. However, as in any surgical and especially endoscopic procedure, safety and success are dependent upon patient selection, thorough knowledge of the surface and surgical anatomy, adequate training, and familiarity with the use and capabilities of the instrumentation. Surgeons who are not familiarized with endoscopic equipment and technique may give rise to major iatrogenic complications.

References

1. Atroshi I, Gummesson C, Johnsson R, Ornstein E, Ranstam J, Rosen I. Prevalence of carpal tunnel syndrome in a general population. JAMA. 1999;282(2):153–8.
2. Learmonth J. The principle of decompression in the treatment of certain diseases of peripheral nerves. Surg Clin North Am. 1933;13:905–13.
3. Palmer DH, Hanrahan LP. Social and economic costs of carpal tunnel surgery. Instr Course Lect. 1995;44:167–72.
4. Vasiliadis HS, Georgoulas P, Shrier I, Salanti G, Scholten RJ. Endoscopic release for carpal tunnel syndrome. Cochrane Database Syst Rev. 2014;(1):CD008265. https://doi.org/10.1002/14651858.CD008265.pub2.
5. Sayegh ET, Strauch RJ. Open versus endoscopic carpal tunnel release: a meta-analysis of randomized controlled trials. Clin Orthop Relat Res. 2015;473(3):1120–32. https://doi.org/10.1007/s11999-014-3835-z.
6. Agee JM, McCarroll HR Jr, Tortosa RD, Berry DA, Szabo RM, Peimer CA. Endoscopic release of the carpal tunnel: a randomized prospective multicenter study. J Hand Surg Am. 1992;17(6):987–95.
7. Jebson PJ, Agee JM. Carpal tunnel syndrome: unusual contraindications to endoscopic release. Arthroscopy. 1996;12(6):749–51.
8. Luria S, Waitayawinyu T, Trumble TE. Endoscopic revision of carpal tunnel release. Plast Reconstr Surg. 2008;121(6):2029–34; discussion 35–6. https://doi.org/10.1097/PRS.0b013e31817123de.
9. Rotman MB, Manske PR. Anatomic relationships of an endoscopic carpal tunnel device to surrounding structures. J Hand Surg Am. 1993;18(3):442–50. https://doi.org/10.1016/0363-5023(93)90089-L.
10. Henry BM, Zwinczewska H, Roy J, Vikse J, Ramakrishnan PK, Walocha JA, et al. The prevalence of anatomical variations of the median nerve in the carpal tunnel: a systematic review and meta-analysis. PLoS One. 2015;10(8):e0136477. https://doi.org/10.1371/journal.pone.0136477.
11. Das SK, Brown HG. In search of complications in carpal tunnel decompression. Hand. 1976;8(3):243–9.
12. MacDonald RI, Lichtman DM, Hanlon JJ, Wilson JN. Complications of surgical release for carpal tunnel syndrome. J Hand Surg Am. 1978;3(1):70–6.
13. Lilly CJ, Magnell TD. Severance of the thenar branch of the median nerve as a complication of carpal tunnel release. J Hand Surg Am. 1985;10(3):399–402.
14. Louis DS, Greene TL, Noellert RC. Complications of carpal tunnel surgery. J Neurosurg. 1985;62(3):352–6. https://doi.org/10.3171/jns.1985.62.3.0352.
15. Kessler FB. Complications of the management of carpal tunnel syndrome. Hand Clin. 1986;2(2):401–6.
16. Terrono AL, Belsky MR, Feldon PG, Nalebuff EA. Injury to the deep motor branch of the ulnar nerve during carpal tunnel release. J Hand Surg Am. 1993;18(6):1038–40. https://doi.org/10.1016/0363-5023(93)90399-N.
17. Brown RA, Gelberman RH, Seiler JG 3rd, Abrahamsson SO, Weiland AJ, Urbaniak JR, et al. Carpal tunnel release. A prospective, randomized assessment of open and endoscopic methods. J Bone Joint Surg Am. 1993;75(9):1265–75.
18. Atroshi I, Larsson GU, Ornstein E, Hofer M, Johnsson R, Ranstam J. Outcomes of endoscopic surgery compared with open surgery

for carpal tunnel syndrome among employed patients: randomised controlled trial. BMJ. 2006;332(7556):1473. https://doi.org/10.1136/bmj.38863.632789.1F.
19. Futami T. Surgery for bilateral carpal tunnel syndrome. Endoscopic and open release compared in 10 patients. Acta Orthop Scand. 1995;66(2):153–5.
20. Jimenez DF, Gibbs SR, Clapper AT. Endoscopic treatment of carpal tunnel syndrome: a critical review. J Neurosurg. 1998;88(5):817–26. https://doi.org/10.3171/jns.1998.88.5.0817.
21. Murphy RX Jr, Jennings JF, Wukich DK. Major neurovascular complications of endoscopic carpal tunnel release. J Hand Surg Am. 1994;19(1):114–8. https://doi.org/10.1016/0363-5023(94)90233-X.
22. Ecker HA Jr. Persistent or recurrent carpal tunnel surgery following prior endoscopic carpal tunnel release. J Hand Surg Am. 1999;24(3):647–8. https://doi.org/10.1053/jhsu.1999.3le03.
23. Forman DL, Watson HK, Caulfield KA, Shenko J, Caputo AE, Ashmead D. Persistent or recurrent carpal tunnel syndrome following prior endoscopic carpal tunnel release. J Hand Surg Am. 1998;23(6):1010–4.
24. Ludlow KS, Merla JL, Cox JA, Hurst LN. Pillar pain as a postoperative complication of carpal tunnel release: a review of the literature. J Hand Ther. 1997;10(4):277–82.
25. Wheatley MJ, Kaul MP. Recurrent carpal tunnel syndrome following endoscopic carpal tunnel release: a preliminary report. Ann Plast Surg. 1997;39(5):469–71.
26. Schonauer F, Varma S, Belcher HJ. Endoscopic carpal tunnel release: practice in evolution. Scand J Plast Reconstr Surg Hand Surg. 2003;37(6):360–4.
27. Trumble TE, Diao E, Abrams RA, Gilbert-Anderson MM. Single-portal endoscopic carpal tunnel release compared with open release: a prospective, randomized trial. J Bone Joint Surg Am. 2002;84-A(7):1107–15.

Complications of Carpal Tunnel Release

7

Panagiotis Giannakopoulos,
Konstantinos Kourkoutas, and George Kasimatis

Introduction

Back in 1980, Giannikas and Touliatos [1], described in their book "The Surgery of the Wounded Hand", the value of the median nerve:

> In primitive mammals, the fifth brain conjugation (the trident) is the primary information gathering center. In human, the primary function of the fifth conjugal was supplanted by the median nerve. Mated with vision, the touch sensor, leads us to trace the truth about the objective world that surrounds us. [1] (originally written in Greek language)

Actually, the median nerve, which gives sensation to the main pinching fingers of our hands, clearly contributed the most in the evolution of the human species. On the contrary, dysfunction of the median nerve leads to a significant reduction in our ability to live in daily life.

The most common pathology of the median nerve is the pressure within the carpal tunnel, called carpal tunnel syndrome (CTS). A great variety of approaches for surgical decompression of the median nerve has been described. The classic open incision, the classic extended, and the mini open are the most often utilized procedures. A transverse incision has also been suggested by a few surgeons. On the other hand, many surgeons prefer to perform minimally invasive techniques, namely endoscopy or using special knifes designed for carpal tunnel release.

Although the procedure is simple, complications following carpal tunnel release, either open or endoscopic, are common. Das and Brown in 1976 [2] and MacDonald et al. [3] in 1978, were reported complications rate 12–15%. Lilly and Magnell, in 1985 found the percentage of complication up to 7% [4], and Mackinnon and Dellon, in 1988 up to 5% [5]. They reported 16 complications in total of 500 cases (3.2%). They had 5 painful scars, 3 CRPS, 2 recurrent CTS, 1 thenar motor branch injury, 1 superficial palmar arch injury and 4 infections [5].

Incomplete release, nerve laceration, painful scar and CRPS, are the most common complications. Nevertheless, a lot of other complications can occur. Knowledge of these complications is very important, since it can help the surgeon to reduce their rate. Correct choice of the surgical approach, adequate and atraumatic surgical technique, use of loupes for magnification, and careful postoperative follow-up are the key factors which will help the surgeon to reduce the rate of complications. Moreover, early recognition of

P. Giannakopoulos (✉) · K. Kourkoutas
Hand, Upper Limb and Microsurgery Center, Athens Medical Center, Athens, Greece
e-mail: pgiannak@otenet.gr; hand@otenet.gr

G. Kasimatis
Athens Medical Center, Athens, Greece

D. G. Sotereanos, L. K. Papatheodorou (eds.), *Compressive Neuropathies of the Upper Extremity*,
https://doi.org/10.1007/978-3-030-37289-7_7

these complications as well as the knowledge for immediate treatment leads to the best possible outcome.

Chronicity of median nerve compression with thenar atrophy is a poor prognostic factor for complete clinical recovery. Neglected atrophy may be irreversible; it is therefore necessary to explain this to the patient. On the other hand, sensory restoration is usually complete, although a small degree of numbness on the pulp of the fingers may persist for a few weeks.

Classification of Carpal Tunnel Surgery Complications

The major question is: what makes carpal tunnel surgery unsuccessful? First, one should exclude having a pathology other than carpal tunnel syndrome. The differential diagnosis of a carpal tunnel syndrome includes cervical spine disorders, brachial plexus abnormalities, thoracic outlet syndrome, pronator syndrome and anterior interosseous syndrome. Careful clinical examination with the aid of imaging and electrodiagnostic studies will help provide the correct diagnosis. A second reason may be incorrect surgical technique, which lead to significant morbidity of the hand. Last but not least, inadequate patient's cooperation, along with other unspecified and unpredictable factors can affect the final result.

For better recognition and easier classification, we can divide complications into three groups: intraoperative, early postoperative and late postoperative.

- *The intraoperative complications* are related to iatrogenic injuries. Complete or partial lacerations of the nerves and tendons are not rare. Minimally invasive techniques increase the intraoperative complication rate, especially during the surgeon's learning curve, but lately, specific endoscopic instruments have reduced the frequency of these injuries.
- *Early postoperative* complications (up to 1 month postoperatively) usually are more serious and increase the patient discomfort dramatically. Incomplete release of the transverse carpal ligament (TCL) will lead to significant deterioration of the symptoms. Wound care problems also need special management.
- Finally, *late postoperative* complications are usually more difficult to recognize and treat. They can last for many months and require special management of the patient. Enhancing patient-doctor confidence is very important. It is prerequisite to extensively explain the problem to the patient and to inform him in detail how you will deal with his problem and what may the expected outcome be.

Intraoperative Complications

Your hands will only achieve what your eyes can see

Intraoperative Magnification Can Minimize Intraoperative Complications!

Intraoperative complications of open (OCTR) or endoscopic (ECTR) carpal tunnel release are usually iatrogenic nerve, tendon and vessels laceration. Although carpal tunnel release is one of the most often performed operations in the world, the occurrence of major neurovascular and tendon injuries associated with both OCTR and ECTR is not rare. The nerves that can be involved are both median and ulnar nerve. The median nerve has the higher incidence of damage as it is found anatomically just below the transverse carpal ligament. Complete or partial laceration of the median nerve, motor branch injury, single digital nerve damage or palmar cutaneous branch can occur (Figs. 7.1 and 7.2) [2, 6]. On the other hand, laceration of the communicating ramus between the median and ulnar nerve or laceration of the ulnar nerve itself may also happen. The high incidence of these injuries, especially of the motor branch, is directly related to the high percentage of anatomical variations that have been reported [7–9]. Lanz, classified the median nerve variations in carpal tunnel in four groups [10]. Group I includes variations in the course of the thenar branch. The second group includes the accessory branches at the distal carpal tunnel. In third group, one can

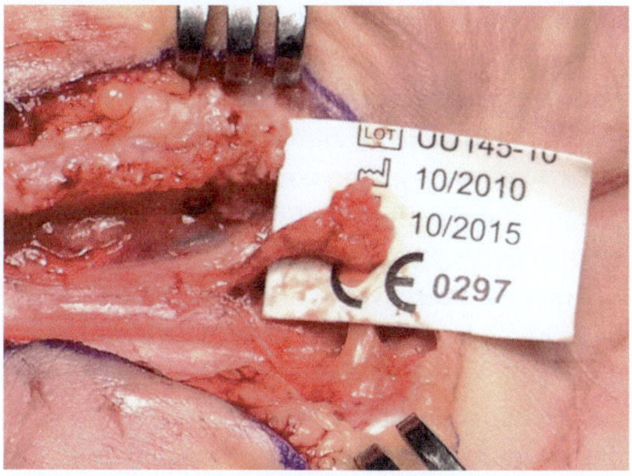

Fig. 7.1 Intra-operative photograph of injury of the motor branch of median nerve after laceration during previous open carpal tunnel release

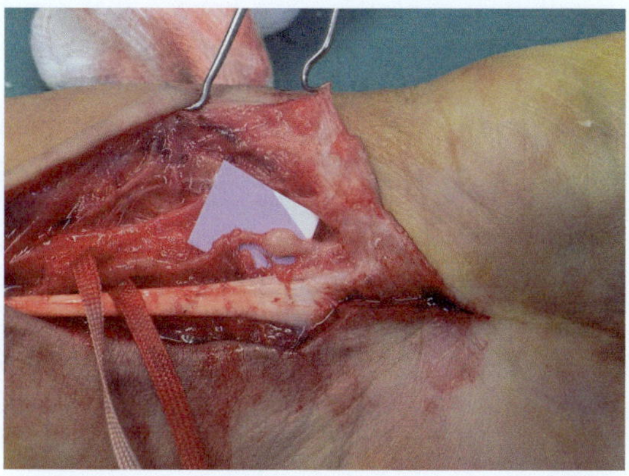

Fig. 7.2 Intra-operative photograph of painful neuroma of palmar cutaneous nerve after open carpal tunnel release

recognize a high division of the median nerve. Finally, the forth group includes the variations with accessory branches proximal to the carpal tunnel. Normally, the motor branch becomes recurrent at the distal margin of the TCL before entering to the thenar muscles. Poise in 1974, reported the relationship of the thenar branch to the transverse carpal ligament (group I). He found three types of variations: 46% extraligamentous, 31% subligamentous, and 23% transligamentous [11]. Other authors have also reported a large number of anatomic variations of the motor branch of the median nerve. Accessory branches (group II) of the motor nerve (double motor branch) at the distal carpal tunnel are not common. More common are the branches from the volar or even the ulnar aspect of the nerve. The high division of the median nerve (group III) is associated with the median artery. In the majority of the cases both parts of the nerve have the same diameter. An accessory lumbrical muscle between the two branches can also be found. Accessory branches proximal to the carpal tunnel (group IV) are rare. The branches run within the transverse carpal ligament distally. The branches can be motor or sensory. All these many variations of the median nerve can be the cause of intraoperative median nerve injury. Ulnar nerve injury is uncommon and usually is the result of improper surgical technique. Release of the TCL in the ulnar side decreases the probability of injury of the median nerve itself and the palmar cutaneous branch. On the other hand, extreme ulnar dissection can lead to ulnar nerve damage. For many years, a lot of surgeons preferred radical decompression of the median nerve with epineural neurolysis and complete tenosynovectomy of the flexor tendons. This technique can increase the possibility for median nerve intra-neural trauma and tendon laceration. Additionally, it can lead to neuroapraxia with median nerve paresthesia. In the long term, various complications as skin and tendon adhesions, neuro-dermodesis phenomenon and painful neuromas have also been reported.

Cases with nerve laceration should be promptly recognized and timely repaired. Direct repair with microsurgery techniques must be the treatment of choice. Any post-operative deficit, motor or sensory, must be evaluated very carefully. Early re-exploration of the median or ulnar nerve is necessary for the evaluation of the injury and its potential reconstruction. Delayed treatment with nerve grafts following internal neurolysis has worse outcome and must be our last solution. Regarding the palmar cutaneous branch injury, we must procced to direct repair in intraoperative cases, while in neuroma cases treatment is performed with excision of the neuroma and relocation of the distal edge into the pronator quadratus muscle. Overall, palmar cutaneous nerve injury must be avoided, as the resulting neuroma is very painful and the treatment is always problematic.

Concerning the vascular structures, the most common injuries are those of the superficial palmar artery arch and its branches and of the median nerve artery. Radial and ulnar artery injury is rare. When vascular injury is the case, recognition and repair of the lesion is necessary. When tourniquet is applied, release of the tourniquet before skin closure is recommended with proper hemostasis to avoid hematoma formation postoperatively. Hematoma, pseudoaneurysm, palmar pain or discoloration can occur if one neglects treatment. Microsurgery techniques are required for vessel reconstruction. For the median nerve artery injury more attention is needed, as the possibility of nerve injury is higher. Intraneural dissection is necessary before median nerve artery cauterization. Drains are not recommended by the majority of surgeons.

Tendon lacerations are also rare and it can be partial or complete. Superficial tendons are most common affected. Profundus tendons are only rarely injured. Direct repair remains the treatment of choice.

Nevertheless, how often is an intraoperative iatrogenic injury? The majority of Orthopaedic and Hand surgeons believe it is impossible to have intraoperative injuries in their practice.

Palmer and Toivonen in 1999 [12], published an article about complications of endoscopic and open carpal tunnel release. The authors sent a questionnaire to 1253 members of the American Society for Surgery of the Hand asking for information on complications resulting from both ECTR or OCTR. Respondents were instructed to report only on intraoperative complications. The question was how many nerve, tendons and vascular injuries they had in their practice and how these injuries were treated. In addition, the respondents were asked which of the intraoperative injuries (nerve, arterial or tendons) they had seen in the last 5 years were their own or referred by another physician. Of the 1253 Hand Surgeons questioned, there were 616 (49%) with open carpal tunnel release and 708 (57%) with use of endoscopic release.

Median nerve injuries were reported with both OCTR and ECTR techniques. There were 283 major complications from the 616 Hand Surgeons following OCTR, including 147 nerve lacerations, 29 ulnar lacerations, 54 digital, 34 vessel and 19 tendon lacerations. On the other hand, there were 455 major complications from surgeons who preferred ECTR, including 100 median nerve, 88 ulnar nerve and 77 digital nerve lacerations. Moreover, there were 121 vessel and 69 tendons lacerations. It should be noted that a large proportion of intraoperative injuries was not recognized during surgery, especially with the endoscopic techniques compared with the open techniques.

The incidence of intraoperative injuries is not low. The surgeon must be prepared to recognize and treat his complications. Based on our clinical experience we believe that some nerve injuries can occur during ECTR due to minimal surgical exploration and limited visualization. In the OCTR group however, there was also a large number of median and ulnar nerve injuries. In fact, there is no significant higher incidence of intraoperative soft tissue damage in ECTR versus OCTR, although open procedures offer better visibility and security. Selection of the surgical method for CTS release must comply with the surgeon's knowledge and surgical experience. Medicolegal implications associated with iatrogenic injuries following carpal tunnel syndrome surgery are common and surgeons should make great effort to avoid them [13, 14].

Early Complications

Early complications after carpal tunnel surgery occur up to 1 month postoperatively. Usually CTS symptoms improve on the first postoperative day. Persistence of symptoms is generally correlated to inadequate median nerve decompression. This is the most common major early complication and usually occurs with aggravation of symptoms.

Wound care problems as hematoma, superficial or deep infection are other early complications.

Inadequate Decompression of the Median Nerve

Incomplete release of the transverse carpal ligament is common in both OCTR and ECTR. It may include incomplete sectioning of the distal or proximal TCL, incomplete sectioning of the distal antebrachial fascia and complete lack of TCL sectioning.

Incomplete sectioning of the distal TCL is probably the most common complication in carpal tunnel surgery (Figs. 7.3 and 7.4), especially with the mini open techniques and in cases with transverse wrist incision [15]. Clinically, Phalen test is often negative, as there is release of the proximal part of TCL, which is responsible for median nerve compression during wrist flexion. On the other hand, Gilliatt and Wilson test is positive due to compression of the nerve in the distal carpal tunnel. Positive Tinel sign also can be seen in the palm, but negative in the wrist flexor region. Negative is also the Bedeschi sign, which evaluates the presence of tension in the anterior wrist region. Nevertheless, the most reliable sign remains the persistence or deterioration of the symptoms. Clinical diagnosis of incomplete distal TCL sectioning can be confirmed by imaging with CT-scan, MRI, or even with electrodiagnostic studies (EMG). Normally, EMG studies improve as early as 2 weeks postoperatively. In cases with incomplete TCL release, EMG values will deteriorate [16–18].

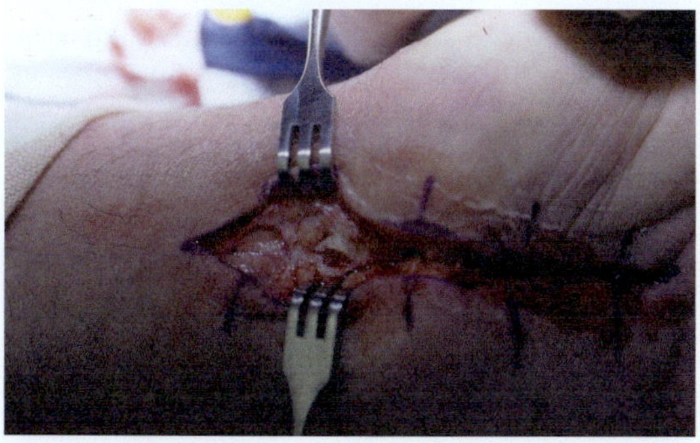

Fig. 7.3 Intra-operative photograph showing incomplete TCL sectioning during revision CTR

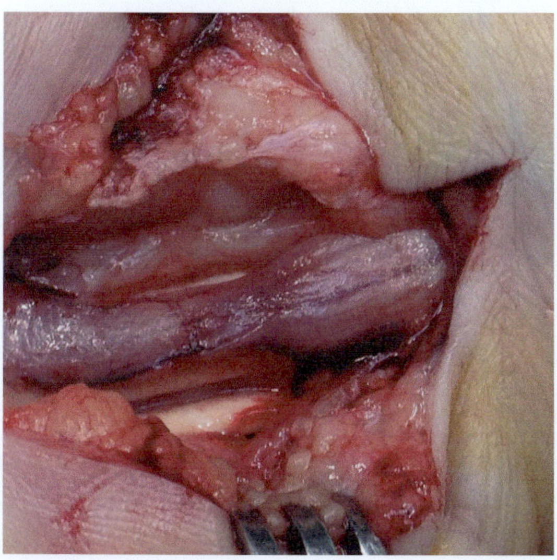

Fig. 7.4 Intra-operative photograph of the median nerve during revision surgery after incomplete TCL sectioning. Note hourglass appearance of the median nerve due to excessive compression

Many authors have reported on their experience following a repeat carpal tunnel release. The majority of them found that incomplete release of the distal TCL was the most common cause for the unsuccessful outcome [15, 19, 20].

Incomplete release of the distal part of the antebrachial fascia is not common. Normally, distal part of the antebrachial fascia does not compress the median nerve. Makinnon suggested that the etiology can be a thickening of the antebrachial fascia as a result from previous trauma of the wrist and forearm [21]. There is usually a persistence of symptoms, but their deterioration is rare. A previous incision not extending proximal to the wrist flexor crease is an indicative element. Phalen and Gilliatt and Wilson tests are positive. Tinel and Bedeschi signs are also positive. CT-scan and/or MRI can be used to confirm the diagnosis. Surgical release of the distal part of the antebrachial fascia is the treatment of choice. Close attention must be paid to perform atraumatic dissection of the subcutaneous tissues from the fascia, otherwise the subcutaneous vessels can be injured and an hematoma may occur. Fascial release must extend approximately 2–3 cm proximal to the wrist flexor crease [19–21].

Complete lack of TCL sectioning is extremely rare, yet not impossible. A few authors have reported such cases. We should however keep in mind the possibility of healing of an incomplete sectioned TCL, in such a way the surgeon who performs the reoperation erroneously considers the TCL as unsectioned [18, 22].

Hematoma

Hematomas after CTS release surgery can arise from severe vascular injuries and from small cutaneous vessels [23]. Atraumatic surgical technique, adequate surgical field, proper hemostasis prior to closure, potential use of drain and the coagulation status of the patient are essential factors to be taken into account, in order to avoid hematoma formation.

Aggressive tenosynovectomy without meticulous hemostasis may also be a reason for postoperative hematoma.

Considering discontinuation of aspirin preoperatively, Brunnetti et al., demonstrated that the continuation of aspirin did not increase the risk of complications [24].

Similarly, AAOS guidelines underline that "Limited evidence supports that the patient might continue the use of aspirin preoperatively" [25]. Based on the same guidelines, no reliable evidence exists for the use of other anticoagulants.

In case of a confirmed hematoma either with clinical evaluation, MRI or ultrasound, the surgeon should consider re-operatation for drainage and irrigation, in order to avoid nerve and tendons adhesions. Once again we recommend dropping the tourniquet prior to closure.

Infection

Post-operative infection following carpal tunnel surgery, whether it's superficial or deep, is quite uncommon in our practice and in the medical literature as well. Several risk factors have been recognized. The necessity of prophylactic antibiotics is being discussed.

Hanssen et al. [26] in their retrospective study of 3620 Carpal Tunnel Syndrome surgeries, reported deep post-operative infection in 17 cases (0.47%). They identified as statistically significant risk factors the intraoperative steroid solution injection into the carpal tunnel, flexor tendon synovectomy, prolonged operative time and the use of surgical drain. Infection rate in males was higher (0.87%) than in females (0.25%). Staphylococcus aureus was the most common pathogen (15 out of 17 cases).

Werner et al. [27] in their analysis of over 450,000 Medicare patients that underwent open carpal tunnel release only 1466 developed postoperative infection (0.32%). They also noted that independent positive risk factors for infection were younger age, male sex, obesity, alcohol, tobacco and comorbidities including diabetes, chronic liver disease, chronic kidney disease, chronic lung disease, peripheral vascular disease, inflammatory arthritis and depression [27].

Harness et al. [28] in a multicenter retrospective review of 3003 patients who underwent uncomplicated carpal tunnel release, identified 11 cases of surgical site infection. From those 11 patients 5 had prophylactic antibiotics and 6 did not, 4 had deep infections and 7 superficial. Infection rate in patients with diabetes was not statistically different from nondiabetic population. They concluded that antibiotic use did not decrease the risk of infection therefore surgeons should carefully consider the risks and benefits of routinely using prophylactic antibiotics in carpal tunnel surgery.

Bykowski et al. [29] in their retrospective review of 8850 cases of clean, elective hand surgery found an infection rate of 0.35%. Surgical site infection did not significantly differ between patients receiving antibiotics (0.54%) and those who did not (0.26%). They also found that, even though diabetes, procedure length and smoking were factors associated with the development of infection, prophylactic antibiotics did not reduce the risk of infection among these patients. Overall, they concluded that antibiotics should not be routinely administered to patients who undergo clean, elective hand surgery.

American Academy of Orthopaedic Surgeons on 2016 published evidence-based clinical practice guidelines concerning the management of carpal tunnel syndrome [25] mentioning that

"Limited evidence supports that there is no benefit for routine use of prophylactic antibiotic prior to carpal tunnel release because there is no demonstrated reduction in postoperative surgical site infection."

In conclusion, infection after carpal tunnel release although uncommon, is a reality which may endanger patient's health. Close postoperative follow up is mandatory, so as to allow for an early diagnosis and treatment of infection.

Rare Major Early Complications

Skin and palmar fascial necrosis following carpal tunnel surgery is extremely rare.

Greco and Curtsinger in 1993, reported necrotizing fasciitis infection as a complication of a carpal tunnel release [30]. A 31 years old diabetic woman presented with the condition following CTS release. Total excision of the palmar skin and fascia was required for the control of the woman's specific condition.

Postsurgical pyoderma gangrenosum following carpal tunnel release has also been reported by Ruebhausen et al., in 2017 [31]. A 33-year-old woman presented on the 2nd postoperative day with wound drainage and pain. Three days later, her symptoms were worse. After a lot of debridements, surgical forearm amputation was selected for the safest and best outcome for the patient.

Another pyoderma gangrenosum after carpal tunnel release was reported by Giugale and Balk, in 2018 [32]. It was treated with multiple debridements and administration of systemic corticosteroids, eventually with hand survival.

Another rear early complication was described by Tiengo et al. [33]. This was a case of critical upper limb ischemia after CTR in patient diagnosed for CTS confirmed by EMG study. This serious complication occurred in the presence of undiagnosed thoracic outlet syndrome obliterating subclavian artery and additionally occlusion of the humeral artery and the final result was necrosis of the distal third of the thumb and index finger. Authors believe that acute occlusion of collaterals due to brachial tourniquet was the reason of limb ischemia. This case underlines the importance of careful clinical examinations knowing that double crush syndromes do exist and that the diagnosis if finally clinical.

The recognition of these rare serious complications is very important, as early diagnosis and adequate treatment can result in hand salvage.

Late Postoperative Complications

We can classify late postoperative complications following carpal tunnel release in two groups. The first one is associated with recurrent symptoms, while the second one with the onset of new symptoms. Recurrence of symptoms is often caused by the fibrotic scar tissue formation around the nerve and by the hypertrophic tenosynovitis of the flexor tendons. The onset of new symptoms may be associated with the surgical procedure and skin incision, or can occur as a result of iatrogenic nerve injury. The complications which are not affected from the incision include pillar pain, piso-triquetral pain syndrome and of course CRPS.

Recurrence of Carpal Tunnel Syndrome

Carpal tunnel surgical release has consistently an excellent outcome. The majority of patients are absolutely free of symptoms after a period of a few months. However, recurrent carpal tunnel syndrome occurs in up to 19% of patients following CTR. There are two major categories where we can classify recurrence. The first one is attributed to pathology unassociated with the primary carpal tunnel syndrome and surgical release, such a distal radius fracture, tumors, pregnancy, diabetes or a systemic disease as rheumatoid arthritis, which lead to a hypertrophic tenosynovitis of the flexor tendons. The second group includes pathologies associated with an extensive scar formation and traction neuropathy following the first operation.

Evaluation and understanding of the causes for recurrence is very critical for the subsequent treatment. Clinical examination is also very important and further studies (computed tomography [CT] scan or magnetic resonance imaging [MRI] and electrodiagnostic studies) may be necessary for correct diagnosis.

The first group requires typical management with revision of carpal tunnel release and synovectomy when needed, as the treatment of choice. Additional procedures may be necessary, such as a correction osteotomy for distal radius malunion or a tumor excision. The second group needs special management. External or internal neurolysis must be followed by vascularized soft tissue coverage or by the vein wrapping technique [34, 35]. The technique of hypothenar fat flap is described in Chap. 9 and the vein wrapping technique is described in Chap. 25.

New Symptoms Appearance

Loss of Hand Grip Strength

Releasing the transverse carpal ligament can results in a decrease of the hand grip and pinch strength. Quite enough studies have estimated the time required for grip and pinch strength to return to the preoperative level. Gellman et al. [36] found that 3 weeks after surgery the strength was at the 28% of the preoperative level, at 6 weeks post-op it was at 73% and it returned to the preoperative level after 3 months. At 6 months after the release, the grip was increased to 116%. The pinch grip had a faster recovery, which was 74%, 96% and 108% of the preoperative level at 3, 6 weeks and 3 months accordingly. Six months post-op, the pinch was 126% of preoperative level [36]. There were a lot of other studies that reporting similar results, although a few authors reported complete recovery after a longer period [37, 38]. There has also been a question whether TCL reconstruction offers faster recovery, and some studies have suggested TCL lengthening-reconstruction. Many techniques have been described for the ligament reconstruction in the first plane, but the results are similar [39, 40]. Overall, TCL lengthening-reconstruction may provide a quicker recovery, but in the long term, restoration of handgrip strength does not seem to have any significant difference compared with patients who didn't undergo this procedure. In everyday practice, the routine need for TCL reconstruction is low and the majority of surgeons does not perform it, as they don't believe it is necessary. In fact, the reduction of the grip strength after carpal tunnel surgery is temporary and rarely leads to significant functional disability. Additionally, the decreased grip power is quite often due to painful scar and pillar pain and this can confuse the diagnosis. The use of a postoperative splint is also controversial. TCL reconstruction for unacceptable reduction of grip power of the hand may be needed in extremely rare cases and only a few methods have been described with the use of local flaps or tendon grafts.

In our practice, we think that a bulky soft dressing for a period of 2–3 weeks, to allow for TCL healing, is enough.

Over the last years, the Hand Surgeons' interest has been to determine whether grip strength recovery differed when open and endoscopic surgical techniques were compared. There is an ongoing debate whether endoscopic methods present advantages. Bande et al. [41] and Brown et al. [42] did not find significant difference between the two methods. On the other hand, MacDermid et al. [43] suggested that endoscopic decompression of the median nerve offers a rapid grip strength recovery compared to the open release.

Tendon Complications

Trigger Finger

Implication of carpal tunnel surgery in the appearance of trigger finger (TF) has been described in the literature. It is believed that the anterior displacement of flexor tendons as a consequence of TCL division during release of median nerve, alters the biomechanics of the tendon-pulley system of the hand and may predispose to trigger finger [44].

Hombal et al. [45] reported trigger finger incidence of 21.9% after CTS surgery. Mackinnon also observed trigger finger after CTR [21].

Fu-Yu et al. [46] in their retrospective, nationwide cohort study of 2605 CTR reported the overall incidence of trigger digits was 3.63-fold greater in the CTR cohort than in non CTR. They also found that the incidence of trigger finger was highest in the first 6 months and then significantly decreased.

In order to avoid this complication immobilization of the wrist in slight extension for 2 weeks, allowing the fingers free to move, may be considered.

Adhesions Between Flexor Tendons

Tenosynovitis and adhesions between flexor tendons into carpal tunnel are common in patients with systemic disease, as rheumatoid arthritis. Carpal tunnel syndrome in these patients can have as a result, apart from the symptoms of the median nerve neuropathy, limited finger and wrist motion due to reduction of flexor tendon gliding. In these cases, carpal tunnel surgical decompression requires synovectomy of flexor tendons in addition to the TCL sectioning. On the other hand, a few surgeons prefer to perform this procedure routinely, when serious tenosynovitis is found. Synovectomy can be followed by adhesions of the flexor tendons due to surgical trauma and the inevitable hematoma [47]. The clinical result is limited hand function with or without recurrence of the median nerve compression symptoms. Diagnosis may be confirmed by MRI or ultrasound.

This complication can be avoided with intraoperative appropriate hemostasis when synovectomy is performed. In most of the cases, intensive rehabilitation program can improve the finger and wrist motion, otherwise a reoperation in needed. Careful tenolysis with diligent hemostasis and drain insertion are necessary. Tenolysis must be performed by local anesthesia for intraoperative control of finger movement. Early intensive finger and wrist rehabilitation is imperative.

Bowstringing of the Flexor Tendons

A rare complication of CTS release surgery is the anterior subluxation of the flexor tendons. TCL proper healing that follows its sectioning during surgery is necessary for the unobstructed functioning of the pulley system at the carpal tunnel and thus the correct positioning of flexor tendons and median nerve in their canal [23].

An increase in the anteroposterior diameter and subsequently of the volume of carpal canal is happening due to TCL sectioning which leads to anterior displacement of its contents [48].

In rare cases, inappropriate TCL healing will lead to bowstringing of the flexor tendons, which will be demonstrated clinically with a cord like appearance when fingers and wrist are actively flexed. Implicated factors are the excision of a part of TCL, the maintenance of the hand in a flexed position postoperatively and the TCL sectioning on its radial side.

A short period of wrist immobilization in slight extension is recommended in order to avoid this rare complication allowing normal healing of TCL.

In a few cases that bowstringing should be addressed surgically, surgeon has to decide among methods of TCL reconstruction [49].

Painful Scar

All surgical scars are painful for the first postoperative period, but after a few weeks they become painless. Some scars have the tendency to become hypertrophic or keloid. Usually, keloid scars are more painful that hypertrophic ones. However, the most important contributor to scar pain intensity variability remains unidentified [47, 50].

Bedeshi [23], suggested three causes for the origin of a painful cutaneous scar. The first one is a neuroma of the palmar cutaneous nerve (usually) or of a branch of the radial nerve. The second reason may be the formation of minineuromas of the cutaneous terminal endings of both median and/or ulnar nerves cutaneous scar formation and adhesions to the median nerve.

Neuroma of palmar cutaneous nerve is the main cause of a painful scar. The most dangerous incisions are the transverse and those, which are located radially, around the thenar eminence [8]. The pain is localized radially over the distal wrist flexor crease. Pressure on the scar causes pain with reflection to the thenar region. Palmer and Toivonen in theirs article [12] which included a questionnaire to the members of the ASSH, reported 117 injuries of the palmar cutaneous branch with OCTR and only 17 with ECTR.

Minineuromas of the cutaneous terminal endings of both median and/or ulnar nerve after open CTS release are common as these branches offer sensation to the palm. Taleisnik [8] has described the safe zone for avoidance the median nerve micro-branches and Engber et al. [51] the corresponding ones for ulnar nerve. Recent studies by Matloub et al. [52], suggested an incision on the central axis of the fourth ray, as it is more secure to avoid injuries of the palmar cutaneous terminal endings. Biyani and Downes [53] suggested two separate small incisions proximal and distal of the TCL to protect the highly innervated skin.

Generally, the postoperative scar can be painful and sensitive, especially during the first weeks. However, the majority of these scars become painless after a period of a few months. For this period, conservative treatment must be followed with scar massage, steroid cream or injections and a program of desensitization. Only in very few cases, revision of the scar is necessary and this may be done after a period of at least 6 months postoperatively.

The scar tissue formation between the median nerve and the scar itself is a more complex, especially in cases where we have subluxation of the median nerve anteriorly. The etiology is a lack of proper healing of the TCL. Predisposition factors are: radial incision and TCL sectioning, removal of a part of TCL and post-operative wrist flexion posture [54]. The symptoms are very intense with pain over the scar even with light touch, Tinel sign and a sensation of electric current. The superficial location of the median nerve can be confirmed by MRI.

For avoidance of this complication, an ulnar palmar incision must be selected. In cases that will be shown, a second surgery was required. Median nerve neurolysis, soft tissue coverage and/or TCL reconstruction may be necessary.

Pillar Pain

Postoperative pain after carpal tunnel release can be located both in the thenar and hypothenar region. The pain becomes worse with pressure over the scar. In addition, grip strength can be limited. The etiology is not clearly defined. Mini neuromas from palmar cutaneous nerve have been implicated. The postsurgical soft tissue edema can also be another cause. Other authors believe that pillar pain has a muscle origin, and it is the result of a transient instability of the aponeurotic insertion of the thenar and hypothenar muscles. There is no relationship with the type of the incision and there is no significant difference between patients operated either with open or endoscopic techniques [55–57].

Pillar pain usually resolves after a period of a few months (normally, this period is between 2 and 12 months). This is the reason why several authors agree with the hypothesis of thenar and hypothenar muscles instability. After healing of the aponeurotic scar, the stability is restored and the symptoms subside. According to this hypothesis, few surgeons have suggested the use of a postoperative splint for a period of 2 months with the wrist in slight extension, in order to favor healing of the transverse carpal ligament, yet there is insufficient documentation.

Piso-Triquetral Pain Syndrome

Although, hypothenar pain after carpal tunnel surgery is not rare, symptoms usually subside within 2–12 months. However, a few patients continue to have tenderness over the piso-triquetral joint. Seradge and Seradge [58] in 1989, suggested as a potential cause for this continuing pain, the subluxation or articular arthrosis of the piso-triquetral joint. The stability of the pisiform is secured by the forces of the flexor carpi ulnaris and abductor digiti minimi ulnarly and the TCL radially. The inadequate healing of the TCL can lead to instability of the pisiform and articular incongruence. Secondly, an asymptomatic chondromalacia can be symptomatic. Lateral radiographs can reveal the subluxation and the arthritic changes and thus yield the diagnosis. Intra-articular local anesthesia positive test will confirm the pathology. For persistent chronic cases, pisiform excision has been suggested.

To avoid the poor or incorrect healing of the transverse carpal ligament, wrist immobilization in extension for 2 weeks is recommended by some authors [59].

Complex Regional Pain Syndrome

Reflex Sympathetic Dystrophy (RSD) or algodystrophy is the old definition for the condition that presents with edema, stiffness, loss of function and vasomotor instability, which today should better be called Complex Regional Pain Syndrome – CRPS. There are two types of CRPS: CRPS-I and CRPS-II. The CRPS-I (previously known as reflex sympathetic dystrophy) is when there no confirmed nerve injury, whereas in CRPS-II (previously known as causalgia) there is an associated confirmed nerve injury. However, although it is unclear if these disorders will always be divided into two types, their treatment is similar.

CRPS-I is well documented as a CTS postoperative complication with a varying rate of 1–5%. Prolonged acute pain postoperatively is considered to be one of the major factors which contribute to this disorder. Moreover, a relationship between psychological and behavioral factors and CRPS-I has been shown and in fact, it is believed that the exacerbation of pain and dysfunction in these patients could help maintain the condition.

The formation of hematoma and/or tight bandages also play an important role for the disorder; some authors have therefore proposed the regular use of drains in order to avoid the hematoma, while others regularly use compressive bandages, despite their potential harmful effect.

CRPS-II causes causalgia, which is a burning sensation of pain, constant and of great severity, which influences patient's life (Fig. 7.5). It is most often encountered after internal neurolysis, where the median nerve forms adhesions with the surrounding tissues. Various authors have therefore advised against internal neurolysis. Reoperations are also considered to increase the likelihood for CRPS-II. If treated late, CRPS-II may sometimes be impossible to treat despite advanced microsurgical techniques. This is especially the case when an iatrogenic injury to the nerve and a painful neuroma is the cause of CRPS-II.

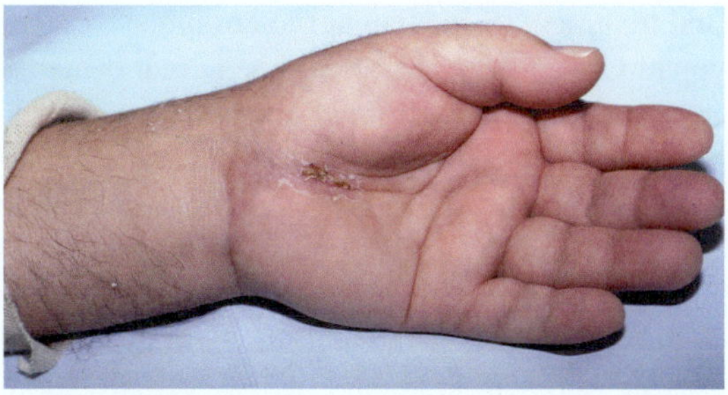

Fig. 7.5 Image of a hand with CRPS II 1 month after open carpal tunnel release

CRPS treatment may require multidisciplinary approach. Different types of medications have been used such as steroids, bisphosphonates, anticonvulsants as well as physiotherapy and behavioral therapy [60]. When conservative treatment fails invasive treatments should be considered [61]. Sympathetic nerve blocks as well as sympathectomy have been described in the literature [62, 63].

It is the principal author's opinion that every factor which continues to cause pain and/or discomfort in the hand should be immediately addressed, so as to stop the vicious cycle which causes CRPS. If there isn't any triggering factor, other than nerve injury, as incomplete release or trigger finger, e.t.c., which should be addressed also surgically, aggressive pain management and/or sympathetic blockade with stellate ganglion injection may be the best treatment.

If encountered late, aggressive pain management and/or sympathetic blockade with stellate ganglion injection may be the best treatment with or without a repeat operation. Overall, prompt identification of the lesion and adequate surgical management is the only way to reduce the possibilities of a permanent debilitating painful condition in these patients.

Conclusions

Carpal tunnel syndrome was first described by Paget in 1854, but it was Phalen in 1966, who reported on his experience regarding diagnosis and treatment of median nerve compressive neuropathy. Ever since, there has been great progress in Hand Surgery. Minimal invasive and endoscopic techniques are now used in everyday practice. However, despite these remarkable achievements in Hand Surgery, the rate of complications remains high; minimally invasive techniques may increase the complication rate due to narrow surgical field and worse visualization. The median nerve laceration is the most common complication in both techniques OCTR and ECTR and tendon laceration is more common after ECTR. The selection of the incision type is of critical importance in order to avoid painful scar formation. Improper TCL healing plays a critical role in the appearance of some types of complications. In conclusion, carpal tunnel surgery is certainly a simple procedure, but the surgeon must be ready to recognize and treat any potential complication.

References

1. Giannikas A, Touliatos A. The surgery of the wounded hand. Athens: Loukatos G Publications; 1982. p. 26.
2. Das SK, Brown HG. In search of complication in carpal tunnel decompression. Hand. 1976;8(3):243–9.
3. MacDonald RI, Lichtman DM, Hanlon JJ, et al. Complications of surgical release for carpal tunnel syndrome. J Hand Surg Am. 1978;3(1):70–6.
4. Lilly CL, Magnell TD. Severance of the thenar branch of the median nerve as a complication of carpal tunnel release. J Hand Surg Am. 1985;10(3):399–402.
5. Mackinnon S, Dellon AL. Surgery of peripheral nerve. New York: Thieme Medical Publishers; 1988. p. 159–63.
6. Boeckstyns MEH, Sorensen AL. Does endoscopic carpal tunnel release have a higher rate of complications than open carpal tunnel release? J Hand Surg. 1999;24B:9–15.
7. Robbins H. Anatomical study of the median nerve in the carpal tunnel and etiologies of the carpal tunnel syndrome. JBJS. 1963;45A(5):953–66.
8. Taleisnik J. The palmar cutaneous branch of the median nerve and the approach to the carpal tunnel. JBJS. 1973;55A(6):1212–7.
9. Schmidt HM, Lanz U. Anatomy of the median nerve in the carpal tunnel. In: Gelberman R, editor. Operative nerve repair and reconstruction. Philadeiphia: Lippincott Williams and Wilkins; 1991. p. 889–98.
10. Lanz U. Anatomical variations of the median nerve in the carpal tunnel. J Hand Surg. 1977;2:44–53.
11. Poisel S. Ursprung und Verlauf des R. Muscolaris des Nervus Digitalis Palmaris Communis. Chir Praxis. 1974;18:471–4.
12. Palmer AK, Toivonen DA. Complications of endoscopic and open carpal tunnel release. J Hand Surg Am. 1999;24(3):561–5.
13. Gil JA, Bokshan S, Genovese T, et al. Medical malpractice following carpal tunnel surgery. Orthopedics. 2018;41(4):e569–71.
14. Ganesh Kumar N, Hricz N, Drolet BC. Litigation following carpal tunnel release. Hand (N Y). 2018;1:1558944718760032.
15. Eaton SY, Belsole RJ, Greene TL. Carpal tunnel release: analysis of suboptimal results. J Hand Surg. 1985;10B:365–9.
16. Phalen G. The carpal tunnel syndrome. JBJS. 1966;48(2):211–28.
17. Gilliatt RW, Wilson TG. A pneumatic tourniquet test in carpal tunnel syndrome. Lancet. 1953;265(6786):595–7.
18. De Smet L. Recurrent carpal tunnel syndrome. Clinical testing indicating incomplete section of the flexor retinaculum. J Hand Surg. 1993;18B:189.
19. Cobb TK, Amadio PC. Reoperation for carpal tunnel syndrome. Hand Clin. 1996;12(2):313–23.
20. Wadsrtoem J, Nigst H. Reoperation for carpal tunnel syndrome. A retrospective analysis of forty cases. Ann Chir Main. 1986;5:54–8.
21. Mackinnon SE. Secondary carpal tunnel surgery. Neurosurg Clin N Am. 1991;2:75–91.
22. Strasberg SR, Novak CB, Mackinnon SE, et al. Subjective and employment outcome following secondary carpal surgery. Ann Plast Surg. 1994;32:485–9.
23. Bedeshi P. Carpal tunnel syndrome surgical complications. In: Luchetti R, Amadio P, editors. Carpal tunnel syndrome. Springer-Verlag Berlin Heidelberg: Springer; 2007. p. 269–89.
24. Brunetti S, Petri GJ, Lucchina S, Garavaglia G, et al. Should aspirin be stopped before carpal tunnel surgery? A retrospective study. World J Othop. 2013;4(4):299–302.
25. AAOS. Management of carpal tunnel syndrome, evidenced-based clinical practice guideline. 2016.
26. Hanssen AD, Amadio PC, et al. Deep postoperative wound infection after carpal tunnel release. J Hand Surg Am. 1989;14(5):869–73.
27. Werner BC, Teran VA, et al. Patient-related risk factors for infection following open carpal tunnel release: an analysis of over 450,000 Medicare patients. J Hand Surg Am. 2018;43(3):214–9.
28. Harness NG, Inacio MV, et al. Rate of infection after carpal tunnel release surgery and effect of antibiotic prophylaxis. J Hand Surg Am. 2010;35(2):189–96.
29. Bykowski MR, Sivak WN, et al. Assessing the impact of antibiotic prophylaxis in outpatient elective hand surgery: a single-center, retrospective review of 8,850 cases. J Hand Surg Am. 2011;36(11):1741–7.
30. Greco RJ, Curtsinger LJ. Carpal tunnel release complicated by necrotizing fasciitis. Ann Plast Surg. 1993;30(6):545–8.

31. Ruebhausen MR, Mendenhall SD, Neumeister W, et al. Postsurgical pyoderma gangrenosum following carpal tunnel release: a rare disease following a common surgery. Eplasty. 2017;17:e10. www.eplasty.com.
32. Giugale JM, Balk ML. Pyoderma gangrenosum following carpal tunnel release. JBJS Case Connect. 2018;8(4):e91.
33. Tiengo C, Monticelli A, Bonvini S, et al. Critical upper limb ischemia due to brachial tourniquet in misdiagnosed thoracic outlet syndrome after carpal tunnel decompression: a case report. World J Plast Surg. 2017;6(3):375–9.
34. Sotereanos D, Giannakopoulos P, Mitsionis G, et al. Vein-graft wrapping for the treatment of recurrent compression of peripheral nerves. Microsurgery. 1995;16(11):752–6.
35. Sarris JK, Sotereanos DG. Vein wrapping for recurrent median nerve compression. J Hand Surg Am. 2004;4(3):189–94.
36. Gellman H, Kan D, Gee V, et al. Analysis of pinch and grip strength after carpal tunnel release. J Hand Surg Am. 1989;14(5):863–4.
37. Katz JN, Fossel KK, Simmons BP, et al. Symptoms, functional status and neuromuscular impairment following carpal tunnel release. J Hand Surg. 1995;20A:549–55.
38. Citron ND, Bendall SP. Local symptoms after open carpal tunnel release. A randomized prospective trial of two incisions. J Hand Surg. 1997;22B:317–21.
39. Karlsson MK, Lindau T, Hagberg L. Ligament lengthening compared with simple division of the transverse carpal ligament in the open treatment of carpal tunnel syndrome. Scand J Reconstr Hand Surg. 1997;31:65–9.
40. Netscher D, Steadman AK, Thornby J, et al. Temporal changes in grip and pinch strength after open carpal tunnel release and the effect of ligament reconstruction. J Hand Surg. 1998;23A:48–54.
41. Bande S, De Smet L, Fabry G. The results of carpal tunnel release: open versus endoscopic technique. J Hand Surg. 1994;19B:14–7.
42. Brown RA, Gelberman RH, Seiler JG, et al. Carpal tunnel release. JBJS. 1993;75A:1265–75.
43. MacDermid JC, Lichtman DM, Hanlon JJ, et al. Endoscopic versus open carpal tunnel release: a randomized trial. J Hand Surg. 2003;28A:475–80.
44. Lee SK, Bae KW, et al. The relationship of trigger finger and flexor tendon volar migration after carpal tunnel release. J Hand Surg (Eur). 2014;39(7):694–8.
45. Hombal JW, Owen R. Carpal tunnel decompression and trigger digits. J Hand Surg (Eur). 1970;2(2):192–6.
46. Fu-Yu L, Manrique OJ, et al. Incidence of trigger digits following carpal tunnel release. Medicine (Baltimore). 2017;96(27):e7355.
47. Kessler FB. Complications of the management of carpal tunnel syndrome. Hand Clin. 1986;2:401–6.
48. Richman JA, Gelberman RH, et al. Carpal tunnel syndrome: morphologic changes after release of the transverse carpal ligament. J Hand Surg Am. 1989;14(5):852–7.
49. Netscher D, Mosharrafa A, et al. Transverse carpal ligament: its effect on flexor tendon excursion, morphologic changes of the carpal canal, and on pinch and grip strengths after open carpal tunnel release. Plast Reconstr Surg. 1997;100(3):636–42.
50. Louis DS, Greene TL, Noellert RC. Complications of carpal tunnel surgery. J Nerosurg. 1985;62: 352–6.
51. Engber WD, Gmeiner JG. Palmar cutaneous branch of the ulnar nerve. J Hand Surg. 1980;5:26–9.
52. Matloub HS, Yan J-G, Van Der Molen M, et al. The detailed anatomy of the palmar cutaneous nerves and its clinical implications. J Hand Surg. 1998;23B:373–9.
53. Biyani A, Downes EM. An open twin incision technique of carpal tunnel decompression with reduced incidence of scar tenderness. J Hand Surg. 1993;18B:331–4.
54. Urbaniak JR. Complications of treatment of carpal tunnel syndrome. In: Gelberman R, editor. Operative nerve repair and reconstruction, vol. 2. Philadelphia: Lippincott; 1991. p. 967–79.
55. Eversmann WW. Entrapment and compression neuropathies. In: Green DP, editor. Operative hand surgery. New York: Churchill Livingstone; 1988. p. 1423–78.
56. Da Silva MF, Moore DC, Weiss AC, et al. Anatomy of the palmar cutaneous branch of the median nerve: clinical significance. J Hand Surg. 1996;21A:639–43.
57. Hunt TR, Osterman AL. Complications of the treatment of carpal tunnel syndrome. Hand Clin. 1994;10:63–71.
58. Seradge H, Seradge E. Piso-triquetral pain syndrome after carpal tunnel release. J Hand Surg. 1989;14A:858–62.
59. Rigoni G. Presentation of 25 cases of the piso-triquetral syndrome occurring in 600 cases of carpal tunnel release. Proceeding of the annual congress if the Swiss Society for Surgery of the Hand, Ann Hand Surg. 1990;9:389.
60. Birklein F, Dimova V. Complex regional pain syndrome-up-to-date. Pain Rep. 2017;2(6):e624.
61. Resmini G, Ratti C, et al. Treatment of complex regional pain syndrome. Clin Cases Miner Bone Metab. 2016;12(Suppl 1):26–30.
62. Singh B, Moodley J, et al. Sympathectomy for complex regional pain syndrome. J Vasc Surg. 2003;37(3):508–11.
63. Toshniwal G, Sunder R, et al. Management of complex regional pain syndrome type I in upper extremity-evaluation of continuous stellate ganglion block and continuous infraclavicular brachial plexus block: a pilot study. Pain Med. 2012;13(1):96–106.

8 Revision Carpal Tunnel Surgical Options

Travis Littleton, Cassidy Costello, and Mark Baratz

Carpal tunnel syndrome (CTS) is one of the most common upper extremity procedures performed. Historically carpal tunnel release (CTR) was reported to have a high success rate. Prior to a study by Langloh and Linscheid in 1972, re-exploration of the carpal canal was not reported on in the literature [1]. The current literature includes studies reporting a failure rate of 2–25% [2–4] with a 3–12% rate of revision surgery [5, 6].

It is important to define "failure" and "recurrence." Failure after nerve surgery can occur for many reasons including a wrong diagnosis, wrong procedure, improperly performed procedure, or following surgery for a patient who, because of age or medical co-morbidities, lacks the capacity to regain normal nerve function in spite of an adequate release. Recurrence is typically defined as a return of numbness after a symptom-free interval following carpal tunnel release. A study of 28 patients by Craft et al. (2007) had an average interval of 7 years between original carpal tunnel release and re-exploration [7]. Zieske et al. (2013) observed a symptom-free interval of approximately 10 years in patients with recurrent CTS [8].

In this chapter we will review the etiology of recurrent carpal tunnel syndrome along with the evaluation, principles of surgical treatment, surgical technique, expected outcome, and outcomes of comparative studies.

Etiology of Recurrent Carpal Tunnel

The causes of recurrent carpal tunnel are most commonly believed to be perineural scarring, reconstitution of the transverse carpal ligament, subsequent trauma or a space occupying lesion such as tenosynovitis or mass that forms within the carpal canal [9] (Fig. 8.1).

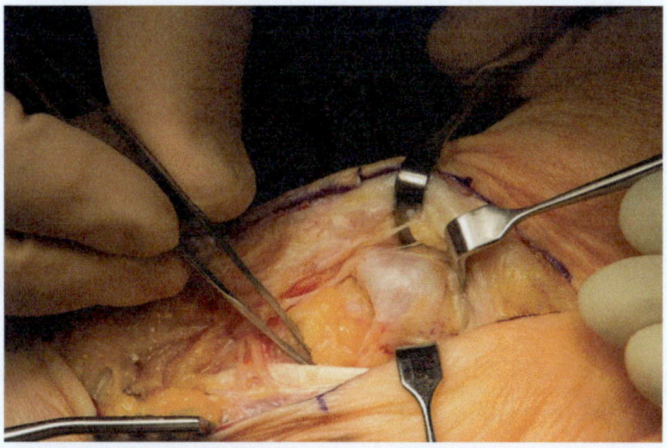

Fig. 8.1 Osteochondroma in the carpal canal

T. Littleton
University of Pittsburgh Physicians, University of Pittsburgh Medical Center (UPMC) Passavant, Pittsburgh, PA, USA

C. Costello
Department of Community Medicine, University of Pittsburgh Medical Center (UPMC) Passavant, Pittsburgh, PA, USA

M. Baratz (✉)
Department of Orthopaedic Specialists, University of Pittsburgh Medical Center (UPMC) Passavant, Pittsburgh, PA, USA
e-mail: baratzme@upmc.edu

D. G. Sotereanos, L. K. Papatheodorou (eds.), *Compressive Neuropathies of the Upper Extremity*, https://doi.org/10.1007/978-3-030-37289-7_8

One of the first studies looking specifically at recurrent CTS was in 1993 by Chang and Dellon. Underlying medical conditions such as diabetic peripheral neuropathy, cervical radiculopathy, multiple sclerosis and Charcot-Marie-Tooth can mimic recurrent carpal tunnel syndrome [10].

Evaluation

The key to an accurate diagnosis is a thorough history. Patients with recurrent carpal tunnel syndrome most commonly present with numbness (60%), paresthesia (50%), and, less commonly, with pain (42%) [7]. Similarly, Zieske et al. (2013) reported that patients with recurrent carpal tunnel were less likely to present with pain [8]. It is our bias that pain alone is rarely sufficient to invoke the diagnosis of recurrent carpal tunnel syndrome. We look for numbness in all or a portion of the median nerve distribution.

A Tinel's, Phalen's, Carpal Compression test may reproduce the symptoms of numbness in a median nerve distribution. The exception is elderly patients who often will not have symptoms with provocative maneuvers.

We typically document two-point discrimination in patients with suspected recurrent CTS even though Semmes-Weinstein monofilament testing has been shown to be more sensitive for compressive neuropathies [11]. We have been ordering fewer electrodiagnostic studies when evaluating primary carpal tunnel syndrome. In suspected recurrent carpal tunnel, we typically order nerve studies.

A diagnostic steroid injection in the carpal tunnel can help confirm the diagnosis of recurrent CTS. Beck et al. (2012) found 87% positive predictive value for successful revision surgery with a corticosteroid injection in the carpal tunnel. They also showed increased sensitivity and specificity when combining preoperative injection results with physical examination findings to 100% and 80% respectively [12].

Imaging studies have been used to evaluate patients with recurrent CTS. The use of MR imaging can be particularly helpful in cases when recurrent symptoms are accompanied by fullness in the region of the carpal canal [13] (Figs. 8.2, 8.3, and 8.4).

Ultrasound can be similarly helpful as a relatively quick, cost-effective tool to look for space

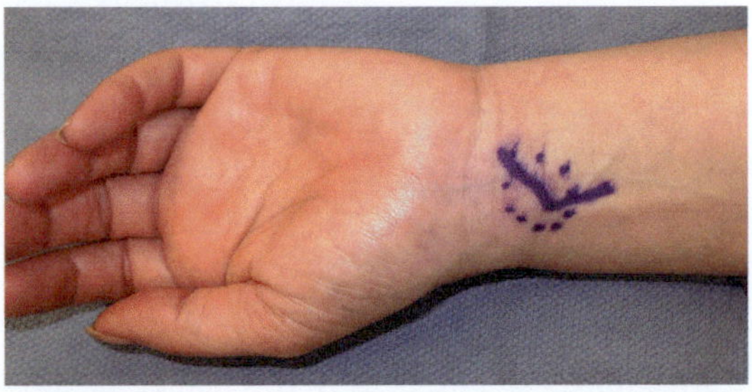

Fig. 8.2 Fullness proximal to carpal canal causing median nerve compression

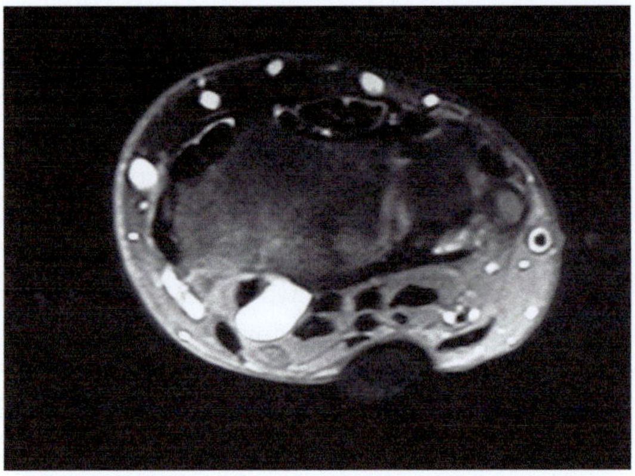

Fig. 8.3 Axial view of fluid filled lesion proximal to the carpal canal

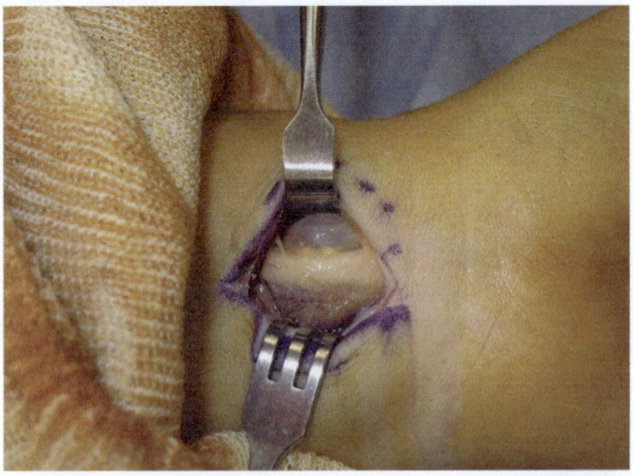

Fig. 8.4 Cyst emanating from the radial carpal joint compressing the median nerve

occupying lesions and to examine the cross-sectional area of the median nerve [14].

Principles of Surgical Treatment for Revision Carpal Tunnel Syndrome

1. Find the median nerve in normal tissue proximal and distal to the carpal canal. We will typically extend our exposure about 2 cm on either end of the existing scar.
2. "Surf the nerve". Most iatrogenic injuries are "side swipe" injuries. It is difficult to injure any longitudinal structure when you expose it from above.
3. Follow the anterior ulnar border of the median nerve. With the exception of aberrant branches, the motor branch exits the radial border of the median nerve (Fig. 8.5).
4. Separate the median nerve from the radial leaflet (Fig. 8.6).
5. Expose all terminal branches of the median nerve (Fig. 8.7).

Techniques with Expected Outcomes

There are numerous techniques that have been proposed for treatment of revision carpal tunnel release. These different "strategies" will be discussed in detail in the techniques section.

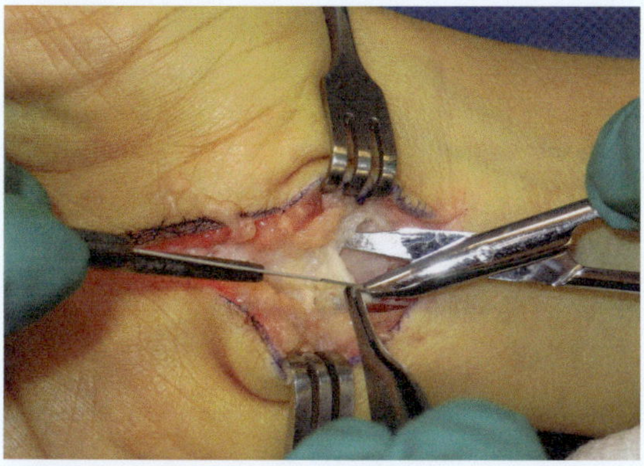

Fig. 8.5 Releasing the median nerve along its ulnar border

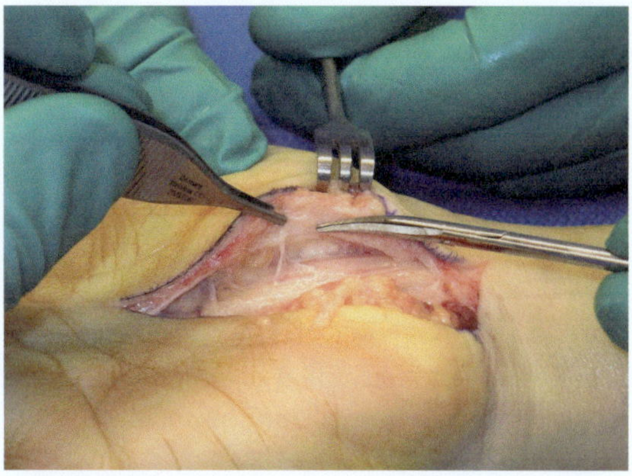

Fig. 8.6 Release adhesions between the median nerve and the radial leaflet

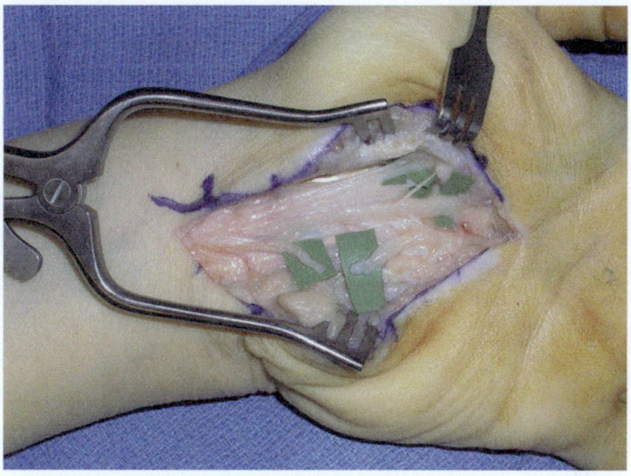

Fig. 8.7 Expose terminal branches of the median nerve

Repeat Simple Decompression

Beck et al. (2012) showed an 82% improvement in symptoms with simple decompression alone in a small sample size of 23 patients [12]. Similar results were found in a large meta-analysis by Soltani et al. in 2013. This study showed a 75% success rate in a heterogeneous cohort of 364 patients who underwent repeat open decompression for recurrent carpal tunnel syndrome. The second cohort included several different types of flaps in 294 patients in 14 different studies. The study concluded that an 86% rate of success could be achieved with decompression in conjunction with a vascularized flap. This was an 11% improvement in symptoms as compared to decompression alone [15]. A recent study by Pace et al. (2018) reviewed revision

CTR with or without hypothenar fat flap and concluded a trend, although not statistically significant, towards improved symptom severity score in patients undergoing simple decompression alone [16].

Historically percutaneous, mini open, and endoscopic carpal tunnel release were believed to have no role in the revision setting. A study by Luria et al. (2008) treated 41 patients with endoscopic revision after failed open release. Of the 41 patients, 37 reported improvement in symptoms, pinch strength and sensation, and reported a decrease in scar sensitivity along with satisfaction [17].

Synovial and Tenosynovial Flap

Revision carpal tunnel release with synovial flap uses locally available tissue with low morbidity. Gannon et al. (2007) described raising a flap of synovium off of the superficial flexors starting on the ulnar aspect of the ulnar canal. The flap is raised from ulnar to radial until the median nerve is encountered. Two transverse limbs are then made from ulnar to radial at the level of the wrist crease proximally and the superficial arch distally (Fig. 8.8). The flap is then laid over the median nerve and sutured to the radial aspect of the transverse carpal ligament (Fig. 8.9). They reviewed 36 patients with a successful outcome in 34/36 [18]. A similar flap is the vascularized tenosynovial flap reported on by Murthy et al. in

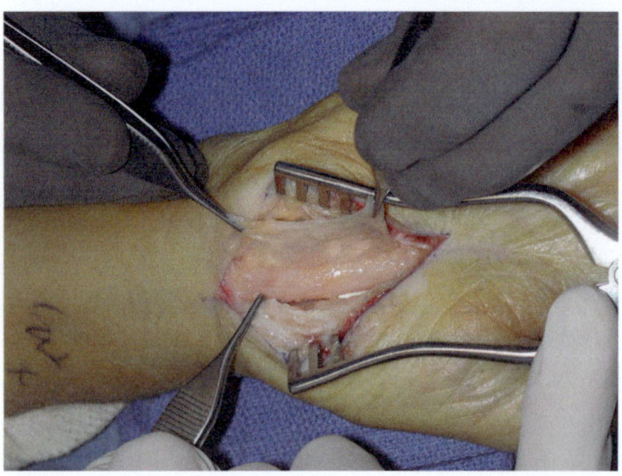

Fig. 8.8 Synovial flap elevated off of the superficial flexor tendons

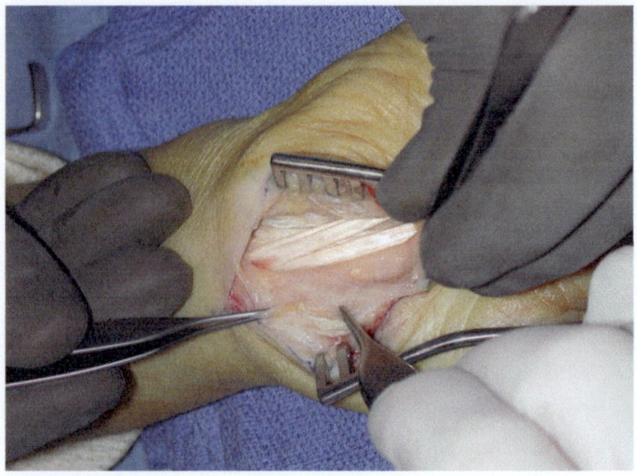

Fig. 8.9 Synovial flap inset between the median nerve and the radial leaflet of the transverse carpal ligament

2013 [19]. This uses the original incision extended in a zig zag fashion ulnarly across the wrist flexion crease. Once the nerve is decompressed attention is turned towards the tenosynovial flap. The ulnar based pedicle of this flap comes from the palmar carpal branches of the ulnar artery. Therefore, this flap is raised from the synovium over the superficial flexors from radial to ulnar until there is enough mobilization of the flap to cover the nerve. Occasionally this requires a back cut to translate the flap proximally or distally. The proposed advantage of this flap is its vascularized nature and ability to allow neovascularization. This study reported good results in their series of 45 cases with complete pain relief in 96% and complete or near complete resolution of numbness and tingling in 80% of patients [19]. One critique of this method is it lacks substantial padding for a hypersensitive median nerve. However, proponents of this technique believe this serves as a barrier over the nerve to prevent the formation of a constrictive scar, which many contend to be the primary cause of recurrent CTS. Post operatively most surgeons recommend a short period of immobilization in a splint.

Hypothenar Fat Pad Flap

Revision carpal tunnel release with a vascularized hypothenar fat flap is one of the most common flaps used in the revision carpal tunnel release. This flap was first described by Cramer in 1985 in a study on four patients and has undergone numerous modifications since that time [20]. The hypothenar fat pad flap receives multiple segmental vessels, usually three vessels, from the ulnar artery in Guyon's canal allowing the flap to be mobilized radially. Some advantages of this flap are that it is locally available, well vascularized, and allows coverage of the median nerve in the carpal tunnel. A limitation of this flap is that it has limited excursion proximally and distally [20]. This fat flap commonly measures three by four cm in size [21]. Once this flap is mobilized it is sutured to the radial leaflet of the transverse carpal ligament. In a study of 28 patients by Craft et al. (2007), they found fibrosis and adherence of the median nerve to the radial leaflet of the transverse carpal ligament in all patients undergoing revision surgery [7].

This technique begins with an incision extending 2 cm proximal and distal to existing zone involved in the initial release (Fig. 8.10). Next, identify the median nerve in the distal forearm (Fig. 8.11) and release it to level of the superficial arch (Fig. 8.12). Afterwards, develop a plane between the ulnar skin and the hypothenar fat tissue. Leave a small layer of adipose tissue on the skin, the subdermal plexus, to avoid skin necrosis (Fig. 8.13). The dissection is carried ulnarly until the dermal attachment of the palmaris brevis muscle is encountered. At this point one must

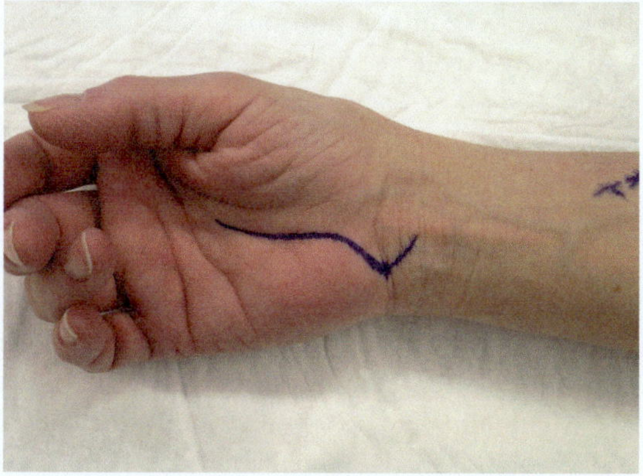

Fig. 8.10 Marked incision for the hypothenar fat pad flap

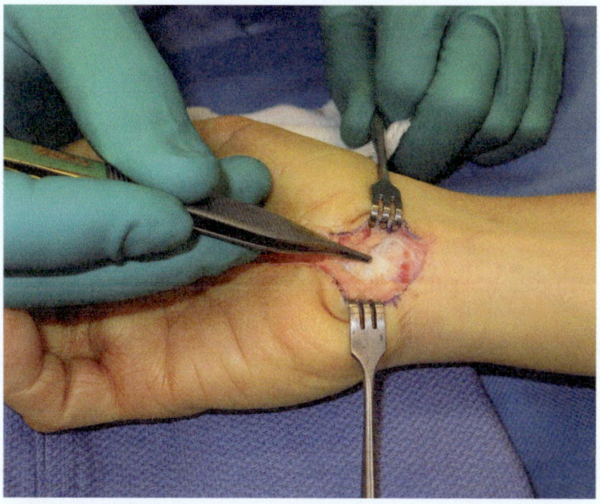

Fig. 8.11 Reconstituted ligament compressing the median nerve

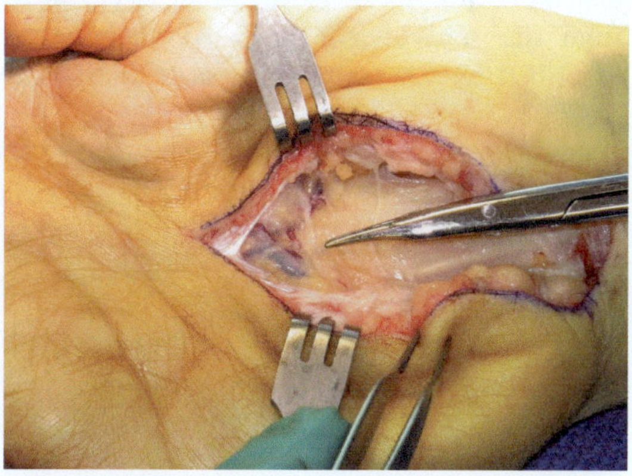

Fig. 8.12 Extending the distal exposure to the superficial arch

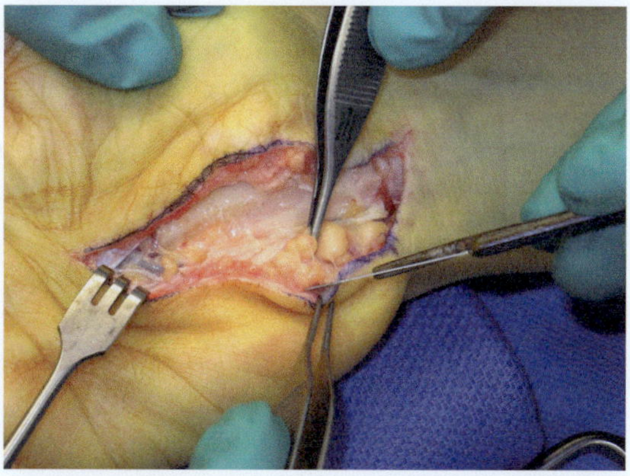

Fig. 8.13 Developing a plane of dissection between the hypothenar fat and the subdermal plexus

identify the digital nerves to the ring and middle finger distally and the ulnar artery and nerve proximally. The dissection then proceeds vertically between the palmaris brevis ulnarly and the ulnar neurovascular bundle radially (Figs. 8.14 and 8.15). This will allow the hypothenar fat pad to be elevated off the hypothenar muscles and translated radially to cover the median nerve. Lastly, use a horizontal mattress with chromic suture to apply the flap to the under surface of the radial leaflet (Figs. 8.16 and 8.17).

Multiple modifications have been described to allow increased mobility of the fat flap so that the flap is not under excess tension. One method is to ligate distally based deep arterial branches of the ulnar artery which allows further radial translation of the ulnar artery away from the ulnar nerve [22]. Another option described by Chrysopoulo et al. (2006) is to

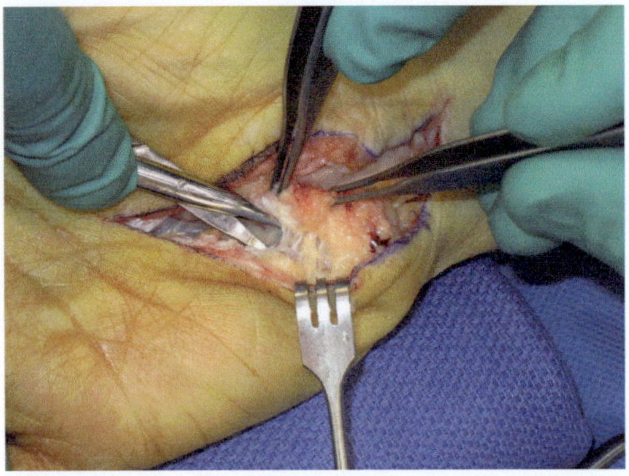

Fig. 8.14 Mobilization of the hypothenar fat pad flap along the course of the superficial arch

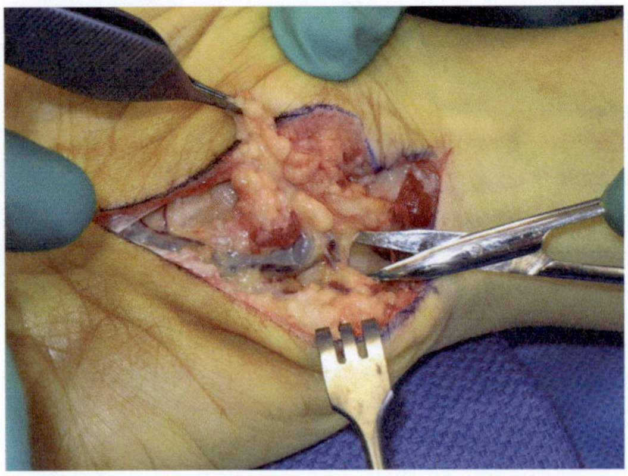

Fig. 8.15 Identifying and protecting the ulnar nerve

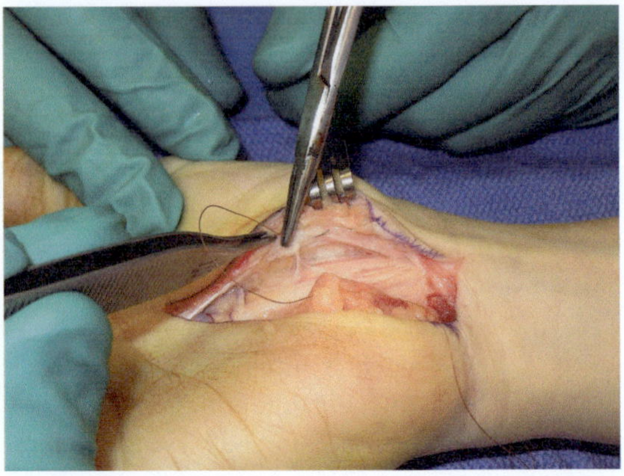

Fig. 8.16 Passing sutures from the flap to the undersurface of the radial leaflet

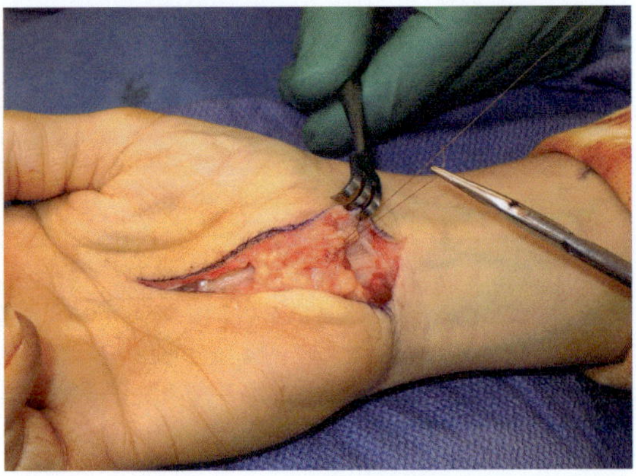

Fig. 8.17 Insetting hypothenar fat flap

also dissect deep to the ulnar neurovascular bundle and to allow separation of the hypothenar fat flap off the underlying transverse carpal ligament. The ulnar portion of the transverse carpal ligament is then resected off of the hamate to allow easier and more complete elevation of the fat pad along with the ulnar neurovascular bundle [23] (Fig. 8.18).

Craft et al. (2007) showed that the hypothenar fat flap was most reliable for reducing pain (83%), and less effective in reducing tingling (50%), and numbness (42%). Importantly, no patients reported being worse off after revision [7]. Mathoulin et al. (2000) reported excellent or good results in 95% of patients (49% and 45% respectively) [22]. Strickland et al. (1996) reported excellent results in 62 patients [24]. More recently Wichelhaus et al. (2015) reported more modest results in a smaller series of 18

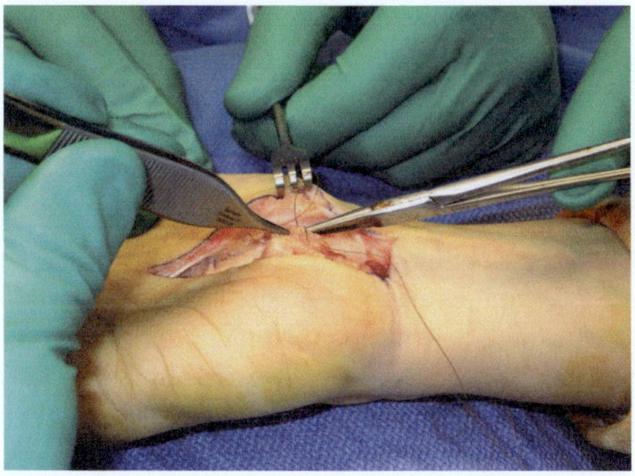

Fig. 8.18 A horizontal mattress suture tucks the flap beneath the radial leaflet

patients with 83% patient satisfaction, and complete pain relief in only 44% [21].

Synthetic Wraps

Another less commonly used technique for median nerve wrapping are the synthetic devices. There are a number of different commercially available synthetic materials that are marketed for revision CTR and nerve wrapping. Some contain an absorbable semipermeable collagen that works by blocking fibroblast and thereby decreasing perineural fibrosis. The synthetic collagen is then broken down by the body's normal metabolic pathways without producing an inflammatory reaction. This not unlike an autologous vein wrapping, in that once the nerve has been decompressed the nerve is wrapped circumferentially along the entire portion of the scarred nerve. Other synthetic nerve wraps are made of polyglycolic acid, placenta, porcine, and caprolactones. The presumed advantage of these synthetic materials is decreased donor site morbidity, and surgical time, compared with the use of local and remote autologous tissues.

Vein Wrapping

Vein wrapping is another option for coverage of the median nerve following revision CTR. The proposed mechanism of vein wrapping is to insulate the peripheral nerve from scar. A second possible benefit derives from placing the intimal side of the vein adjacent to the nerve to enhance nerve gliding. See Chap. 25 for vein wrapping technique. Varitimidis et al. (2001) presented on 15 patients treated with autologous vein insulator in the setting of revision CTR. They reported improved pain and sensation in all patients. They also noted improved objective parameters: nerve conduction velocities in eight patients and improved two-point discrimination in 14/15 patients [25].

Muscle Flaps

A number of local muscle flaps have been studied for coverage of the median nerve. These include pronator quadratus, palmaris brevis and abductor digiti minimi. Tung and Mackinnon (2001) described the pronator quadratus flap [6]. Palmaris brevis has been shown to be effective in the setting of revision CTR [26]. However, Strickland et al. (1996) stated that more often than not the palmaris brevis muscle was either absent or too small to provide adequate coverage.

Abzug et al. (2012) described the flexor digitorum superficialis muscle flap. Once the median nerve has been decompressed the incision is extended proximally past the myotendinous junction of the flexor digitorum superficialis. The muscle belly of the superficial flexor digitorum to either the ring or long finger is elevated off of the flexor digitorum carefully to preserve the myotendonous junction. The muscle belly is rotated 180° and used to cover the median nerve distally. This muscle flap should cover approximately 75% of the circumference of the median nerve and is then tacked down both radially and ulnarly [27].

Vascularized Fascial Flaps

The reversed radial artery fascial flap is a pedicle flap described for recurrent CTS by Tham et al. (1996). This technique requires sacrificing the radial artery which could lead to cold intolerance or ischemia. A pre-operative Allen test is critical to ensure adequate ulnar arterial blood supply [28]. This flap has more recently been modified to a perforator-based radial forearm fascial flap. This can be done in either a single or two-incision technique with the use of an arm tourniquet. After performing an external neurolysis and epineurotomy of the median nerve dissection proceeds to the middle of the forearm by extending the carpal tunnel incision proximally or by making a second incision over the planned flap. The radial artery has 6–10 septocutaneous distal perforators off the radial artery. The most proximal perforator is reliably located five to eight centimeters proximal to the radial styloid and this is most commonly the pivot point for this flap. This perforator usually allows coverage of the median nerve in the forearm all the way to the distal end of the scarred median nerve in the palm. This can be modified and pivoted off of a more distal perforator if needed as these perforators are reliably located approximately every 0.4–1.5 cm distally ending 1.5 cm proximal to the radial styloid. The flap is raised ulnarly from the fascia over the flexor carpi ulnaris and extended laterally raising the fascia over the extensor carpi radialis brevis until the perforators off of the radial artery are encountered. The lateral antebrachial cutaneous nerve must be protected in the forearm. Mahmoud et al. (2013) reported good medium-term results in a small series of eight patients [29].

Remote Pedicle or Free Flaps

There have also been a number of remote pedicle or free flaps proposed for median nerve coverage in revision CTR. Goitz and Steichen (2005), reviewed a long term follow up in a small series of nine patients who underwent microvascular omental transfer. They reported on nine extremities in six patients who had previously failed a minimum of two procedures including a failed local pedicle flap coverage. The technique requires a large extensile open approach to the carpal tunnel extending approximately 7 cm proximal to the wrist crease with an external neurolysis, flexor tenosynovectomy, and exposure of the cephalic vein and radial artery in the proximal forearm. The omental flap is harvested from the gastroepiploic vessels by an abdominal or peripherial vascular surgeon. A microvascular anastamosis is then performed in the forearm with an end-to-end technique from the gastroepiploic vein to the cephalic vein. Additionally, the gastroepiploic artery is sutured end-to-side into the radial artery. Lastly the omentum in the forearm is then covered by a partial-thickness skin graft. They showed patient satisfaction and improved quality of life in five of the six patients. There were four complications, all relating to the omental harvest site, in this small series of nine extremities [30].

Outcomes Including Comparative Studies

Outcomes following revision carpal tunnel surgery are less predictable compared to primary CTR. Cobb et al. (1996) reported on 131 patients who underwent reoperation for CTS. This included a heterogeneous group of revision procedure ranging from simple decompression to flap coverage. They concluded no difference in outcomes based on the type of surgical procedure. They also found poor outcomes in one quarter of the patients with over 10% requiring a third operation [5].

When comparing the results of CTR following previous open verses endoscopic surgery, Hulsizer et al. (1998) found that patients having undergone previous endoscopic release had significantly better results than those who underwent open release. A total of 23 patients (30 wrists) were included in this study. Of the 23 patients, 14 (17 wrists) had a previous open CTR surgery and 9 patients (13 wrists) had a previous endoscopic CTR surgery. All patients underwent a standard open CTR for revision surgery. In the open surgery group, 47% reported improved or completely resolved symptoms, whereas, 77% patients in the endoscopic group had improved or completely resolved symptoms [31].

Numerous studies demonstrate that open revision carpal tunnel release is successful in treating patients after failed endoscopic CTR [31, 32]. In 22 patients (24 wrists) that underwent open revision CTR for recurrent CTS after primary endoscopic release, Varitimidis et al. (1999), found that 20 patients (22 wrists) had an incomplete release of the flexor retinaculum. Pre-revision, 22 patients did not return to work after primary endoscopic release. After open revision 15 patients (16 wrists) returned to their previous employment and 5 patients (6 wrists) began working at different jobs with lighter duties. These results demonstrate that patients with persistent carpal tunnel syndrome after incomplete endoscopic release can experience improvement of symptoms with expected return to work after open revision [32].

In conclusion, revision carpal tunnel surgery has modest results as compared to primary carpal tunnel release. However, many authors have shown improvement in 50–85% of revision cases in small retrospective studies. O'Malley et al. (1992) showed 60–70% improvement in a study in 1998 [33]. Simple decompression alone has shown to be effective for treatment of revision carpal tunnel syndrome. Often the nerve shows significant scarring, and many recommend some type of coverage or interoposition to provide a barrier to scar tissue and to help with tendon gliding.

Our senior author's preference is a hypothenar fat flap in most cases of revision carpal tunnel release. The advantage of this flap is that it is locally available vascularized flap with low morbidity and good reproducibility. Post operatively early range of motion is initiated to help with nerve gliding. One other consideration is our senior author performs the majority of carpal tunnel surgery utilizing a Wide Awake Local Anesthesia No Tourniquet (WALANT) technique. The locally available hypothenar fat pad flap as well as the synovial flaps can easily be performed under WALANT.

References

1. Langloh ND, Linscheid RL. Recurrent and unrelieved carpal-tunnel syndrome. Clin Orthop Relat Res. 1972;83:41–7.
2. Bande S, De Smet L, Fabry G. The results of carpal tunnel release: open verse endoscopic technique. J Hand Surg. 1994;19B:14–7. https://doi.org/10.1016/0266-7681(94)90039-6.
3. Jones NF, Ahn HC, Eo S. Revision surgery for persistent and recurrent carpal tunnel syndrome and for failed carpal tunnel release. Plast Reconstr Surg. 2012;129:683–92. https://doi.org/10.1097/PRS.0b013e3182402c37.
4. Tollestrup T, Berg C, Netscher D. Management of distal traumatic median nerve painful neuromas and of recurrent carpal tunnel syndrome: hypothenar fat pad flap. J Hand Surg. 2010;35A:1010–4. https://doi.org/10.1016/j.jhsa.2010.03.035.
5. Cobb TK, Amadio PC, Leatherwood DF, Schleck CD, Ilstrup DM. Outcome of reoperation for carpal tunnel syndrome. J Hand Surg. 1996;21A:347–56. https://doi.org/10.1016/S0363-5023(96)80341-8.
6. Tung TH, Mackinnon SE. Secondary carpal tunnel surgery. Plast Reconstr Surg. 2001;107:1830–43.
7. Craft RO, Duncan SFM, Smith AA. Management of recurrent carpal tunnel syndrome with microneurolysis and the hypothenar fat pad flap. Hand. 2007;2:85–9. https://doi.org/10.1007/s11552-007-9025-7.
8. Zieske L, Ebersole GC, Davidge K, Fox I, Mackinnon SE. Revision carpal tunnel surgery: a 10-year review of intraoperative findings and outcomes. J Hand Surg. 2013;38A:1530–9. https://doi.org/10.1016/j.jhsa.2013.04.024.
9. Stütz N, Gohritz A, Van Schoonhoven J, Lanz U. Revision surgery after carpal tunnel release- analysis of the pathology in 200 cases during a 2-year period. J Hand Surg. 2006;31B:68–71. https://doi.org/10.1016/j.jhsb.2005.09.022.
10. Chang B, Dellon AL. Surgical management of recurrent carpal tunnel syndrome. J Hand Surg. 1993;18B:467–70.
11. Padua L, Coraci D, Erra C, Pazzaglia C, Paolasso I, Loreti C, et al. Carpal tunnel syndrome: clinical features, diagnosis, and management. Lancet Neurol. 2016;15:1273–84. https://doi.org/10.1016/S1474-4422(16)30231-9.
12. Beck JD, Brothers JG, Maloney PJ, Deegan JH, Tang X, Klena JC. Predicting the outcome of revision carpal tunnel release. J Hand Surg Br. 2012;37A:282–7. https://doi.org/10.1016/j.jhsa.2011.10.040.
13. Taghizadeh R, Tahir A, Stevenson S, Barnes DE, Spratt JD, Erdmann MW. The role of MRI in the diagnosis of recurrent/persistent carpal tunnel syndrome: a radiographical and intraoperative correlation. J Plast Reconstr Aesthet Surg. 2011;64:1250–2. https://doi.org/10.1016/j.bjps.2011.03.019.
14. Duetzmann S, Tas S, Seifert V, Marguardt G, Dombert T, Staub F. Cross-sectional area of the median nerve before revision carpal tunnel release – a cross-sectional study. Oper Neurosurg. 2018;14:20–5. https://doi.org/10.1093/ons/opx079.
15. Soltani AM, Allan BJ, Best MJ, Mir HS, Panthaki ZJ. A systematic review of the literature on the

outcomes of treatment for recurrent and persistent carpal tunnel syndrome. Plast Reconstr Surg. 2013;132:114–21. https://doi.org/10.1097/PRS.0b013e318290faba.
16. Pace GI, Zale CL, Gendelberg D, Taylor KF. Self-reported outcomes for patients undergoing revision carpal tunnel surgery with or without hypothenar fat pad transposition. Hand. 2018;13(3):292–5. https://doi.org/10.1177/1558944717701243.
17. Luria S, Waitayawinyu T, Trumble TE. Endoscopic revision of carpal tunnel release. Plast Reconstr Surg. 2008;121:2029–36. https://doi.org/10.1097/PRS.0b013e31817123de.
18. Gannon C, Baratz K, Baratz M. The synovial flap in recurrent and failed carpal tunnel surgery. Oper Tech Orthop. 2007;17:102–5. https://doi.org/10.1053/j.oto.2007.01.010.
19. Murthy PG, Abzug JM, Jacoby SM, Culp RW. The tenosynovial flap for recalcitrant carpal tunnel syndrome. Tech Hand Up Extrem Surg. 2013;17:84–6. https://doi.org/10.1097/BTH.0b013e318281d0e8.
20. Cramer LM. Local fat coverage for the median nerve. ASSH Corresp. Newsl. 1985;35:246.
21. Wichelaus A, Mittlmeier T, Gierer P, Beck M. Vascularized hypothenar fat pad flap in revision surgery for carpal tunnel syndrome. J Neurol Surg. 2015;76:438–42. https://doi.org/10.1055/s-0035-1551831.
22. Mathoulin C, Bahm J, Roukoz S. Pedicled hypothenar fat pad flap for median nerve coverage in recalcitrant carpal tunnel syndrome. J Hand Surg. 2000;5:33–40. https://doi.org/10.1142/S0218810400000120.
23. Chrysopoulo MT, Greenberg JA, Kleinman WB. The hypothenar fat pad transposition flap: a modified surgical technique. Tech Hand Up Extrem Surg. 2006;10:150–6. https://doi.org/10.1097/01.bth.0000225004.56982.42.
24. Strickland JW, Idler RS, Lourie GM, Plancher KD. The hypothenar fat pad flap for management of recalcitrant carpal tunnel syndrome. J Hand Surg. 1996;21A:840–8. https://doi.org/10.1016/S0363-5023(96)80201-2.
25. Varitimidis SE, Vardakas DG, Goebel F, Sotereanos DG. Treatment of recurrent compressive neuropathy of peripheral nerves in the upper extremity with an autologous vein insulator. J Hand Surg. 2001;26A:296–302. https://doi.org/10.1053/jhsu.2001.22528.
26. Rose EH, Norris MS, Kowalski TA, Lucas A, Flegler EJ. Palmaris brevis turnover flap as an adjunct to internal neurolysis of the chronically scarred median nerve in recurrent carpal tunnel syndrome. J Hand Surg. 1991;16A:191–201. https://doi.org/10.1016/S0363-5023(10)80096-6.
27. Abzug JM, Jacoby SM, Osterman AL. Surgical options for recalcitrant carpal tunnel syndrome with perineural fibrosis. Hand. 2012;7:23–9. https://doi.org/10.1007/s11552-012-9391-7.
28. Tham SK, Ireland DC, Riccio M, Morrison WA. Reverse radial artery fascial flap: a treatment for the chronically scarred median nerve is recurrent carpal tunnel syndrome. J Hand Surg. 1996;21:849–54. https://doi.org/10.1016/S0363-5023(96)80202-4.
29. Mahmoud M, Shafie SE, Coppola EE, Elfar JC. Perforator-based forearm fascial flap for management of recurrent carpal tunnel syndrome. J Hand Surg. 2013;38A:2151–8. https://doi.org/10.1016/j.jhsa.2013.06.034.
30. Goitz RJ, Steichen JB. Microvascular omental transfer for the treatment of severe recurrent median neuritis of the wrist: a long-term follow-up. Plast Reconstr Surg. 2005;115:163–71. https://doi.org/10.1097/01.PRS.0000138808.77038.D7.
31. Hulsizer DL, Stabler MP, Weiss APC. The results of revision carpal tunnel release following previous open verses endoscopic surgery. J Hand Surg. 1998;23A:865–9. https://doi.org/10.1016/S0363-5023(98)80164-0.
32. Varitimidis SE, Herndon JH, Sotereanos DG. Failed endoscopic carpal tunnel release: operative findings and results of open revision surgery. J Hand Surg Br. 1999;24B(4):465–7. https://doi.org/10.1054/jhsb.1999.0243.
33. O'Malley MJ, Evanoff M, Terrono AL, Millender LH. Factors that determine re-exploration treatment of the carpal tunnel syndrome. J Hand Surg. 1992;17A:638–41. https://doi.org/10.1016/0363-5023(92)90307-B.

Hypothenar Fat Pad Flap: Surgical Technique

9

James W. Strickland and Gary M. Lourie

Introduction

Carpal Tunnel Syndrome remains the most common compression peripheral neuropathy treated. Conservative treatment is usually successful, with the remaining unsuccessful 10% of patients relieved of symptoms with simple release [1]. Unfortunately 10–25% of patients undergoing primary carpal tunnel release will fail. The etiology of this occurrence is multifactorial including incomplete release of the transverse carpal ligament or distal antebrachial fascia, tenosynovitis, postoperative development of adhesions surrounding the nerve, and intraneural fascicular scarring [2, 3]. Scarring of the median nerve with adherence to the radial leaf of the released transverse carpal ligament creates a neurodesis that often cannot be treated successfully with conservative treatment. These dysesthetic symptoms can become incapacitating and often require a surgical procedure to affect a successful outcome. Simple repeat release of the nerve has been met with universal failure. The literature is replete with surgical procedures to address the scar adhesions surrounding the median nerve. The procedures vary but all strive to create a barrier to epineural scarring. Soft tissue flaps including fat, fascia, muscle, and vein along with inert and non-inert commercial products comprised of allograft collagen and even small intestine submucosa have been described with encouraging clinical results [3–6]. The desired procedure must meet four requisites; it should be reproducible, safe, clinically effective, and in this day and age cost effective.

The hypothenar fat pad flap (HTFPF) procedure mobilizes a generous pad of vascularized fat from the hypothenar eminence as a pedicled pad and interposes the flap between the neurolysed median nerve and remaining radial leaf of the transverse carpal ligament. The fat pad flap serves to cover the nerve, prevent readherence, and return a smooth gliding bed for the median nerve. First described in 1985, this flap was refined by the senior author (JWS), his series published in the Journal of Hand Surgery in 1996 [1]. In this retrospective review of 62 hands with an average follow-up of 33 months, patient satisfaction was high with successful relief of persistent dysesthetic pain and low complication rate. Ensuing published reports confirmed equal results solidifying the hypothenar fat pad flap (HTFPF) as a viable, safe, efficacious, and cost effective procedure to alleviate recalcitrant idiopathic carpal tunnel syndrome [1, 2]. This chapter will discuss

J. W. Strickland
St. Francis Hospital, Indianapolis, IN, USA

Department of Orthopaedics-Emeritus, Indiana University School of Medicine, Indianapolis, IN, USA

G. M. Lourie (✉)
The Hand and Upper Extremity Center of Georgia, Atlanta, GA, USA

D. G. Sotereanos, L. K. Papatheodorou (eds.), *Compressive Neuropathies of the Upper Extremity*,
https://doi.org/10.1007/978-3-030-37289-7_9

the vascular basis and surgical technique in stepwise fashion of this flap highlighting and emphasizing the salient point to affect a successful outcome.

Anatomic Dissections and Vascular Basis for the Hypothenar Fat Pad Flap

Anatomic dissections and clinical observations have shown that the hypothenar eminence consistently includes a generous layer of adipose tissue of sufficient width and thickness to provide coverage of the median nerve within the carpal tunnel. Cadaveric studies have documented that in latex-injected hypothenar tissue there is a consistent supply of arterial branches to the fat pad arising directly from the medial side of the ulnar artery in Guyon's canal and more distally from branches of the ulnar artery to the small finger and fourth web space [1]. These transverse branches originate from the ulnar artery in a ladder type fashion separated 1 cm apart beginning at the distal wrist flexion crease. Additional branches to the fat pad arose from arterial branches to the hypothenar muscles and palmaris brevis muscles. Dissection of skin overlying the hypothenar fat pad revealed a rich plexus of arteries running through the superficial adipose tissue. An important observation in dissecting the fat pad was that the ulnar digital nerve of the small finger and the common digital nerve to the fourth web space ran deep to the distal third of the fat pad after branching from the ulnar nerve in Guyon's canal. This has clinical importance for the surgeon dissecting the flap to avoid inadvertent neuropraxic injury to these nerve branches.

Surgical Technique

The procedure is carried out under regional or general anesthesia. Intravenous antibiotics are not given routinely unless the patient demonstrates co-morbidities or risk factors. A linear incision was made in the midpalmar crease lateral to the hypothenar eminence crossing the wrist in a zig-zag fashion in line with the radial aspect of the ring finger. An extended incision is often recommended to decompress the median nerve starting in the distal forearm in more native unscarred tissue. In the palm the dissection is carried down through the palmar aponeurosis and reconstituted transverse carpal ligament. The median nerve is identified and, if the nerve is found to be adherent within the carpal canal, often seen to be tethered to the released radial leaf of the transverse carpal ligament, then an external neurolysis is performed. In those patients having preoperative clinical hypersensitivity of the median nerve at the wrist or intraoperative findings of neurodesis, a HTFPF is performed. A surgical plane is developed by sharp dissection just deep to the subdermal plexus between the skin overlying the hypothenar eminence and the underlying adipose tissue (Fig. 9.1). Care must be taken not to make this cutaneous flap too thin so as not to devascularize the overlying skin. The superficial dissection is continued ulnar to the dermal insertion of the palmaris brevis. Care is taken to identify the digital nerves to the ring and small fingers distally and the ulnar artery and nerve proximally (Fig. 9.1). From the ulnar edge of the fat pad, the deep dissection elevates the flap from the thenar muscles. The deep dissection is carried in a lateral direction until the ulnar nerve and vessels are visualized in Guyon's Canal. The Guyon's canal can be initially released and the ulnar nerve and artery are identified and protected throughout the dissection of the flap. A segment of the ulnar leaf of the transverse carpal ligament is excised to aid in mobilization of the flap during this part of the deep dissection. The flap is then transposed to determine if it could be easily advanced over the median nerve to the radial wall of the carpal canal (Fig. 9.2). If it had not been sufficiently mobilized, additional undermining is carried out, with care taken to preserve the vascular pedicles of the flap and to not damage the ulnar artery or nerve. When sufficiently mobilized, the HTFPF is placed palmar to the median nerve and deep to the radial leaf of the transverse carpal ligament. With the contents of the canal retracted ulnarly, three horizontal sutures are placed from the edge of the HTFPF

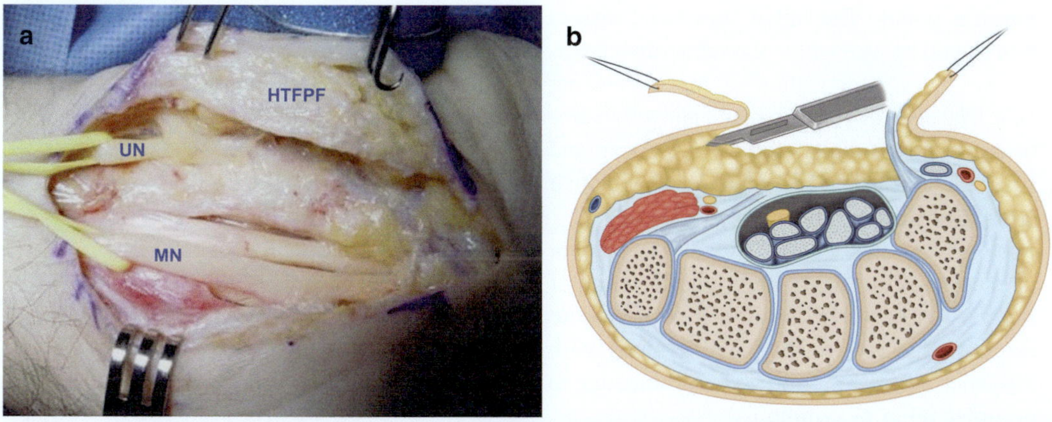

Fig. 9.1 (**a**) The hypothenar fat pad flap (HTFPF) is raised by subcutaneous dissection in an ulnar direction. MN: median nerve, UN: ulnar nerve. Photo courtesy of Dr. Dean Sotereanos. (**b**) A corresponding axial illustration

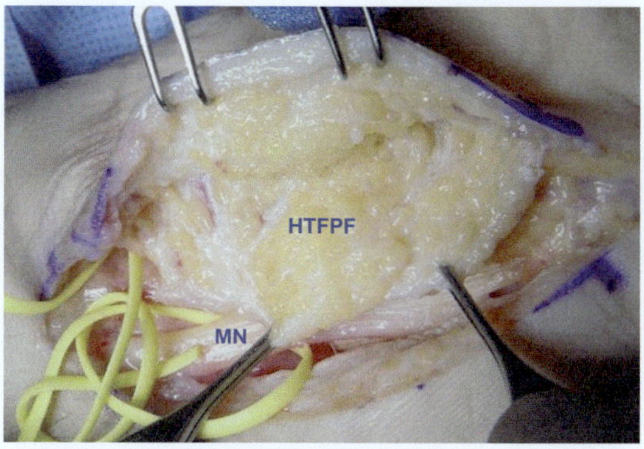

Fig. 9.2 The hypothenar fat pad flap (HTFPF) is tested to see if it advances easily over the median nerve (MN). (Photo courtesy of Dr. Dean Sotereanos)

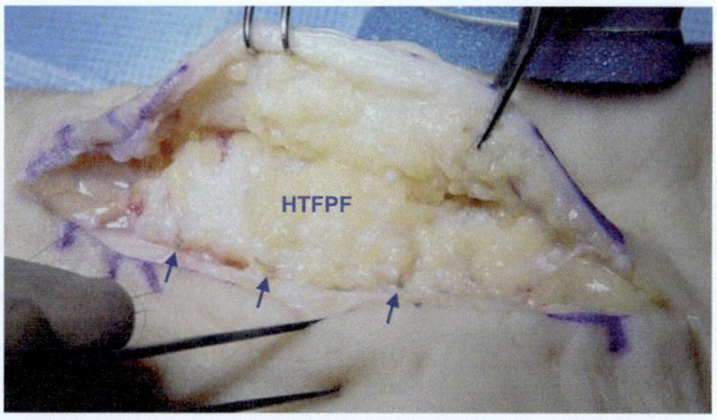

Fig. 9.3 The hypothenar fat pad flap (HTFPF) is sutured to the radial remnant of transverse carpal ligament (arrows) without tension covering the median nerve. (Photo courtesy of Dr. Dean Sotereanos)

into the radial wall of the carpal tunnel adjacent to the flexor pollicis longus tendon and back through the HTFPF (Fig. 9.3). Sutures are tagged to facilitate the placement of all stitches prior to tying them in sequence.

As the sutures are tied, the radial and ulnar borders of the hand are gently compressed to ease the delivery of the flap well down into the radial side of the carpal canal. A layered skin closure is then performed in usual fashion. After surgery, gentle transverse compression is applied within the dressing across the palm, with the thumb adducted to minimize tension on the HTFPF. The wrist is placed in slight dorsiflexion, with the fingers free for immediate postoperative motion. The surgical dressing and sutures are removed at 10–14 days after surgery. Patients are instructed in scar massage and desensitization. Wrist motion is commenced with interval splinting for an additional 2 weeks. At 6 weeks after surgery, unrestricted use is permitted and a formal strengthening program is commenced.

Pearls

1. Patient selection. The indications for this procedure need to be met by patient and the surgeon. Persistent and or recurrent symptoms of median nerve compression thought to be due to tethering or neurodesis of the nerve to the released radial leaf of the transverse carpal ligament unresponsive to conservative treatment remains the main indication for the HTFPF.

2. Surgical points. The initial superficial dissection should be well within the subdermal plexus to avoid devascularization of the hypothenar skin. The deep dissection should allow for identification of the digital nerves to the ring and small finger distal and the ulnar nerve and ulnar artery proximal to avoid iatrogenic damage.
3. Postoperative recommendations. The patient is encouraged to begin early digital range of motion in the early postoperative period to prevent adhesions to the HTFPF, along with diligence to wrist motion and scar massage to optimize relief of symptoms.

Conclusion

Recalcitrant or recurrent carpal tunnel syndrome can be incapacitating for the patient. Many techniques for alleviating symptoms have been advocated including repeat release, along with introduction of tissue or materials to wrap and protect the nerve from adhesion formation. A successful procedure should be reproducible, safe, clinically effective, and cost effective. The hypothenar fat pad flap (HTFPF), developed and refined by James W Strickland MD has met these 4 tenets and should be part of the hand surgeon's armamentarium in treating this challenging clinical condition [1, 2].

References

1. Strickland JW, Idler RS, Lourie GM, Plancher KD. The hypothenar fat pad for management of recalcitrant carpal tunnel syndrome. J Hand Surg Am. 1996;21A(5):840–8.
2. Plancher KD, Idler RS, Lourie GM, Strickland JW. Recalcitrant carpal tunnel: the hypothenar fat pad flap. Hand Clin. 1996;12(2):337–49.
3. Dy CJ, Aunins B, Brogan DM. Barriers to epineural scarring: role in treatment of traumatic nerve injury and chronic compressive neuropathy. J Hand Surg Am. 2018;43:360–7.
4. Tollestrup T, Berg C, Netscher D. Management of distal traumatic median nerve painful neuromas and of recurrent carpal tunnel syndrome: hypothenar fat pad flap. J Hand Surg. 2010;35A:1010–4.
5. Zieske L, Ebersole GC, Davidge K, Fox I, Mackinnon SE. Revision carpal tunnel surgery: a 10-year review of intraoperative findings and outcomes. J Hand Surg. 2013;38A:1530–9.
6. Sarris IK, Sotereanos DG. Vein wrapping for recurrent median nerve compression. J Am Soc Surg Hand. 2004;4(3):189–94.

10 Tumors and Tumor-Like Lesions Mimicking Peripheral Neuropathies

Zoe H. Dailiana and Vasileios A. Kontogeorgakos

Upper extremity peripheral neuropathies may be idiopathic or due to occupational, systemic, and local factors including trauma and subsequent scar-tissue formation, anatomic variances and aberrant muscles, tumors and tumor like lesions [1–3]. Although upper extremity peripheral neuropathies are common, involving in declining order the median, ulnar, posterior interosseous, sensory branch of radial nerve, musculocutaneous, and suprascapular nerves, tumor related compressive neuropathies are rare, and their diagnosis is easily overlooked, resulting to relapsing symptoms in the case that the causative factor is not addressed. In a study of 1110 patients treated for carpal tunnel syndrome (CTS), less than 3% was related to a tumor or tumor-like lesion [1].

General Aspects

Diagnostic Approach

A high index of suspicion is required in patients suffering from peripheral neuropathies, with atypical characteristics concerning their gender, age, and occupation, e.g. CTS in young patients, male patients, non-manual workers, without endocrine disorders [1].

The diagnostic workup includes a detailed history, physical examination including the evaluation of peripheral nerve compression and the investigation for palpable masses that may be evident in high percentages (up to 65%) of patients [1], nerve conduction studies, and appropriate imaging studies. Although plain radiographs may reveal nonspecific soft-tissue masses, ultrasound and MRI have a high sensitivity in diagnosing peripheral nerve compression [4], and in detecting space-occupying lesions that may be related to peripheral nerves, providing useful information about the position (inside or outside the nerve), the ascending point and the dimensions of the lesions, and their correlation with the respective nerves and surrounding structures [5, 6].

Differential Diagnosis

These space occupying lesions may be intra- or extra-neural, benign or malignant. The differentiation of neoplastic conditions (benign or malignant) from tumor like masses is not always an easy case. Sometimes, biopsy of the mass should precede a definite surgical treatment, as a negative tissue margin is mandatory for malignant

Z. H. Dailiana (✉)
Department of Orthopaedic Surgery, Faculty of Medicine, University of Thessaly, Larissa, Greece
e-mail: dailiana@med.uth.gr

V. A. Kontogeorgakos
Department of Orthopaedic Surgery, Attikon University Hospital, National and Kapodistrian University of Athens, Athens, Greece

D. G. Sotereanos, L. K. Papatheodorou (eds.), *Compressive Neuropathies of the Upper Extremity*,
https://doi.org/10.1007/978-3-030-37289-7_10

tumors versus marginal resections for benign and reactive tumor like lesions.

The most common extraneural tumors and tumor like lesions are lipomas, ganglion cysts, tenosynovitis, rheumatoid nodules, calcium and uric acid deposits and abnormal muscles. Intraneural peripheral nerve tumors are rare and include schwannomas, neurofibromas, sarcomas, and intraneural tumors of non-neural origin. The tumors of peripheral nerves are benign in at least 85–90% of clinically symptomatic cases, while malignant peripheral nerve sheath tumors and other malignant lesions, such as lymphoma and metastases are rare. This low general incidence of malignant tumors should not be underestimated in patients with type 1 neurofibromatosis. Among these patients, 8–10% will develop a malignant peripheral nerve sheath tumor during their lifetimes [7].

Treatment

Apart of surgical nerve decompression according to the nerve entrapped, the characteristics of the tumor/tumor like lesion, including the location (intra- or extraneural), the extent, and the aggressiveness (benign or malignant) dictate the approach and subsequent procedure (biopsy, neurolysis, excision of mass). After excision of extraneural benign lesions, the outcome is usually favourable. In intraneural lesions the preservation of nerve function and continuity are of utmost importance and thus, a biopsy ruling out malignancy, is often necessary [8]. According to the biopsy results, the lesion may be left in place (Fig. 10.1), undergo microsurgical dissection leaving intact the nerve fascicles or resecting the involved fascicles (Fig. 10.2) and, in confirmed malignancy, the lesion may be resected aggressively. In all cases nerve grafting of the respective fascicle/nerve gap is necessary.

Categorization

According to their histologic characteristics these tumors and tumor like lesions are presented in specific categories, with concurrent presentation of the diagnostic and therapeutic approach:

Lipomatous Tumors

Lipomas are composed of mature white adipocyte cells, and these are the most common soft tissue mesenchymal neoplasm in adults. Benign lipomatous tumors have a low metabolic rate and increase their size slowly. Neighboring peripheral nerves in close proximity to lipomas accommodate to the slow size increase of lipomas. Thus, lipomas are an uncommon cause of chronic compressive neuropathies and even more rarely an acute motor neuropathy can develop.

Lipomas

Intraneural or extraneural lipomas are rare, focal, usually well-defined benign lipomatous masses. The mass does not infiltrate the nerve. However,

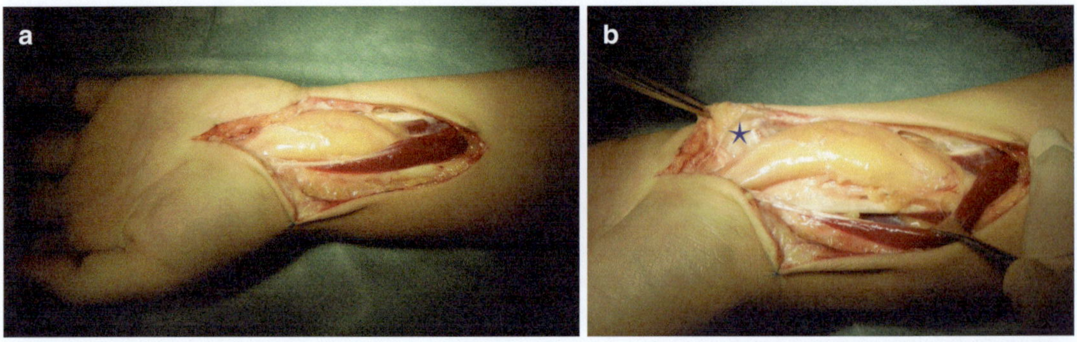

Fig. 10.1 (**a**) Neurofibroma of the median nerve in a 17-year-old female patient presenting with carpal tunnel syndrome. (**b**) Normal nerve fibers are difficult to separate from the tumor and surgical treatment is limited to nerve decompression (asterisk on divided transverse carpal ligament)

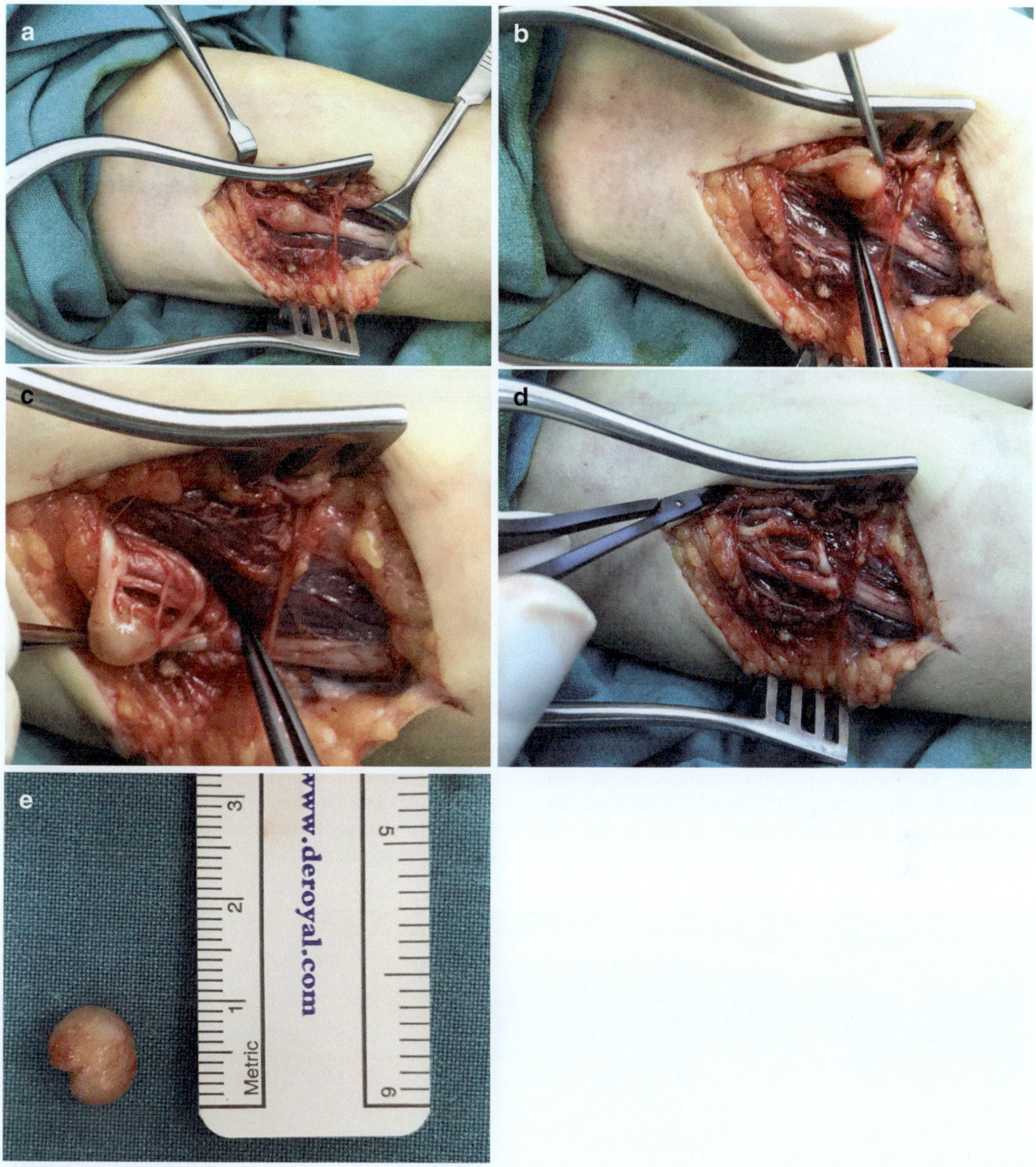

Fig. 10.2 (**a**) Ulnar nerve schwannoma proximal to the elbow, in a 17-year-old male, with motor and sensory deficits. The tumor is enveloped by the ulnar nerve perineurium. (**b–d**) After microsurgical dissection the tumor, arising from one fascicle of the ulnar nerve, is shelled out from the nerve trunk. (**e**) Gross specimen

due to size of the lipoma the nerve may be displaced and compressed [9–13]. Median nerve at the carpal tunnel is typically affected but ulnar and sciatic nerve involvement is reported. Because of the defined morphology of the mass, lipomas can be resected resulting in symptom improvement (Figs. 10.3 and 10.4).

Nerve Lipomatosis

Nerve lipomatosis is also known as intraneural lipoma or fibrolipomatous hamartoma of the nerve [14]. Nerve lipomatosis is characterized by diffuse epineurial and interfascicular infltrate of mature fatty or fibroadipose tissue [10]. The size of the affected nerve is considerably increased,

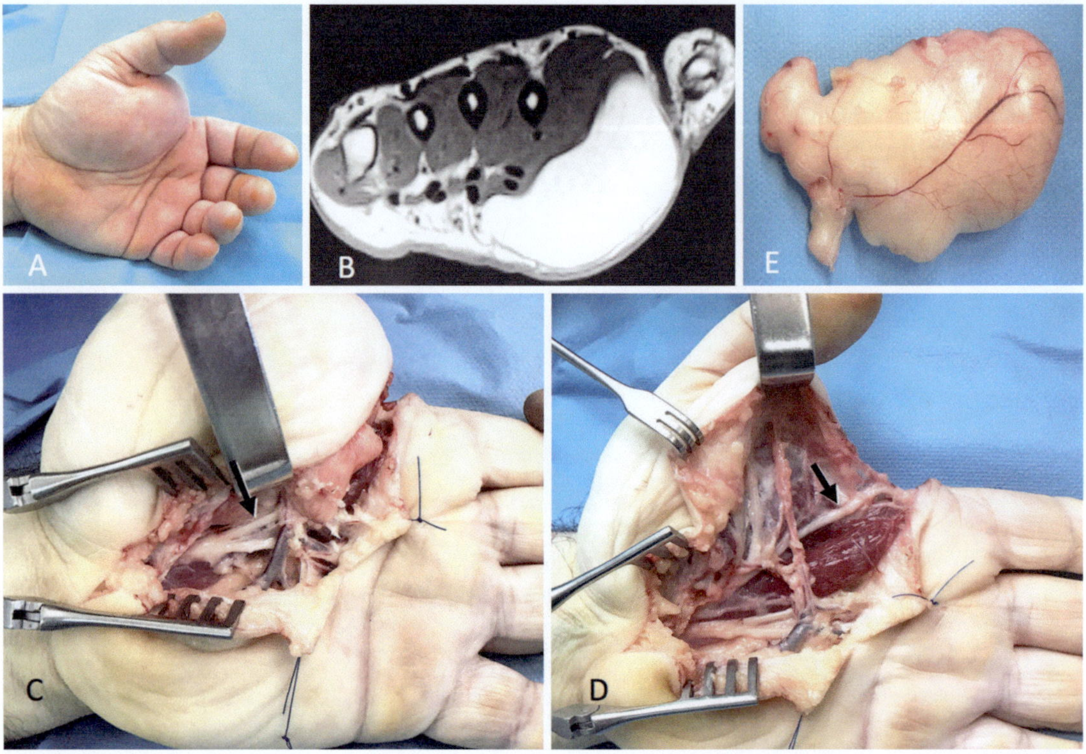

Fig. 10.3 (**a**) Large size lipoma located at the deep thenar area. The patient reported dysesthesia at the radial side of index finger. (**b**) MRI axial view depicting a lipomatous tumor at the palmar side of the thenar area extending to mid-palm. (**c**) Deep dissection reveals compression of the radial palmar index digital nerve under the lipoma mass and the superficial arterial arch (black arrow). (**d**) Intraoperative view after lipoma resection. Black arrow points to the index palmar radial nerve. (**e**) The lipoma gross specimen

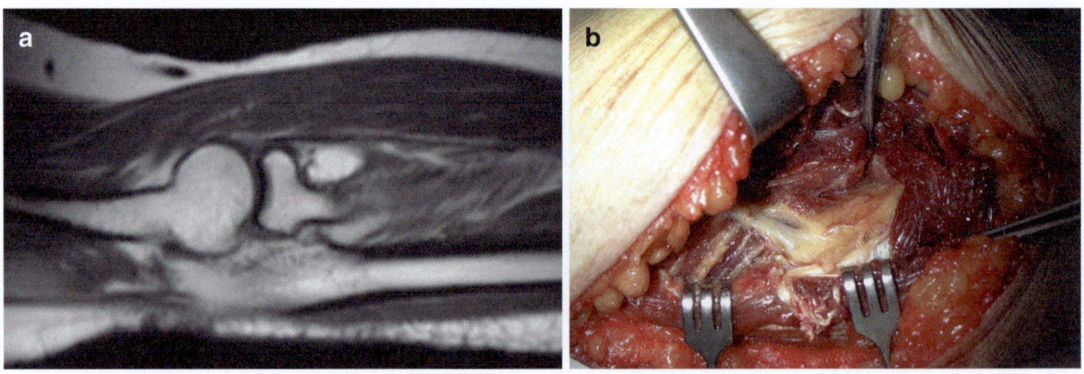

Fig. 10.4 (**a**) Elbow MRI depicting a lipoma at the radial neck, in a 59-year-old female patient with acute palsy of the posterior interosseous nerve (PIN). (**b**) Superficial dissection of the PIN. (**c**, **d**) Deep dissection reveals compression of the PIN from a lipoma

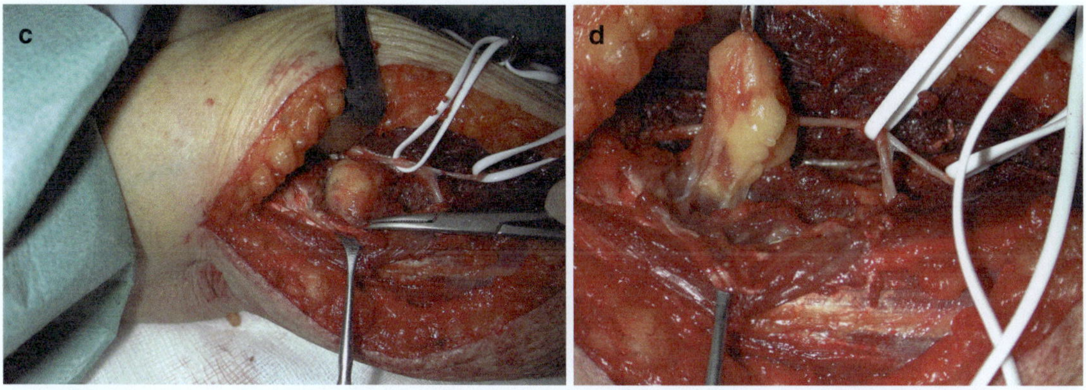

Fig. 10.4 (continued)

but the entrapped nerve fascicles are macroscopically normal. The median nerve is most commonly involved (85%) followed by the ulnar nerve. More than one nerve may be affected and frequently a contralateral lesion, symmetrical [15] or asymmetrical, is present [16].

About 20–66% of patients with nerve lipomatosis have a variable degree of accompanying overgrowth of mesenchymal elements in the distribution of the affected nerve, typically including fibroadipose tissue and bone [10, 14, 17].

MRI of nerve lipomatosis is very characteristic, with a fusiform nerve enlargement. Imaging characteristics include serpiginous low-intensity structures representing thickened nerve fascicles, surrounded by evenly distributed fat, high signal intensity on T1 sequences and low signal intensity on T2 sequences. The nerve has a cable-like appearance on axial planes and a spaghetti-like appearance on coronal planes [17].

Surgical treatment regarding compression neuropathy is limited to nerve decompression, resulting in symptom relief. Nerve resection and cable nerve graft reconstruction has been described but the indications for such a procedure are very limited.

Parosteal Lipomas

Parosteal lipomas are benign fatty tumors located on a bone surface, intimately related to the periosteum. At the upper extremity, these lesions often develop around the proximal radius. In a review of 32 cases of parosteal lipomas, 50% had osseous reaction, including osseous bowing, focal cortical hyperostoses or cortical erosion [18]. In the study by Moon et al. [19], 55% (11 of 20 patients) presented with posterior interosseous nerve palsy. Intraoperatively the tumor is encapsulated and strongly adhered to the periosteum requiring a subperiosteal dissection or an osteotome for the removal of the neoplasm [20] (Fig. 10.5).

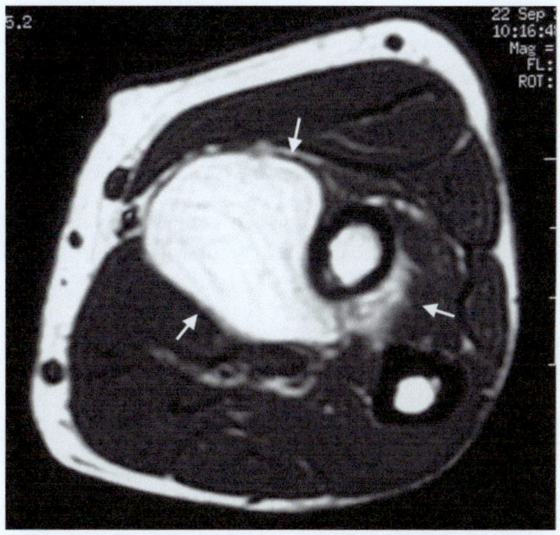

Fig. 10.5 A 55-year-old woman presented with painless PIN palsy over 2 weeks. MRI T1 axial image reveals a lipoma in close proximity to proximal radius. Intraoperatively, the lipoma was strongly adhered to the underlying periosteum. Gradual restoration of muscle strength was noticed 4 months later after tumor removal

Ganglion and Synovial Cysts

The word ganglion comes from a Greek word that, simply translated, means knot [3]. Ganglions are mucin filled cysts and rarely are the cause of

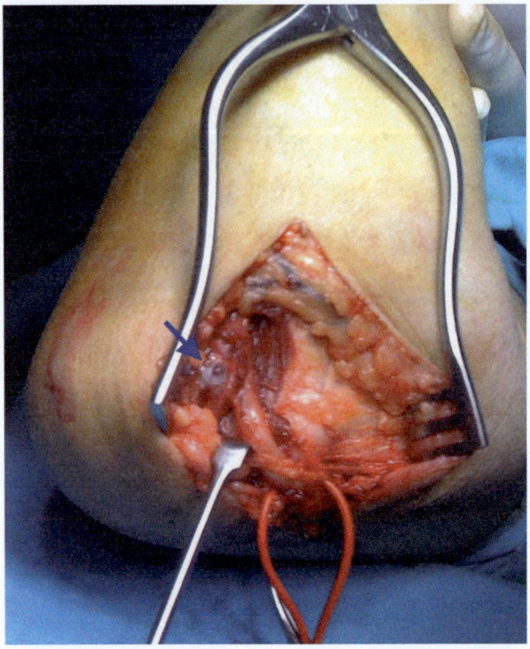

Fig. 10.6 Ganglion cyst (arrow) compressing the ulnar nerve in a 65-year-old male patient with cubital tunnel syndrome

a peripheral nerve compression (Fig. 10.6). They are sometimes painful and frequently fluctuate in size. Ganglions can exert pressure over a nerve either as an extraneural or as an intaneural cyst. The pathogenesis of intraneural ganglia is an issue of debate for 200 years. Three major theories have been proposed to explain their existence, namely, degenerative, synovial (articular), and tumoral theories. In 2009, Spinner et al proposed the unifying theory [21, 22]. In their study, all intraneural cysts, even in a remote location from a joint had joint connections. Ligation of the articular branch connecting the cyst to nearby joint, is an important surgical step in order to avoid recurrence of the cyst.

Intraneural cyst of the peroneal nerve is well known and described entity. Usually the patients present with motor and sensory deficit and a positive Tinel's sign [23]. Several case reports appear in the literature regarding ganglion cysts compressing the ulnar nerve [24, 25] (Fig. 10.6). Beauchene in 1810 described an intraneural cyst of the ulnar nerve at the cubital tunnel [26, 27]. Clinically the patients present with progressive pain, numbness, and weakness along the distribution of the ulnar nerve.

MRI is very useful in preoperative diagnosis. Ganglions present as non-enhancing soft tissue lesions with low and high intensity signal on T1 and T2 images respectively. Usually, microsurgical resection of the cyst can be performed resulting in significant resolution of preoperative symptoms. However, motor recovery may not be complete if the ganglion cyst extensively involves the nerve and symptoms have been present for more than 1 year [25].

Chang et al reported on 184 patients with cubital tunnel syndrome who underwent surgical treatment [28]. Of these patients, 16 had extraneural cysts and 3 had intraneural ganglion cysts (10.33%). All 19 patients had elbow osteoarthritis. For patients with mild neural compression, the ulnar nerve was decompressed and released in situ. But for space occupying lesion or severe neural compression or entrapment in the cubital tunnel, routine anterior transposition of the ulnar nerve was performed. Wang et al reported on nine patients with pure deep ulnar nerve branch compression by a ganglion [29]. All patients presented with no sensory loss but with different degrees of muscular atrophy and weakness of the interossei and adductor pollicis muscles. Ganglion excision and decompression of Guyon's canal was performed in all patients. The ganglion compressing the deep branch originated from the pisohamate joint in eight cases. Grip strength improved from a mean of 63% of the unaffected side preoperatively to 88% of the unaffected side postoperatively. Tip pinch strength improved from a mean of 61% to 87%. According to the modified Bishop's scoring system, six patients (67%) obtained excellent results, two (22%) had good results.

Special mention should be made for the acute palsy of the posterior interosseous nerve (PIN) from rheumatoid synovial cysts (bursa) around the elbow, in the rheumatoid patients [30]. Only 18 cases of PIN palsy secondary to rheumatoid arthritis in 17 patients have been reported in the English literature [31]. There were 13 female and 4 male patients with a mean age of 53 years.

The average duration of symptoms at presentation was 3.8 weeks.

Compression of the PIN presents with painless finger extension paresis associated with wrist extension in radially deviated position. Differential diagnosis of entrapment neuropathy of PIN should be made from vasculitic neuropathy and degenerative rupture of the extensor tendons. Vasculitic neuropathy patients usually have painful, sensory loss and weakness of the peripheral nerves. The onset is usually sudden and asymmetrical if multiple peripheral nerves are involved. In entrapment neuropathy, the onset is subacute and painless [31]. Degenerative extensor rupture in rheumatoid patients is a well-known condition [32]. Tendon rupture usually is asymptomatic and begins at the ulnar side of the hand. The patients are not able to perform active metacarpophalangeal (MCP) joint extension. When the wrist is placed in passive flexion, the MCP joints remains flexed. However, in the case of PIN nerve palsy, when the wrist is placed in passive flexion, thumb and finger extension at MCP joints occur (tenodesis effect).

Treatment with oral or steroid injection into the elbow may not produce lasting recovery [31, 33]. Nerve decompression and elbow synovectomy, sometimes combined with radial head excision, is the preferred method of treatment [31, 33, 34]. An anterolateral approach for division of the arcade of Frohse is effective in cases with diffuse synovitis, while in the case of a local cystic swelling, a posterolateral approach provides better access [33].

Compression of the median nerve from a ganglion, at the carpal tunnel is an uncommon diagnosis [35, 36]. Anterior wrist ganglion, which mainly originates from the radiocarpal joint, accounts for 15–20% of wrist ganglions [37, 38]. The recurrence rate for cases treated with aspiration is 83% and for those treated by surgical resection is 20% [38]. Because of the high recurrence rate of the ganglion, a careful dissection of the stalk from the anterior wrist capsule has been suggested [35, 38].

Kerrigan et al reported on 12 cases of ganglion cyst with carpal tunnel syndrome in 11 patients [36]. One half of the cysts were associated with direct trauma, usually with wrist hyperextension. Treatment included open carpal tunnel release with ganglion resection, resulting in symptom relief.

The suprascapular nerve can be compressed at the suprascapular or spino-glenoid notch. Compression at the suprascapular notch generally leads to weakness of both the supraspinatus and infraspinatus muscle. The suprascapular ligament is often the offending agent and must be released. In contrast, compression at the spinoglenoid notch leads to isolated infraspinatus weakness, and it is often caused by a cyst with an associated labral lesion [39]. The most common symptom is deep, posterior shoulder pain (97.8%), with a mean duration of symptoms before decompression of 19 months [39]. Memon et al identified 40 studies including 259 patients with suprascapular neuropathy, treated arthroscopically [40]. The most common etiology of suprascapular neuropathy was suprascapular nerve compression by a cyst at the spinoglenoid notch (42%). Overall, 97% of patients reported significant improvement or complete resolution of their pre-operative symptoms (including pain, strength, and subjective function of the shoulder) over a mean follow-up period of 23.7 months.

Reactive and Inflammatory Lesions

Tenosynovitis

Tenosynovitis from occupational disorders, rheumatoid arhtritis or gout may lead to nerve compression syndromes. Flexor tenosynovitis is a common cause of median nerve compression and development of CTS [1], while De Quervain's tenosynovitis has been described as a cause of compression of the superficial branch of the radial nerve [41]. Ultrasound is used to confirm the clinical finding of a palpable mass that is moving with finger flexion/extension and surgical treatment includes synovectomy in combination to division of the transverse ligament or neurolysis, according to the entrapped nerve (Fig. 10.7).

Neuritis Ossificans

Neuritis ossificans is a very rare reactive lesion occurring mostly in the peripheral nerves. Both

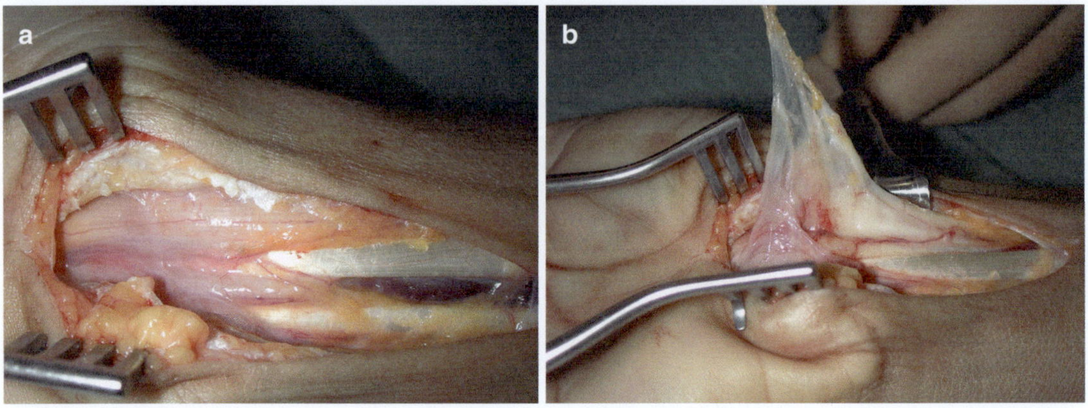

Fig. 10.7 (**a**) Intraoperative view of the carpal tunnel content after division of the transverse carpal ligament, in a 34-year-old female patient presenting with carpal tunnel syndrome and a palpable distal radius mass. (**b**) Dissection of the synovial tissue surrounding the finger flexors and the median nerve

upper and lower peripheral nerves can be offended. The architecture of this lesion is distinctly zonal. Under low microscope magnification there is a central fibroblastic core, an intervening zone of osteoid production, and a peripheral layer of ossification. This histologic pattern is remarkably similar to that of myositis ossificans [42–44]. Repetitive microtrauma, burns and central nervous system injury have been considered as predisposing factors for neuritis ossificans [43, 45–48].

Clinically, neuritis ossificans resembles peripheral nerve mononeuropathy, causing pain and paresthesias along its distribution [46]. A painful palpable mass may be found on clinical examination. Imaging characteristics are related to the stage of maturity of the mass. A histologically mature mass demonstrates a ring of ossification (according to the zonation phenomenon histologically) that can be depicted on radiographs and more clearly on CT scan.

When a calcified soft tissue mass is identified, biopsy is usually needed to rule out malignancy. Synovial sarcomas are well known malignant lesions that can have a long-standing course and demonstrate intra-tumoral calcifications. However, the final decision to perform a core needle biopsy of the mass is based on several parameters. For small size lesions needle biopsy may not be feasible and excisional biopsy may be considered.

Surgical resection of the mass is recommended with microsurgical technique in order to separate the mass from the nerve. However, the mass is firmly attached to the nerve and frequently nerve fascicles are within the lesion and have to be sacrificed. Thus, a nerve-sparing resection is not always possible [43]. Recurrence of the lesion is very uncommon.

Inflammatory Pseudotumor of Peripheral Nerve (IPPN)

Inflammatory pseudotumors represent a heterogeneous group of tumefactive lesions composed of largely chronic inflammatory cells, proliferating fibroblasts with collagen deposition and occasionally an element of increased vascularity [49, 50]. Although inflammatory pseudotumors of peripheral nerves are clearly associated with inflammation, there is no documented correlation to systemic inflammatory disease, infection, neoplasia, or trauma [51, 52].

This lesion presents clinically as a progressive axonal mononeuropathy with weakness, sensory loss, and pain. The symptoms may be induced acutely or may be slowly progressive over a long period. The lesions are often palpable and manipulation typically induces pain [51, 52].

Maurmann et al reported of five patients diagnosed with IPPN [52]. In their study, the involved nerves were the musculocutaneous, the median and the ulnar nerve in two patients and the peroneal and sciatic nerves in three patients. Histologically, all lesions had reactive features of inflammation, increased epineural vascularity, and marked fibrosis with increased collagen content, comprising 50–75% of the nerve area. The lesions demonstrated increased epineural perivascular inflammatory cell collections (CD-45) consisting of >100 lymphocytes/collection (large collection). No biopsies exhibited changes suggestive of inflammatory demyelination [52]. MRI demonstrated irregular, large masses involving and surrounding nerve with heterogenous signal characteristics on T1- and T2-weighted and post-contrast sequences. Three patients were treated with weekly courses of intravenous steroids for 3 months, resulting in significant improvement in pain and weakness.

Peripheral Nerve Sheath Tumors

Schwannomas (or neurilemomas) and neurofibromas are benign peripheral nerve sheath tumors (PNSTs).

Schwannomas

Schwannomas are the most frequent benign PNST overall, with upper extremity involvement occurring in 19% of patients with a PNST [53]. They are well circumscribed and usually grow eccentrically within a peripheral nerve. The ulnar nerve is frequently involved. The characteristic clinical presentation is of a solitary painless mass with occasional radiating pain. Schwannomas need differential diagnosis from malignant PNSTs. Ancient schwannomas are longstanding schwannomas demonstrating degenerative changes, seen histologically and on imaging, that may raise the suspicion of malignancy [54, 55]. In the study from Ogose et al, all benign lesions showed a smooth tumoral margin, while half the malignant PNSTs showed an invasive margin on CT or MRI [56]. The authors concluded that absence of severe motor weakness and a central enhancement pattern strongly suggest a benign nature, while severe rest pain and invasive tumor margins suggest malignant lesions in peripheral nerve tumors.

Schwannomas are enveloped by a true capsule formed by the perineurium of the nerve bundle of origin [57] (Fig. 10.2a). Intraoperatively the tumor is shelled out from the nerve trunk (Fig. 10.2b–e). Post-operative nerve dysfunction has been reported in 2.5–30% of patients [57, 58]. Young et al reported on 291 patients with a schwannoma [59]. Pain was the chief complaint in 55% and dysesthesia's in 4.8% of patients. Complete pain relief following excision was reported in 76%.

Neurofibromas

In contrast to schwannomas, neurofibromas arise within the nerve fascicles and their excision is much more difficult than schwannomas (Fig. 10.1a). Intraoperatively, normal nerve fibers are difficult to separate from the tumor and post-operative neurological deficits can occur [60]. Surgical treatment regarding compression neuropathy may be limited to nerve decompression (Fig. 10.1b).

Peripheral Nerve Compression and Malignancy

Compression from Lymph Nodes & Peripheral Nerve Lymphomatosis

Upper extremity peripheral nerve compression by enlarged lymph nodes at the elbow [61] or brachial plexus compression at the axillary region has been described, while neurolymphomatosis is a rare manifestation of non-Hodgkin lymphoma characterized by infiltration of neurotropic neoplastic cells into peripheral nerves, nerve roots and plexus, in the setting of an unknown or a known hematologic malignancy [62, 63]. The brachial plexus and the lumbosacral plexus are frequently involved. Histologically, the nerves are infiltrated by B-large and rarely by T lymphoma cells [63, 64]. Lymphomatous cell invasion induces demyelination and subsequent axonal degeneration distal to the infiltration site. The International Primary CNS Lymphoma Collaborative Group retrospectively analyzed 50 patients [65]. Nerve lymphomatosis was related to non-Hodgkin lymphoma in 90% and to acute leukemia in 10%. Peripheral nerves were the most frequently involved site [66]. The manifestation of painful neuropathy was recorded in 38 (76%) patients, with sensorimotor neuropathy being the most common type (36 cases). Pure motor neuropathy was described in 20% of the patients. PET/CT seems to be more sensitive than MRI in the diagnosis of nerve lymphomatosis [67] and treatment consists of chemotherapy alone or in combination to radiotherapy.

Metastatic Disease to Brachial Plexus and Peripheral Nerves

Metastatic disease to peripheral nerves is extremely rare [68]. The axonal environment of the peripheral nervous system is isolated from the extracellular space by a diffusion barrier called the blood-nerve barrier, which is similar to the blood-brain barrier [69]. It appears that the blood-nerve barrier is responsible for the resistance to metastatic implantation [70] of the circulating metastatic tumor cells into the peripheral nerve system. Most commonly peripheral nerves are compressed from a tumoral mass. Typical sites of malignant compression include the ulnar nerve at the axilla or elbow, the intercostals due to rib metastasis, the sciatic nerve in the pelvis, and the peroneal nerve near the fibular head [71, 72].

The brachial plexus is either invaded by direct extension from regional organs or is compressed or infiltrated by regional metastatic lymph nodes. Most tumors affecting the brachial plexus are from the lung or breast [73]. Breast cancer is associated with brachial plexopathy with an incidence of 1.8–4.9% at 5 years after treatment [74]. Brachial plexopathy is rarely the initial manifestation of cancer, with the exception of Pancoast tumors [71]. Pain is the most common presenting symptom in patients presenting with neoplastic brachial plexopathies [73]. The patients will often experience shoulder and axillary pain radiating along the medial aspect of the arm and forearm [74]. With lower-plexus (C8–T1) involvement, patients frequently develop pain, weakness, and atrophy along the ulnar side of hand and arm. Horner syndrome in neoplastic brachial plexopathy results from infiltration of the sympathetic ganglia near the T1 vertebrae. In patients with Horner syndrome, one-third will have epidural disease [74]. It is important to differentiate neoplastic brachial plexopathies from radiation- induced plexopathies. In a long-term follow-up study of 71 breast cancer patients who had received 4500–5000 cGy of radiation, plexopathy was identified in 17% [75]. Horner syndrome and lower- trunk brachial plexopathy commonly has neoplastic etiology whereas upper-trunk plexopathies are more often radiation induced. Pain at rest followed by weakness and numbness supports neoplastic plexopathy, while in radiation induced plexopathies, pain in not the predominant symptom and patients complain of numbness and dysesthesia [76].

Soft Tissue Sarcomas

Soft tissue sarcomas (STS) are malignant mesenchymal tumors that arise within the soft tissue. STSs usually grow within a tissue compartment at their poles and only at late stages they extend out of their compartment. During their growth STS push off surrounding nerves and vessels and only in rare cases they encapsulate the neurovascular bundles (Fig. 10.8). Neurological symptoms from nerve compression is not the rule and when present the patients report mild sensory symptoms.

Common primary malignant intra-neural sarcomas are the Malignant Peripheral Nerve Sheath Tumors (MPNST), while the synovial sarcoma is an STS histologic subtype that rarely rises within a peripheral nerve.

MPNST

MPNSTs are uncommon sarcomas compromising 5–10% of all soft tissue sarcomas. Patients with Neurofibromatosis NF-1 have a life time risk of 10% of developing MPNST [77]. Although the exact histogenesis remains unclear, MPNSTs present as high-grade sarcomas with a tendency to locally recur and mestasize hematogenous commonly to the lungs.

In the study by Kim et al the common clinical presentation was painful paresthesias in the distribution of the involved nerve with or without progressive loss of function [78]. Neural function loss was more likely with malignant tumors than with benign ones. The cornerstone of treatment is complete surgical resection of the tumor.

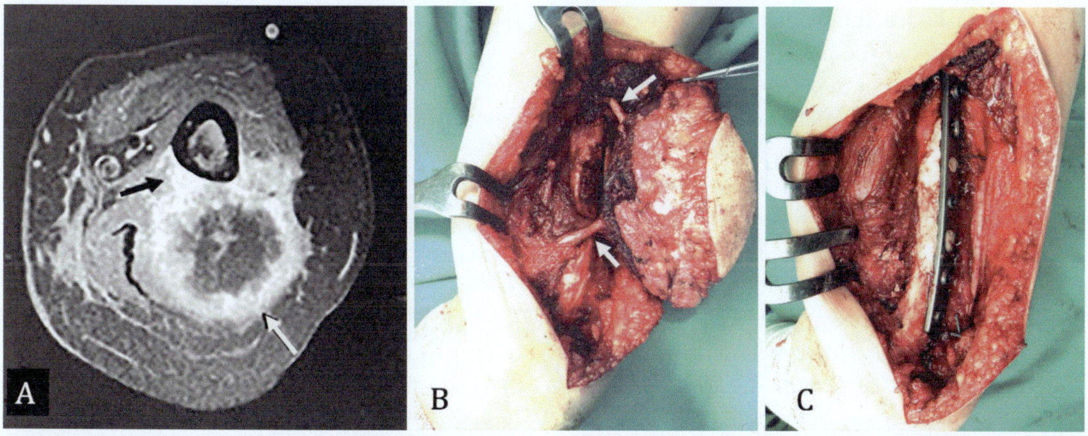

Fig. 10.8 (**a**) A 60-year-old woman presented with a palpable and painful mass of the posterior left humerus and radial nerve dysesthesia. MRI revealed a soft tissue mass with indistinct margin. Core needle biopsy was consistent with high grade pleomorphic sarcoma and the patient underwent 3 cycles of pre-operative chemotherapy. (**b**) Intraoperatively the radial nerve was encapsulated from the sarcoma and strongly adhered to the posterior cortex of the humerus. The tumor was resected to negative margins. However, the radial nerve, as well as a piece 5 cm long of the posterior cortex (arrows) was resected en-block with the tumor. (**c**) The bone defect was filled with PMMA and a 4.5 mm plate was used to protect the humerus. Boyes radial nerve tendon transfers were performed to restore wrist, thumb and finger extension. One year later the patient had protective sensation over the first dorsal web and a functional hand. No local tumor recurrence was noted

MPNSTs tend to have an infiltrative pattern to the adjacent soft tissue and extend along the nerve trunk in a long distance. Thus, resection to negative margin may be not feasible. The cornerstone of treatment is surgical resection to negative margins. Amputation may be indicated for extensive tumors and for MPNSTs that recur after apparently adequate excision [79, 80]. Cable nerve grafting for bridging the nerve defect can be considered in cases were functional recovery is anticipated within anticipated life expectancy and adjuvant treatment context.

Radiation therapy is delivered frequently in order to reduce the local recurrence rate. Preoperative chemotherapy may be useful in cases with large tumors as tumor size reduction and pseudocapdule stabilization may facilitate surgical resection [81]. In the EORTC STBSG trial, 175 MPNST patients received chemotherapy. In a median follow up of 4.1 years the median overall survival for the MPNST group was 48 weeks [82].

Synovial Sarcoma of Nerves

Synovial sarcomas are malignant soft tissue tumors that account for approximately 10% of all STS. These tumors can produce distant metastasis, and the 5-year survival rate is only 50–60% [76].

Primary intraneural synovial sarcomas are similar histologically to their more common soft tissue counterparts. The identification of the characteristic for synovial sarcoma translocation (X;18) is very helpful in difficult cases [83].

Hashimoto et al in 2018 reported on the 40th published patient diagnosed with intraneural synovial sarcoma located at the tibial nerve [84]. However, only few cases with synovial sarcoma of the peripheral nerves at the upper extremity are reported in the literature. The common clinical presentation is a painful mass and motor/sensory disturbance may be present. The patient may recall vague symptoms even years before diagnosis [85].

Scheithauer et al reported on ten patients with primary intraneural synovial sarcomas with a mean age of 40 years (range11–68 years) [86]. Only in three patients the tumor was located at the upper extremity and the median nerve, ulnar and the brachial plexus (C7) were involved. In their study, they reviewed another 12 patients from the English literature. In the combined study of 22 patients with intraneural synovial sarcoma of the upper and lower extremity, 73% of the patients had a tumor size of 5 cm or less. Clinically, 75% of the patients experienced sensorimotor loss and/or pain [80]. On imaging, soft tissue synovial sarcomas are often mistaken for benign nerve sheath tumors given their oval shape and frequent longitudinal orientation relative to surrounding soft tissue. In the study of Scheithauer et al, MRI revealed an isointense to muscle on T1-weighted imaging, hyperintense on T2-weighted sequences, and avid gadolinium enhancement [86]. However, the lesions had irregular margins and were clearly associated with individual nerves. Treatment includes tumor resection to negative margins. The nerve usually has to be sacrificed as the tumor invades the nerve. Intraneural synovial sarcomas tend to have a more favorable prognosis, probably related to the small tumor size at diagnosis.

References

1. Dailiana ZH, Bougioukli S, Varitimidis S, Kontogeorgakos V, Togia E, Vlychou M, Malizos KN. Tumors and tumor-like lesions mimicking carpal tunnel syndrome. Arch Orthop Trauma Surg. 2014;134:139–44.
2. Mathoulin C, Dailiana Z. Palmaris profundus associé a un syndrome du canal carpien. A propos d'un cas et revue de la bibliographie. La Main. 1998;3:261–5.
3. Sherman CE, Murray PM. Tumor-like conditions of the hand and upper extremity. J Hand Surg Am. 2017;42:1009–17.
4. Horng YS, Chang HC, Lin KE, Guo YL, Liu DH, Wang JD. Accuracy of ultrasonography and magnetic resonance imaging in diagnosing carpal tunnel syndrome using rest and grasp positions of the hands. J Hand Surg Am. 2012;37:1591–8.
5. Höglund M, Muren C, Engkvist O. Ultrasound characteristics of five common soft tissue tumors in the hand and forearm. Acta Radiol. 1997;38:348–54.
6. Peh WC, Truong NP, Totty WG, Gilula LA. Pictorial review: magnetic resonance imaging of benign soft tissue masses of the hand and wrist. Clin Radiol. 1995;50:519–25.
7. Valeyrie-Allanore L, Ismaïli N, Bastuji-Garin S, Zeller J, Wechsler J, Revuz J, Wolkenstein P. Symptoms associated with malignancy of peripheral nerve sheath tumours: a retrospective study of 69 patients with neurofibromatosis I. Br J Dermatol. 2005;153:79–82.
8. Russell SM. Preserve the nerve: microsurgical resection of peripheral nerve sheath tumors. Neurosurgery. 2007;61:113–7.
9. Flores LP, Carneiro JZ. Peripheral nerve compression secondary to adjacent lipomas. Surg Neurol. 2007;67:258–63.
10. Spinner RJ, Scheithauer BW, Amrami KK, Wenger DE, Hébert-Blouin MN. Adipose lesions of nerve: the need for a modified classification. J Neurosurg. 2012;116:418–31.
11. Al-Qattan MM. Lipfibromatous hamartoma of the median nerve and its associated conditions. J Hand Surg Br. 2001;26:368–72.
12. Al-Qattan MM, Al-Lazzan AM, Al Thunayan A, Al Namiah A, Mahmoud S, Hashem F, Tulbah A. Classification of benign fatty tumours of the upper limb. Hand Surg. 2005;10:43–59.
13. Oster LH, Blair WF, Steyers CM. Large lipomas in the deep palmar space. J Hand Surg. 1989;14A:700–4.
14. Amadio PC, Reiman HM, Dobyns JH. Lipofibromatous hamartoma of nerve. J Hand Surg Am. 1988;13:67–75.
15. Jung SN, Yim Y, Kwon H. Symmetric lipo bromatous hamartoma affecting digital nerves. Yonsei Med J. 2005;46:169–72.
16. Salon A, Guero S, Glicenstein J. Fibrolipoma of the median nerve. Review of 10 surgically treated cases with a mean re- call of 8 years. Ann Chir Main Memb Super. 1995;14:284–95.
17. Marom EM, Helms CA. Fibrolipomatous hamartoma: pathognomonic on MR imaging. Skelet Radiol. 1999;28:260–4.
18. Fleming AJ, Alpent M, Garcia A. Panosteal lipoma. AJR. 1962;87:1075–84.
19. Moon N, Manmor L. Parosteal lipoma of the proximal part of the radius: a clinical entity with frequent radial-nerve injury. J Bone Joint Surg Am. 1964;46A:608–14.
20. Murphey MD, Johnson DL, Bhatia PS, Neff JR, Rosenthal HG, Walker CW. Parosteal lipoma: MR imaging characteristics. AJR Am J Roentgenol. 1994;162:105–10.
21. Spinner RJ, Scheithauer BW, Amrami KK. The unifying articular (synovial) origin of intraneural ganglia: evolution-revelation-revolution. Neurosurgery. 2009;65A:115–24.
22. Desy NM, Wang H, Elshiekh MA, et al. Intraneural ganglion cysts: a systematic review and reinterpretation of the world's literature. J Neurosurg. 2016;125:615–30.
23. Spinner RJ, Atkinson JL, Scheithauer BW, et al. Peroneal intraneural ganglia: the importance of the articular branch. Clinical series. J Neurosurg. 2003;99:319–29.
24. Boursinos LA, Dimitriou CG. Ulnar nerve compression in the cubital tunnel by an epineural ganglion: a case report. Hand (NY). 2007;2:12–5.
25. Sharma RR, Pawar SJ, Delmendo A, Mahapatra AK. Symptomatic epineural ganglion cyst of the ulnar nerve in the cubital tunnel: a case report and brief review of the literature. J Clin Neurosci. 2000;7:542–3.

26. Spinner RJ, Vincent JF, Wolanskyj AP, Scheithauer BW. Intraneural ganglion cyst: a 200-year-old mystery solved. Clin Anat. 2008;21:611–8.
27. Beauchene M. Considerations sur l'organisation de l'oeil et sur l'operation de la cataracte appliquee au traitement des animaux domestiques/presentees et soutenues a la Faculte de medecine de Paris le 19 janvier 1809 par M. Beauchene fils. A Paris: de l'Imprimerie de Didot jeune, imprimeur, Theses Medecine 01311. 1809.
28. Chang WK, Li YP, Zhang DF, Liang BS. The cubital tunnel syndrome caused by the intraneural or extraneural ganglion cysts: case report and review of the literature. J Plast Reconstr Aesthet Surg. 2017;70:1404–8.
29. Wang B, Zhao Y, Lu A, Chen C. Ulnar nerve deep branch compression by a ganglion: a review of nine cases. Injury. 2014;45:1126–30.
30. Ishikawa H, Hirohata K. Posterior interosseous nerve syndrome associated with rheumatoid synovial cysts of the elbow joint. Clin Orthop Relat Res. 1990;254:134–9.
31. Malipeddi A, Reddy VR, Kallarackal G. Posterior interosseous nerve palsy: an unusual complication of rheumatoid arthritis: case report and review of the literature. Semin Arthritis Rheum. 2011;40:576–9.
32. Hsueh JH, Liu WC, Yang KC, Hsu KC, Lin CT, Chen LW. Spontaneous extensor tendon rupture in the rheumatoid wrist: risk factors and preventive role of extended tenosynovectomy. Ann Plast Surg. 2016;76(Suppl 1):S41–7.
33. White SH, Goodfellow JW, Mowat A. Posterior interosseous nerve palsy in rheumatoid arthritis. J Bone Joint Surg Br. 1988;70:468–71.
34. Westkaemper JG, Varitimidis SE, Sotereanos DG. Posterior in- terosseous nerve palsy in a patient with rheumatoid synovitis of the elbow: a case report and review of the literature. J Hand Surg Am. 1999;24:727–31.
35. Okada K, Miyake J, Kataoka T, Moritomo H, Murase T, Yoshikawa H. Median nerve neuropathy in the forearm due to recurrence of anterior wrist ganglion that originates from the scaphotrapezial joint: case report. J Brachial Plex Peripher Nerve Inj. 2012;7(1):1.
36. Kerrigan JJ, Bertoni JM, Jaeger SH. Ganglion cysts and carpal tunnel syndrome. J Hand Surg Am. 1988;13:763–5.
37. Johnson J, Kilgore E, Newmeyer W. Tumorous lesions of the hand. J Hand Surg Am. 1985;7:284–6.
38. Wright TW, Cooney WP, Ilstrup DM. Anterior wrist ganglion. J Hand Surg Am. 1994;7(6):954–8.
39. Momaya AM, Kwapisz A, Choate WS, Kissenberth MJ, Tolan SJ, Lonergan KT, Hawkins RJ, Tokish JM. Clinical outcomes of suprascapular nerve decompression: a systematic review. J Shoulder Elb Surg. 2018;27:172–80.
40. Memon M, Kay J, Ginsberg L, Simunovic N, Bak K, Lapner P, Ayeni OR. Arthroscopic management of suprascapular neuropathy of the shoulder improves pain and functional outcomes with minimal complication rates. Knee Surg Sports Traumatol Arthrosc. 2018;26:240–66.
41. Lagueny A, Julien J, Bullier R. De Quervain's tenosynovitis: a cause of compression of the superficial branch of the radial nerve. Nouv Press Med. 1981;10:2590.
42. Wasman JK, Willis J, Makley J, Abdul-Karim FW. Myositis ossificans-like lesion of nerve. Histopathology. 1997;30:75–8.
43. George DH, Scheithauer BW, Spinner RJ, et al. Heterotopic ossification of peripheral nerve ("neuritis ossificans"): report of two cases. Neurosurgery. 2002;51:244–6.
44. Kontogeorgakos VA, Papachristou DJ, Varitimidis S. Fibro-Osseous Pseudotumor of the hand. J Hand Surg Asian Pac Vol. 2016;21:269–72.
45. Wainapel SF, Rao PU, Schepsis AA. Ulnar nerve compression by heterotopic ossification in a head-injured patient. Arch Phys Med Rehabil. 1985;66:512–4.
46. Muzaffar N, Ahmad N, Bhat A, Shah N. Neuritis ossificans of the radial nerve. Orthopedics. 2012;35(4):589–91.
47. Vorenkamp SE, Nelson TL. Ulnar nerve entrapment due to heterotopic bone formation after a severe burn. J Hand Surg. 1987;12:378–80.
48. Spinner RJ, Scheithauer BW. Neuritis ossificans of the common peroneal nerve. Skelet Radiol. 2010;39:311–2.
49. Weiland TL, Scheithauer BW, Rock MG, Sargent JM. Inflammatory pseudotumor of nerve. Am J Surg Pathol. 1996;20:1212–8.
50. Beer T, Carr NJ, Weller RO. Inflammatory pseudotumor of peripheral nerve. Am J Surg Pathol. 1998;22:1035–6.
51. Perez-Lopez C, Gutierrez M, Isla A. Inflammatory pseudotumor of the median nerve. Case report and review of the literature. J Neurosurg. 2001;95:124–8.
52. Mauermann ML, Scheithauer BW, Spinner RJ, Amrami KK, Nance CS, Kline DG, O'Connor MI, Dyck PJ, Engelstad J, Dyck PJ. Inflammatory pseudotumor of nerve: clinicopathological characteristics and a potential therapy. J Peripher Nerv Syst. 2010;15(3):216–26.
53. Das Gupta TK, Brasfield RD, Strong EW, Hajdu SI. Benign solitary schwannomas (neurilemomas). Cancer. 1969;24:355–6.
54. Vlychou M, Dailiana ZH. Ancient schwannoma of the hand. J Hand Surg Am. 2011;36:2030–3.
55. Malizos K, Ioannou M, Kontogeorgakos V. Ancient schwannoma involving the median nerve: a case report and review of the literature. Strategies Trauma Limb Reconstr. 2013;8:63–6.
56. Ogose A, Hotta T, Morita T, Yamamura S, Hosaka N, Kobayashi H, Hirata Y. Tumors of peripheral nerves: correlation of symptoms, clinical signs, imaging features, and histologic diagnosis. Skelet Radiol. 1999;28:183–8.
57. Knight DM, Birch R, Pringle J. Benign solitary schwannomas: a review of 234 cases. J Bone Joint Surg Br. 2007;89:382–7.

58. Kang HJ, Shin SJ, Kang ES. Schwannomas of the upper extremity. J Hand Surg Br. 2000;25:604–7.
59. Young ED, Ingram D, Metcalf-Doetsch W, Khan D, et al. Clinicopathological variables of sporadic schwannomas of peripheral nerve in 291 patients and expression of biologically relevant markers. J Neurosurg. 2017;8:1–10.
60. Donner TR, Voorhies RM, Kline DG. Neural sheath tumors of major nerves. J Neurosurg. 1994;81:362–73.
61. Desta K, O'Shaughnessy M, Milling MA. Non-Hodgkin's lymphoma presenting as median nerve compression in the arm. J Hand Surg Br. 1994;19:289–91.
62. Kinoshita H, Yamakado H, Kitano T, Kitamura A, Yamashita H, Miyamoto M, Hitomi T, Okada T, Nakamoto Y, Sawamoto N, Takaori-Kondo A, Takahashi R. Diagnostic utility of FDG-PET in neurolymphomatosis: report of five cases. J Neurol. 2016;263:1719–26.
63. Baehring JM, Damek D, Martin EC, Betensky RA, Hochberg FH. Neurolymphomatosis. Neuro-Oncology. 2003;5:104–15.
64. Levin N, Soffer D, Grissaru S, Aizikovich N, Gomori JM, Siegal T. Primary T-cell CNS lymphoma presenting with leptomeningeal spread and neurolymphomatosis. J Neuro-Oncol. 2008;90:77–83.
65. Grisariu S, Avni B, Batchelor TT, van den Bent MJ, Bokstein F, Schiff D, et al. Neurolymphomatosis: an International Primary CNS Lymphoma Collaborative Group report. Blood. 2010;115:5005–11.
66. Foo TL, Yak R, Puhaindran ME. Peripheral nerve lymphomatosis. J Hand Surg Asian Pac Vol. 2017;22:104–7.
67. Capek S, Hébert-Blouin MN, Puffer RC, Martinoli C, Frick MA, Amrami KK, Spinner RJ. Tumefactive appearance of peripheral nerve involvement in hematologic malignancies: a New Imaging Association. Skelet Radiol. 2015;44:1001–9.
68. Matsumine A, Kusuzaki K, Hirata H, Fukutome K, Maeda M, Uchida A. Intraneural metastasis of a synovial sarcoma to a peripheral nerve. J Bone Joint Surg Br. 2005;87:1553–5.
69. Hirakawa H, Okajima S, Nagaoka T, Takamatsu T, Oyamada M. Loss and recovery of the blood-nerve barrier in the rat sciatic nerve after crush injury are associated with expression of intercellular junctional proteins. Exp Cell Res. 2003;284:196–210.
70. Meller I, Alkalay D, Mozes M, Geffen DB, Ferit T. Isolated metastases to peripheral nerves: report of five cases involving the brachial plexus. Cancer. 1995;76:1829–32.
71. Gwathmey KG. Plexus and peripheral nerve metastasis. Handb Clin Neurol. 2018;149:257–79.
72. Ramchandren S, Dalmau J. Metastases to the peripheral nervous system. J Neuro-Oncol. 2005;75:101–10.
73. Kori SH, Foley KM, Posner JB. Brachial plexus lesions in patients with cancer: 100 cases. Neurology. 1981;31:45–50.
74. Jaeckle KA. Plexopathies. In: Levin VA, editor. Cancer in the nervous system. 2nd ed. New York: Oxford University Press; 2002. p. 413–22.
75. Johansson S, Svensson H, Larsson LG, et al. Brachial plexopathy after postoperative radiotherapy of breast cancer patients – a long-term follow-up. Acta Oncol. 2000;39:373–82.
76. Jaeckle KA. Neurological manifestations of neoplastic and radiation-induced plexopathies. Semin Neurol. 2004;24:385–93.
77. Evans DG, Baser ME, McGaughran J, Sharif S, Howard E, Moran A. Malignant peripheral nerve sheath tumours in neurofibromatosis 1. J Med Genet. 2002;39:311–4.
78. Kim DH, Murovic JA, Tiel RL, Kline DG. Operative outcomes of 546 Louisiana State University Health Sciences Center peripheral nerve tumors. Neurosurg Clin N Am. 2004;15:177–92.
79. Ferner RE, Gutmann DH. International consensus statement on malignant peripheral nerve sheath tumors in neurofibromatosis. Cancer Res. 2002; 62:1573–7.
80. Cashen DV, Parisien RC, Raskin K, Hornicek FJ, Gebhardt MC, Mankin HJ. Survival data for patients with malignant schwannoma. Clin Orthop Relat Res. 2004;426:69–73.
81. Carli M, Ferrari A, Mattke A, Zanetti I, Casanova M, Bisogno G, Cecchetto G, Alaggio R, De Sio L, Koscielniak E, Sotti G, Treuner J. Pediatric malignant peripheral nerve sheath tumor: the Italian and German soft tissue sarcoma cooperative group. J Clin Oncol. 2005;23:8422–30.
82. Kroep JR, Ouali M, Gelderblom H, Le Cesne A, Dekker TJ, Van Glabbeke M, Hogendoorn PC, Hohenberger P. First- line chemotherapy for malignant peripheral nerve sheath tumor (MPNST) versus other histological soft tissue sarcoma subtypes and as a prognostic factor for MPNST: an EORTC soft tissue and bone sarcoma group study. Ann Oncol. 2011;22:207–14.
83. Coindre JM, Hostein I, Benhattar J, Lussan C, Rivel J, Guillou L. Malignant peripheral nerve sheath tumors are t(X;18)-negative sarcomas. Molecular analysis of 25 cases occurring in neurofibromatosis type 1 patients, using two different RT-PCR-based methods of detection. Mod Pathol. 2002;15:589–92.
84. Hashimoto K, Nishimura S, Fujii K, Kakinoki R, Akagi M. Intraneural synovial sarcoma of the tibial nerve. Rare Tumors. 2018;24:10.
85. Rinehart GC, Mustoe TA, Weeks PM. Management of synovial sarcoma of the median nerve at the elbow. Plast Reconstr Surg. 1989;83:528–32.
86. Scheithauer BW, Amrami KK, Folpe AL, Silva AI, Edgar MA, Woodruff JM, Levi AD, Spinner RJ. Synovial sarcoma of nerve. Hum Pathol. 2011;42:568–77.

11 Clinical Presentation and Diagnosis of Cubital Tunnel Syndrome

Claudius D. Jarrett

Introduction

Since the early description of Cubital tunnel syndrome, the diagnosis remains primarily based on the history of the present illness and the physical examination. Recent advances in research have provided additional information into demographic risk factors, occupational and recreational hazards, as well as subtleties in presentation that adds clarity in ones diagnosis. The physical examination can delve deep from the surface when provocative examination are utilized and weighted to their strengths. The value of imaging studies continues to evolve. Numerous studies have been performed to provide insight on the utility of elctrodiagnostic studies, ultrasound, and magnetic resonance images (MRIs). When used appropriately, these tools can supplement the surgeon's examination, treatment, as well as discussion of prognosis with patients. This chapter will discuss classic and novel aspects of the presentation and diagnosis of Cubital tunnel syndrome that the clinician can bring to their daily practice.

C. D. Jarrett (✉)
Division of Orthopaedic Surgery, Wilmington Health Associates, Wilmington, NC, USA

Presentation

Patients with Cubital tunnel syndrome classically present with painful paresthesias radiating from the medial elbow down the forearm into the ulnar one and a half digits. A substantial portion of patients may also describe weakness in their grip strength. Some may complain of their small finger getting caught while attempting to place their hand in their pants pocket. The length of symptoms can range from weeks to years. Clarifying whether a patient's symptoms are constant or intermittent is an important aspect of the history [1]. Intermittent symptoms can be a sign of transient nerve ischemia that can help guide type and prognosis of treatment. At times, patients will present with purely motor complaints of hand weakness, loss of dexterity, and subtle ulnar sided digital clawing deformity. This unique patient population presents an ominous prognostic dilemma, as intrinsic muscle atrophy can be rather severe without any antecedent sensory complaints.

One should inquire about specific occupational demands and recreational activities. Repetitive or protracted elbow hyperflexion, whether performed at work or in the gym, can be associated with exacerbation of symptoms. Some patients also report prolonged use of vibratory tools at work. Occasionally, patients may describe an antecedent traumatic event to the medial elbow as well.

D. G. Sotereanos, L. K. Papatheodorou (eds.), *Compressive Neuropathies of the Upper Extremity*,
https://doi.org/10.1007/978-3-030-37289-7_11

Nighttime symptoms are common. The clinician should ask about positional sleeping habits. Typically, paresthesias are more prominent at night, as a result of unintentional elbow flexion, but can progress resulting in dense daytime numbness. Exacerbating factors can include elevated cellphone use, prolonged driving, and reading. Some may describe worsening symptoms with weight lifting such as overhead triceps extensions, closed fist bench press, and triceps pull-down.

Physical Examination

The physical exam should begin with assessing the overall appearance of symptomatic arm. The clinician should observe how the patient moves and uses the arm during conversation, writing, shaking hands, as well as the normal resting position and tone. One should assess for the presence of muscle atrophy in comparison to the contralateral arm. The presence of intrinsic muscle atrophy should be noted as it likely reveals a more advanced form of the disease process (Fig. 11.1). The clinician should evaluate for masses, swelling, wounds, and/or prior incisions. One should document the range of both active and passive motion in the shoulders, elbows, wrists, and hands. Motor function should be assessed by grading resisted digital flexion as well as intrinsic strength. In comparison to the intrinsic muscles, the fascicles innervating the flexor digitorum profundus to the ring and small fingers are more centrally located within the ulnar nerve and unlikely to be involved until the later stages of the disease process. Sensory testing should be performed, at the minimum, by assessing light touch as well as both static and dynamic two-point discrimination. During early stages of neuropathy, the Semmes Weinstein monofilament test and vibratory testing can be effective in detecting sensory impairment. Alternation of normal sensation along the dorsal ulnar hand (i.e. dorsal sensory branch of the ulnar nerve) can help distinguish between pathologic ulnar nerve compression at the elbow versus at the wrist. Additionally, ulnar nerve compression at the wrist typically does not lead to weakness of the ring and small finger flexor digitorum profundus. Digital perfusion and distal pulses should also be evaluated. Evidence of perfusion abnormalities (i.e. loss of radial pulse) may hint towards a different etiology such as thoracic outlet syndrome.

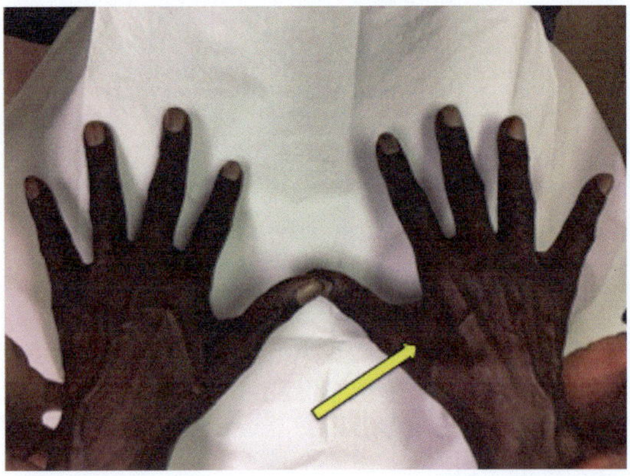

Fig. 11.1 Patient with advanced Cubital tunnel syndrome with evidence of intrinsic atrophy (arrow)

The presence of Wartenberg and/or Froment sign also correlates with motor weakness in patients with Cubital tunnel syndrome. Wartenberg sign occurs when the patient is unable to fully adduct the small finger secondary to the weakened interosseous muscles and the overpowering pull of the small finger extensors (Fig. 11.2a). Froment sign results secondary to weakness of the intrinsic muscle adductor pollicis. The sign is positive when a patient is unable to hold a piece of paper between the thumb and index finger without flexing the thumb at the interphalangeal joint (Fig. 11.2b).

Several provocative maneuvers remain the core of the physical examination and allow distinguishing Cubital tunnel syndrome from other sites of nerve compression (i.e. C8 radiculopathy) [2] (Table 11.1). A Tinel's test, direct compression test, or placement of the elbow in a position of hyperflexion test (i.e. elbow flexion test) may all reproduce the patient's symptoms. The Tinel's test is performed by repeatedly tapping or percussing over the Cubital tunnel. The direct compression test is executed simply applying direct continuous pressure over the Cubital tunnel. The elbow flexion test is completed by

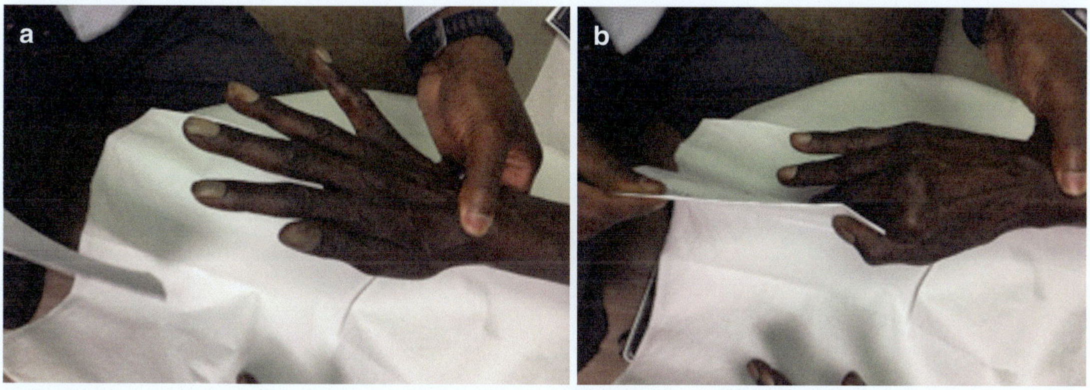

Fig. 11.2 (**a**) Patient with a positive Wartenberg's sign. He is unable to fully adduct the small finger secondary to the weakened interosseous muscles and the overpowering pull of the small finger extensors. (**b**) Patient with a positive Froment's sign. He is unable to hold a piece of paper between the thumb and index finger without flexing the thumb at the interphalangeal joint

Table 11.1 Reported sensitivity and specificity of commonly applied provocative maneuvers for Cubital tunnel syndrome

Name	Examination maneuver	Sensitivity/ specificity
Tinel's	4–6 taps on the ulnar nerve just proximal to the cubital tunnel	70%/98% [3]
Elbow Flexion	Elbow placed in maximum flexion with forearm supinated and wrist in neutral	75%/99% [3]
Direct Pressure	Place index and middle finger directly on subject's ulnar nerve proximal to cubital tunnel with elbow in 90° of flexion	89%/98% [3]
Combined Elbow flexion – Direct Pressure	Elbow placed in maximum flexion while directly pressing on ulnar nerve just proximal to cubital tunnel	98%/95% [3]
Elbow flexion-shoulder abduction/internal rotation	Elbow in hyperflexion with shoulder abducted to 90° and in maximum internal rotation	58%/100% [4, 5]
Modified elbow flexion-shoulder abduction/internal rotation	Elbow in hyperflexion, shoulder abducted to 90° and internally rotated, forearm supinated, and wrist extended	87%/98% [4, 5]

The sensitivity and specificity may vary based on length of duration of exam [3–5]

passively flexing the elbow to the maximum angle for 1–3 min. The sensitivity and specificity of these tests do vary in the literature (Table 11.1) [3–5]. The clinician should remain cognizant of the varying rates of false positives for these tests published in the literature. The author recommends limiting the duration of provocation to no more than 1 min as longer time periods may lead to positive findings in asymptomatic controls [3, 6–9]. Rayan et al and Kuschner et al reported a positive percussion test in approximately 24% and 34% of normal volunteers, respectively [6, 7]. Combining or slightly modifying these exams may increase their sensitivity and specificity (Fig. 11.3a, b). A combination of the elbow flexion test with the direct pressure while adding additional tension to the ulnar nerve by shoulder abduction/internal rotation, forearm supination, and wrist extension has been found by investigators to do such that. By doing this, Ochi and colleagues increased the sensitivity and specificity of the elbow flexion test to 85% and 98%, respectively [5]. However, one must be aware that these additions may also increase the false-positive results of the provocative maneuver.

The scratch collapse test is another described provocative maneuver for Cubital tunnel syndrome. The exam is done by first placing the patient's flexed elbow at their side and acquiring a baseline their shoulder external rotation strength. Next, the clinician lightly scratches over the Cubital tunnel then re-evaluates the patient's

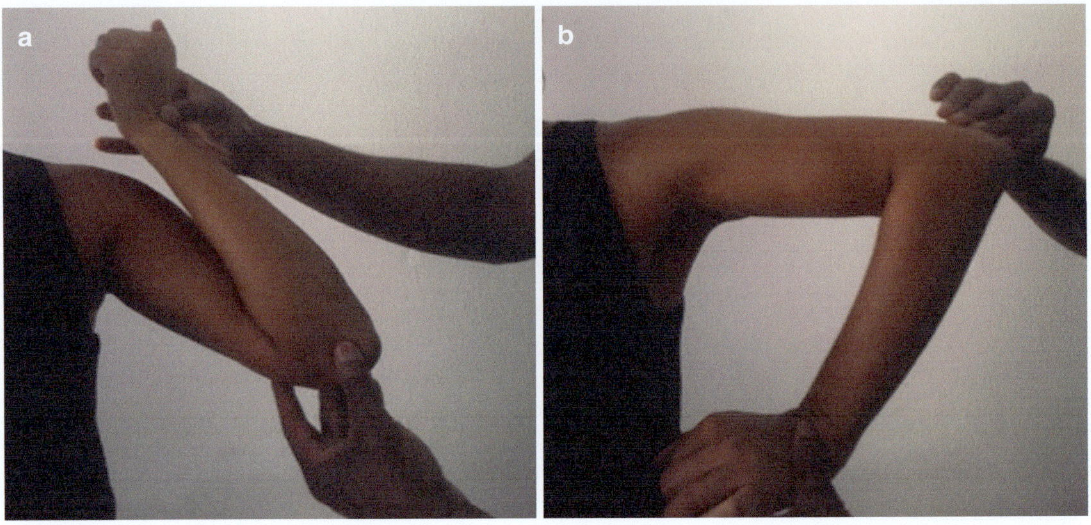

Fig. 11.3 (**a**) Example of the combined elbow flexion and direct pressure test (**b**) Example of modified elbow flexion test including shoulder internal rotation, elbow flexion, wrist extension, and direct pressure test

shoulder external rotation strength. In patients with Cubital tunnel syndrome, a positive test will produce temporary diminished shoulder external rotation strength. Investigators have reported a 69% sensitivity and 99% specificity for Cubital tunnel syndrome [8].

The ulnar nerve should also be assessed for stability. This can be assessed by placing one or two fingers on the medial epicondyle and taking the elbow from full extension to full flexion. The ulnar nerve will slide underneath ones fingers if unstable. This assessment should be performed on both sides as up to approximately a third of patients have physiologic subluxation on exam [6, 10, 11].

The physical exam should be completed by full examination of cervical spine and shoulder girdle to rule out other potential sites of nerve compression or injury.

Classification

Cubital tunnel syndrome is commonly categorized based on the physical examination by the McGowan classification system [12]. Patients with McGowan Grade I Cubital tunnel syndrome present with sensory changes but no objective motor weakness on exam. Grade II is delineated by the presence of motor weakness. Patients are considered Grade IIa if the motor weakness is mild and Grade IIb if moderate (i.e. 3 out of 5). Patients with McGowan Grade III present with profound motor weakness and intrinsic atrophy upon examination. Dellon later modified the McGowan classification to include the severity of sensory changes [13]. Based on the Dellon modification, patients with mild Cubital tunnel syndrome have intermittent paresthesias. Moderate Cubital tunnel syndrome results in a decrease to vibratory sensation on exam. Severe Cubital tunnel syndrome is marked by abnormal two-point discrimination.

Electrodiagnostic Studies

Electrodiagnostic studies continue to be used as a supplemental tool to confirm the diagnosis of Cubital tunnel syndrome [1]. However, innate limitations including patient discomfort, precise localization, detection of structural abnormalities, as well as risk of false-negatives prevent it broad utilization [14–16]. Current criteria used to confirm pathologic nerve conduction at the elbow include a ulnar nerve conduction velocity <50 m/s, a 10-m/s difference from the contralateral side, and/or a 20% reduction in amplitude in comparison to the contralateral side [1, 17]. Electrodiagnostic testing can reliably confirm abnormal nerve conduction in patients with moderate to severe (e.g. McGowan II or III) Cubital tunnel syndrome. However, these tests can be unpredictable in patients with mild disease (e.g. McGowan I) [15, 18]. Hence, the results of electrodiagnostic testing should not take precedence over ones history and physical examination.

Imaging

Plain Radiographs

The acquisition of plain radiographs should not be routine but dictated by history, examination, and planned surgical approach. A history of trauma, limited elbow range of motion, an abnormal carrying angle, and/or presence of elbow swelling are just some of the clinical findings that warrant acquisition of plain x-rays of the elbow. Three views of the elbow (anteroposterior [AP], oblique, and lateral) are typically sufficient. When surgical intervention is anticipated, preoperative radiographs should be acquired to evaluate the bony anatomy, alignment, presence or absence of arthritis, post-traumatic changes, and articular congruency.

Ultrasound

The exact role of ultrasonography for the diagnosis of ulnar neuropathy at the elbow continues to be refined [19]. Technological advances have allowed for improved the visualization of structural abnormalities. The inexpensive nature and ability to perform dynamic evaluation are some of its unique touted advantages. However, consistent correlation with clinically significant disease remains variable [14, 20–22]. This may be in part secondary to the technician dependency of the study. Most ultrasound studies provide estimates on the appearance and size of the ulnar nerve in and around the Cubital tunnel. The cross sectional area (CSA) and largest diameter on transverse scans are frequently doc-

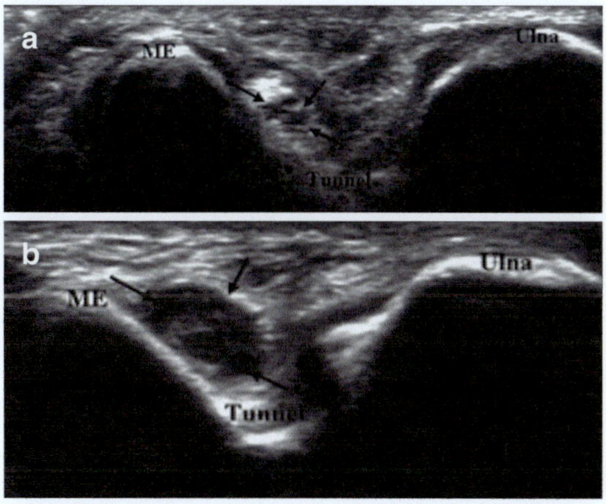

Fig. 11.4 (**a**) Ultrasound of the elbow in an asymptomatic volunteer with an ulnar nerve cross-sectional area of 0.08 cm^2. The cross-section of the ulnar nerve is depicted by arrows outlining its periphery. ME, medial epicondyle; Tunnel, ulnar tunnel. (**b**) Ultrasound of the elbow in a patient with Cubital tunnel syndrome with an ulnar nerve cross-sectional area of 0.29 cm^2. Similarly, the cross-section of the ulnar nerve is depicted by arrows outlining its periphery. (From Wiesler et al. [19] with permission)

umented exam findings (Fig. 11.4a, b) [14, 19, 23–25]. Substantial nerve enlargement on ultrasound has been shown to coincide with electrodiagnostic studies and clinical symptoms by some investigators [25, 26]. Volpe et al prospectively compared the CSA and electrodiagnostic studies in 50 elbows with Cubital tunnel syndrome to 50 controls. The authors reported an 88% sensivity and specificity for diagnosing electrodiagnostic confirmed Cubital tunnel syndrome using ultrasound when using a cut-off of $\geq$10 mm^2 CSA [27]. However, there remains no standard guideline on what is considered significant enlargement and the ideal location to measure it [14, 21–25].

MRI

Magnetic resonance imaging (MRI) continues to be investigated as a potentially attractive noninvasive alternative to assist in the diagnosis of Cubital tunnel syndrome. The improved resolution of modern 3 Tesla scans allows a clearer detection of morphological changes of the ulnar nerve. The technique for acquisition of the MRI should be performed with care. The elbow ought be held in extension during the scan, and the ulnar nerve should be to be aligned within 10^0 relative to the direction of the main magnetic field B_0. This precaution minimizes the artificial contribution to the T2 signal by the magic angle effect [28, 29]. On MRI scans, the ulnar nerve is most visibly seen on axial slices posterior to the medial epicondyle. A normal nerve should appear as a round hypointense structure surrounded by fat [30]. Increased signal of as well as increase in caliber of the ulnar nerve within the Cubital tunnel on T2-weighted or Diffusion weighted images can correlate with clinical diagnosis and electrophysiological testing [30–34]. The longitudinal extension of the increased signal as seen on several axial slices proximally and distally improves the clinical relevance. Altun and colleagues compared traditional MRI scans and diffusion weighted – MRI scans in patients with 24 symptomatic elbows with 26 controls. Electrophysiological testing and clinical criteria for the diagnosis for Cubital tunnel syndrome were used to assess both cohorts. All 24 elbows with Cubital tunnel syndrome had increased pathologic signaling on diffusion-weighted imaging and 20 of the 24 elbows had increased signal on T2-weighted imaging. None of the controls had pathologic signaling on their MRI scans [33]. In a similar study, Iba et al compared traditional MRI scans and diffusion weighted – MRI scans in 11 elbows with clinically diagnosed Cubital tunnel syndrome to 6 normal controls. Again, none of the normal elbows were found to have pathologic signally within the ulnar nerve. Diffusion-weighted MRI revealed positive signals in all 11 elbows and T2-weighted imaging revealed high signal intensity in 8 of the 11 elbows [32]. However, caution must remain on relying to heavily on imaging alone. Others have reported up to 60% of asymptomatic elbows may how increased signal on MRI [35].

Conclusion

The diagnosis of Cubital tunnel syndrome will continue to heavily rely on a thorough inquiry and a detailed physical examination. Secondary to varieties in presentation, the diagnosis can be difficult to confirm. An array of provocative maneuvers arms the clinician with several ways to clarify the diagnosis. Advances in electrodiagnostic studies and imaging can provide supplemental tools for selective patients. An appreciation of the important aspects of the history of the presenting illness as well as a firm grasp on the physical examination will continue to direct timely diagnosis, prognosis, and treatment of Cubital tunnel syndrome.

References

1. Palmer BA, Hughes TB. Cubital tunnel syndrome. J Hand Surg WB Saunders. 2010;35(1):153–63.
2. Jarrett CD, Papatheodorou LK, Sotereanos DG. Cubital tunnel syndrome. Instr Course Lect. 2017;66:91–101.
3. Novak CB, Lee GW, Mackinnon SE, Lay L. Provocative testing for cubital tunnel syndrome. J Hand Surg Elsevier. 1994;19(5):817–20.
4. Ochi K, Horiuchi Y, Tanabe A, Morita K, Takeda K, Ninomiya K. Comparison of shoulder internal rotation test with the elbow flexion test in the diagnosis of cubital tunnel syndrome. J Hand Surg Am. 2011;36(5):782–7.
5. Ochi K, Horiuchi Y, Tanabe A, Waseda M, Kaneko Y, Koyanagi T. Shoulder internal rotation elbow flexion test for diagnosing cubital tunnel syndrome. J Shoulder Elb Surg. 2012;21(6):777–81.
6. Rayan GM, Jensen C, Duke J. Elbow flexion test in the normal population. J Hand Surg. 1992;17(1):86–9.
7. Kuschner SH, Ebramzadeh E, Mitchell S. Evaluation of elbow flexion and linel tests for cubital tunnel syndrome in asymptomatic individuals. Orthopedics. 2006;29(4):305–8.
8. Cheng CJ, Mackinnon-Patterson B, Beck JL, Mackinnon SE. Scratch collapse test for evaluation of carpal and cubital tunnel syndrome. J Hand Surg Am. 2008;33(9):1518–24.
9. Beekman R, Schreuder AHCML, Rozeman CAM, Koehler PJ, Uitdehaag BMJ. The diagnostic value of provocative clinical tests in ulnar neuropathy at the elbow is marginal. J Neurol Neurosurg Psychiatry BMJ Publishing Group Ltd. 2009;80(12):1369–74.
10. Childress HM. Recurrent ulnar-nerve dislocation at the elbow. Clin Orthop Relat Res. 1975;108:168–73.
11. Calfee RP, Manske PR, Gelberman RH, Van Steyn MO, Steffen J, Goldfarb CA. Clinical assessment of the ulnar nerve at the elbow: reliability of instability testing and the association of hypermobility with clinical symptoms. J Bone Joint Surg Am Journal of Bone and Joint Surgery, Inc. 2010;92(17):2801–8.
12. McGOWAN AJ. The results of transposition of the ulnar nerve for traumatic ulnar neuritis. J Bone Joint Surg Br. 1950;32-B(3):293–301.

13. Dellon AL. Review of treatment results for ulnar nerve entrapment at the elbow. J Hand Surg. 1989;14(4):688–700.
14. Cho C-H, Lee Y-H, Song K-S, Lee K-J, Lee S-W, Lee S-M. Accuracy of preoperative ultrasonography for cubital tunnel syndrome: a comparison with intraoperative findings. Clin Orthop Surg. 2018;10(3):352–7.
15. Greenwald D, Blum LCI, Adams D, Mercantonio C, Moffit M, Cooper B. Effective surgical treatment of cubital tunnel syndrome based on provocative clinical testing without electrodiagnostics. Plast Reconstr Surg. 2006;117(5):87e–91e.
16. Yoon JS, Walker FO, Cartwright MS. Ulnar neuropathy with normal electrodiagnosis and abnormal nerve ultrasound. Arch Phys Med Rehabil WB Saunders. 2010;91(2):318–20.
17. Hutchison RL, Rayan G. Diagnosis of cubital tunnel syndrome. J Hand Surg Elsevier. 2011;36(9):1519–21.
18. Tomaino MM, Brach PJ, Vansickle DP. The rationale for and efficacy of surgical intervention for electrodiagnostic-negative cubital tunnel syndrome. J Hand Surg W.B. Saunders. 2001;26(6):1077–81.
19. Wiesler ER, Chloros GD, Cartwright MS, Shin HW, Walker FO. Ultrasound in the diagnosis of ulnar neuropathy at the cubital tunnel. J Hand Surg. 2006;31(7):1088–93.
20. Beekman R, Visser LH, Verhagen WI. Ultrasonography in ulnar neuropathy at the elbow: a critical review. Muscle Nerve Wiley-Blackwell. 2011;43(5):627–35.
21. Mondelli M, Filippou G, Frediani B, Aretini A. Ultrasonography in ulnar neuropathy at the elbow: relationships to clinical and electrophysiological findings. Neurophysiol Clin. 2008;38(4):217–26.
22. Gruber H, Glodny B, Peer S. The validity of ultrasonographic assessment in cubital tunnel syndrome: the value of a cubital-to-humeral nerve area ratio (CHR) combined with morphologic features. Ultrasound Med Biol. 2010;36(3):376–82.
23. Bayrak AO, Bayrak IK, Turker H, Elmali M, Nural MS. Ultrasonography in patients with ulnar neuropathy at the elbow: comparison of cross-sectional area and swelling ratio with electrophysiological severity. Muscle Nerve Wiley-Blackwell. 2010;41(5):661–6.
24. Ozturk E, Sonmez G, Çolak A, Sildiroglu HO, Mutlu H, Senol MG, et al. Sonographic appearances of the normal ulnar nerve in the cubital tunnel. J Clin Ultrasound. 2008;36(6):325–9.
25. Yoon JS, Hong S-J, Kim B-J, Kim SJ, Kim JM, Walker FO, et al. Ulnar nerve and cubital tunnel ultrasound in ulnar neuropathy at the elbow. Arch Phys Med Rehabil. 2008;89(5):887–9.
26. Zhong W, Zhang W, Zheng X, Li S, Shi J. The high-resolution ultrasonography and electrophysiological studies in nerve decompression for ulnar nerve entrapment at the elbow. J Reconstr Microsurg Thieme Medical Publishers. 2012;28(5):345–8.
27. Volpe A, Rossato G, Bottanelli M, Marchetta A, Caramaschi P, Bambara LM, et al. Ultrasound evaluation of ulnar neuropathy at the elbow: correlation with electrophysiological studies. Rheumatology (Oxford) Oxford University Press. 2009;48(9):1098–101.
28. Chappell KE, Robson MD, Stonebridge-Foster A, Glover A, Allsop JM, Williams AD, et al. Magic angle effects in MR neurography. AJNR Am J Neuroradiol. 2004;25(3):431–40.
29. Kästel T, Heiland S, Bäumer P, Bartsch AJ, Bendszus M, Pham M. Magic angle effect: a relevant artifact in MR neurography at 3T? AJNR Am J Neuroradiol. 2011;32(5):821–7.
30. Andreisek G, Crook DW, Burg D, Marincek B, Weishaupt D. Peripheral neuropathies of the median, radial, and ulnar nerves: MR imaging features. Radiographics. 2006;26(5):1267–87.
31. Bäumer P, Dombert T, Staub F, Kaestel T, Bartsch AJ, Heiland S, et al. Ulnar neuropathy at the elbow: MR neurography—Nerve T2 signal increase and caliber. Radiology Radiological Society of North America, Inc. 2011;260(1):199–206.
32. Iba K, Wada T, Tamakawa M, Aoki M, Yamashita T. Diffusion-weighted magnetic resonance imaging of the ulnar nerve in cubital tunnel syndrome. Hand Surg World Scientific Publishing Company. 2010;15(1):11–5.
33. Altun Y, Aygun MS, Cevik MU, Acar A, Varol S, Arıkanoglu A, et al. Relation between electrophysiological findings and diffusion weighted magnetic resonance imaging in ulnar neuropathy at the elbow. J Neuroradiol Elsevier Masson. 2013;40(4):260–6.
34. Breitenseher JB, Kranz G, Hold A, Berzaczy D, Nemec SF, Sycha T, et al. MR neurography of ulnar nerve entrapment at the cubital tunnel: a diffusion tensor imaging study. Eur Radiol Springer Berlin Heidelberg. 2015;25(7):1911–8.
35. Husarik DB, Saupe N, Pfirrmann CWA, Jost B, Hodler J, Zanetti M. Elbow nerves: MR findings in 60 asymptomatic subjects—Normal anatomy, variants, and pitfalls. Radiology Radiological Society of North America. 2009;252(1):148–56.

In Situ Decompression of Cubital Tunnel

12

Thomas Hughes

Introduction

Entrapment of the ulnar nerve is the second most common compression neuropathy in the upper extremity after carpal tunnel syndrome [1, 2]. The most common site of compression is at the elbow, although compression at Guyon's canal must always be considered as a potential cause for the patient's symptoms. A thorough knowledge of the anatomy of the ulnar nerve can assist with diagnosis and guide treatment. Patients often present with paresthesias in the ulnar nerve distribution and weakness or atrophy of the intrinsic musculature of the hand. Pain is usually not the predominant feature early in the development of ulnar nerve symptoms. Various surgical techniques for decompression of the ulnar nerve have been described in the literature and a definitive "gold standard" does not exist. A thorough understanding of the pathology of cubital tunnel syndrome will help guide treatment and lead to successful outcomes.

T. Hughes (✉)
Department of Orthopaedic Surgery, UPMC Passavant Hospital, University of Pittsburgh, Pittsburgh, PA, USA
e-mail: hughestb2@upmc.edu

Operative Treatment

Surgical treatment of cubital tunnel syndrome is indicated with motor weakness or when conservative measures have failed [3]. Even prior to weakness, constant numbness may be an indication for surgical intervention. It is not uncommon for patients with constant numbness to have persistent symptoms after decompression, and so it may be helpful to decompress the nerve earlier in the course of the disease. A discussion should be had pre-operatively with patients regarding the expectations of surgical intervention. In patients that have intermittent symptoms, rapid, or immediate, resolution of symptoms may follow surgical decompression. With constant numbness (usually accompanied by intermittent or positional dysesthesias) and weakness, there may be an initial improvement from decompression, but it is not typically complete. It can take many months for the symptoms to improve and final outcomes from the surgery may not be noted for over a year. Patients should be made aware of this, as it certainly improves patient satisfaction when there is a complete understanding of the objectives and expectations of the procedure.

A valuable tool in assessing the patient's degree of numbness is the use of Semmes-Weinstein monofilament examination pre-operatively [4, 5]. Obtaining an objective measure of numbness can be very valuable in helping patients appreciate the improvements they obtain

D. G. Sotereanos, L. K. Papatheodorou (eds.), *Compressive Neuropathies of the Upper Extremity*,
https://doi.org/10.1007/978-3-030-37289-7_12

through surgical intervention. When patients present with intrinsic wasting and dense numbness, the improvement post-operative is incredibly slow. This ability to demonstrate an improvement in the monofilament exam can help to demonstrate complete decompression and validate the decision to proceed with surgery. It can also be very encouraging to patients to see these improvements over time.

When surgical treatment has been decided upon, there are multiple techniques available. These include in situ decompression, transposition, and medial epicondylectomy. In cases of transposition, the nerve can be placed subcutaneously, intramuscularly, and sub-muscularly. In situ decompression can be performed in an open or endoscopic fashion. There is ongoing controversy as to which is the optimal surgical treatment of this nerve entrapment [6–15].

In Situ Decompression

In situ decompression has been proposed by various authors as a treatment for cubital tunnel syndrome [5, 16–20]. For in situ decompression, a skin incision is made along the course of the ulnar nerve between the medial epicondyle and the olecranon. The length of the incision can be made to the surgeon's preference. The author prefers a small incision through which a complete decompression can be performed. The skin incision is used as a mobile window to visualize the cubital tunnel along the entire course of the ulnar nerve (Fig. 12.1). Through a 3 cm incision, the nerve can be decompressed along an 11–12 cm interval. Dissection is taken through the subcutaneous tissues to the fascia. The author prefers to identify the ulnar nerve by making a small opening into Osborne's ligament to confirm the nerve's location.

Once the nerve is identified, the tunnel is not opened yet, but the subcutaneous tissues are dissected proximally and distally along the course of the nerve beneath the skin. The subcutaneous dissection is performed directly on the fascia of Osborne's ligament enclosing the nerve, so that any superficial nerve branches are lifted up directly with the subcutaneous fat. The long end of an Army-Navy retractor is placed first distally, then proximally. This pulls the skin window along the course through which the nerve is to be decompressed. When the retractor is placed proximally, there is a coronal fascial band that may push the retractor anterior or posterior to the course of the nerve. This is an extension of the medial intermuscular septum (from the septum to the skin) and should be disrupted through blunt dissection so that the retractor can be maintained directly over the course of the nerve.

The advantages to this small incision are more than just cosmetic. Any branches of the medial antebrachial cutaneous nerve (MABC) will be in the subcutaneous fat between the skin and the fascia (Fig. 12.2) [21]. These are lifted from the fascia with this small incision technique. Lifting them in this way precludes the skeletalization that is required to protect them if a longer incision is used. There is also less skin scar to remain tender after surgery, although it is worth mentioning to patients that they will be sore over an area much longer then the skin incision itself. Additionally, there is no scarring between the skin and the MABC branches, as this plane is never developed.

Osborne's ligament is released directly over the nerve. Most authors suggest release the nerve as dorsally as possible to avoid subluxation of the ulnar nerve after decompression. The nerve always lies directly posterior to the medial epicondyle, except in cases of subluxation, where it may lie upon the medial epicondyle. It can typically be palpated by running a finger over the nerve and feeling the nerve structure roll under the finger. There is a tendency in larger elbows for surgeons to drift posteriorly, mistaking the edge of the triceps fascia for the ulnar nerve. By frequent re-orientation to the medial epicondyle, this error can be avoided, and the nerve found efficiently. Once the nerve is palpated, the fascia must be entered. One technique for this is to carefully grasp the fascia with and Adson toothed forceps, taking care not to grasp the nerve at the same time. The fascia is pulled taught and the tip of a tenotomy scissor is carefully plunged into the fascia, taking care not to plunge into the nerve

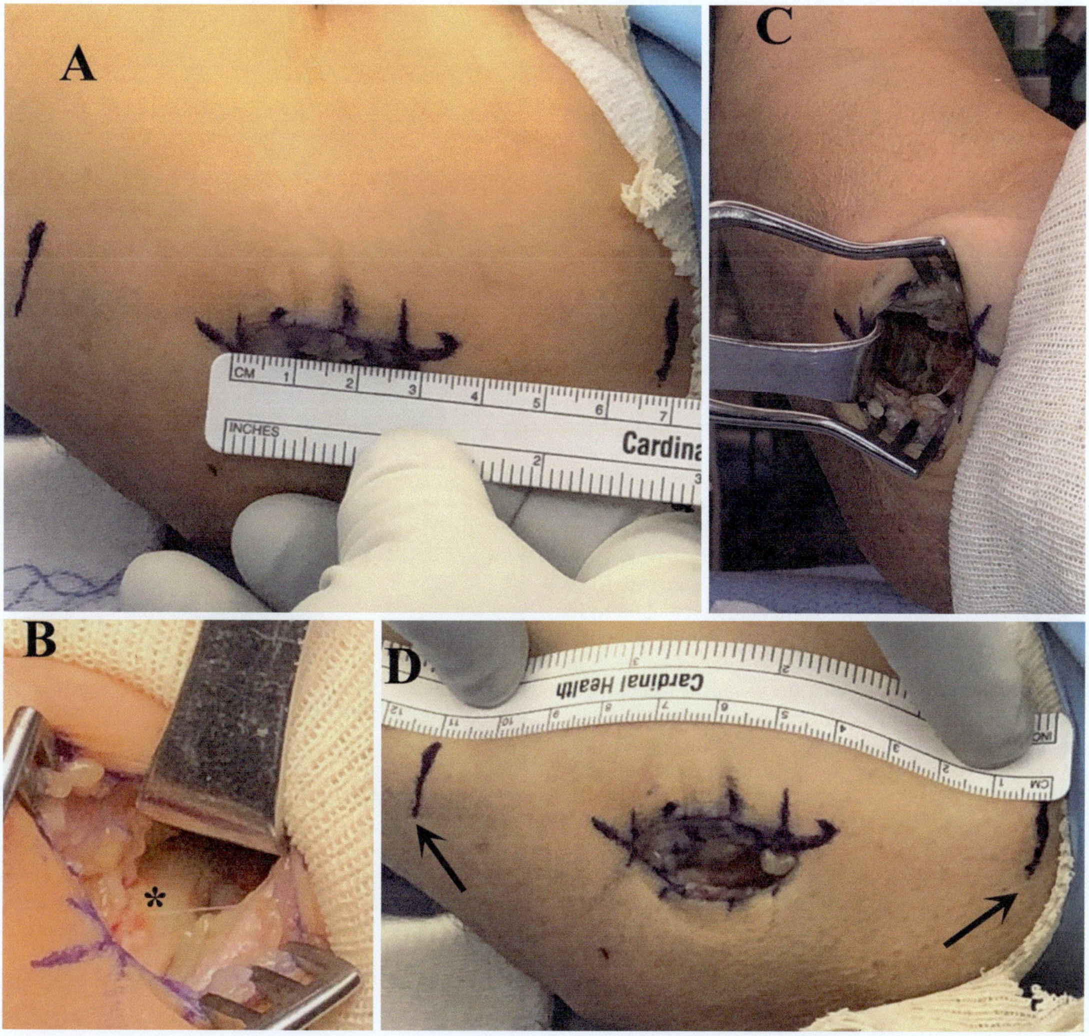

Fig. 12.1 An *in situ* nerve decompression performed through a small incision. (**a**) While an approximately 5 cm incision line is marked, only a 3 cm incision was used in this case. (**b**) The longer end of an army-navy retractor is placed just above the fascia containing the cubital tunnel. In this image, the ulnar nerve (asterisk) can be seen to have been decompressed at the cubital tunnel and under the retractor. (**c**) The retractor is the placed distally, superficial to the FCU. In this image, the superficial fascia of the FCU has been released, but the deep fascia has yet to be released. (**d**) The blue lines proximal and distal to the incision (marked with an arrow) were drawn at the proximal and distal edge of the retractor. The nerve was decompressed at least to that level

(Fig. 12.3). Alternatively, the fascia can be spread, but care must be taken when spreading not to place undue stretch upon the nerve.

Next, the Flexor Carpi Ulnaris (FCU) is identified just distal to Osborne's ligament. The superficial fascia can be released initially by small cuts, but then eventually by sliding the scissors along the fascia. This slide technique becomes safe once there is a layer of muscle between the superficial and deep fascia. This muscle layer protects the nerve from injury when sliding the scissors. The muscle is bluntly separated. The deep fascia is then released. In contrast to the superficial fascia, the scissors should not be slid along this fascial layer. Rather, the fascia should be carefully separated from the nerve and cut in small segments. Wide spreads deep to this fascia should also be avoided, as this will

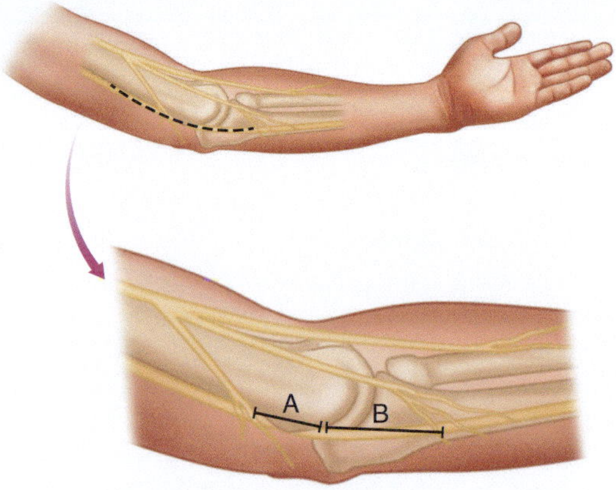

Fig. 12.2 Branches of the medial antebrachial cutaneous nerve (MABC) cross from anterior to posterior in the region of ulnar nerve decompression surgery. Proximal crossing branches (**a**) were identified in 61% of cases, while distal crossing branches (**b**) were found in 100%. The average distance from the medial epicondyle to the proximal branches (**a**) was 1.8 cm and to the distal branches was 3.1 cm. Note that the interval between the two points (**a** and **b**) is similar to the small incision proposed by the author. By lifting the subcutaneous tissues with an Army-Navy retractor, most branches of the MABC can be avoided entirely. Certainly, when developing the subcutaneous window, branches of the MABC may still be present and must be identified. (Lowe et al. [21]; with permission)

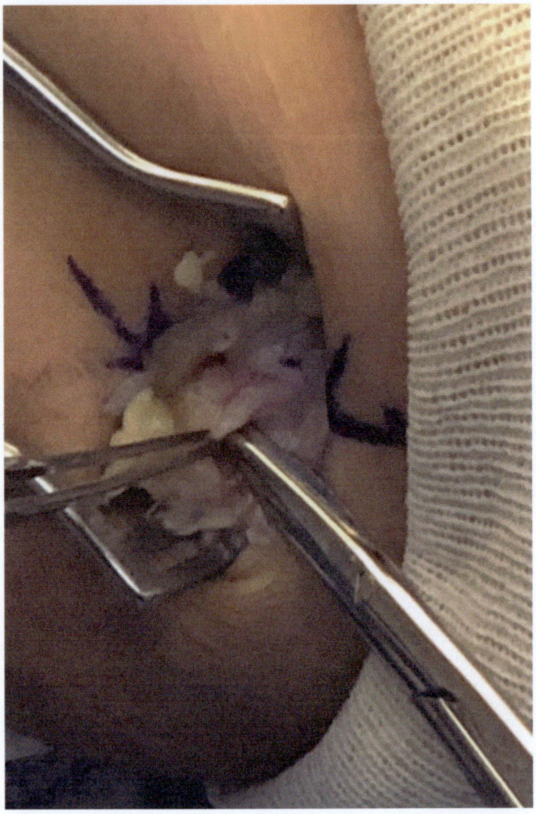

Fig. 12.3 To enter the cubital tunnel with less trauma to the nerve, the following technique can be used. The fascia overlying the nerve is grasped with an Adson forceps. Care is taken not to grab the epineurium. Once tension is applied to the fascia, the tip of a tenotomy is "poked" into the cubital tunnel. Care should be taken not to plunge into the nerve, but it is a reasonable forceful push to enter the fascia

frequently put excessive pressure on the nerve, which is made evident by stimulation of the motor branch and twitching the of the hand distally. As the dissection proceeds distally, the motor branch will frequently be identified. While the surgeon should be careful and aware of its presence, in most cases of in situ decompression, identification is not necessary. If a decision is later made to transpose the nerve, the motor branch may need to be identified and freed from surrounding tissues in order to aid in transposition.

Following the distal dissection, the nerve is followed proximally. It is traced along the intramuscular septum. To gain visualization through a small incision, it may be necessary to almost lift the arm with the army-navy retractor. This both retracts the skin window vigorously, but also aligns the subcutaneous tunnel that is formed with the surgeon's eyes and scissors. Seven-inch scissors and Debakey, or some other longer forceps, may be needed to reach into this tunnel to help manipulate the soft tissues. Again, the fascia here is carefully lifted from the nerve before cutting with the scissors. Sliding of the scissors in this location is not safe.

The nerve is not removed from its bed, nor is it circumferentially dissected free of the surrounding connective tissue. If the soft-tissues are dissected circumferentially, the nerve is more likely to become unstable after in situ decompression. If there is evidence of compression in some region, this should be released wherever necessary, but routine circumferential dissection is not necessary and should not be performed routinely.

At this point, the ulnar nerve should be completely decompressed. If any portion of the decompression is limited by the skin incision, the incision should be extended. While the small incision has some minor advantages, it should not be used at the expense of a well-executed in situ decompression.

The elbow should then be placed through a full range of motion while the ulnar nerve is observed. It should remain within the cubital tunnel. It may appear to "perch" or push medial as it comes under tension around the medial epicondyle. If it truly subluxates, the author recommends transposition (Fig. 12.4). If it only perches, the author does not typically transpose, although this is a judgment call that is made on an individual basis. There is little evidence to define how much "perching" is acceptable, though some studies have attempted to define it. However, developing differences in outcomes based on these assessments will be difficult. In the author's experience, when in situ decompression was initially adopted, there was a trend towards allowing any amount of "perching" that did not snap. This may have been in an effort to adopt a newer technique to all patients. Some of these patients went on to develop true subluxation post-operatively. Since that experience, the author as transposed a greater number of patients, which he estimates is in the range of 10–15% of all decompressions. One trend the author and others have noticed is a trend towards instability in younger patients, although this is by no means a universal finding. This data is very anecdotal, and each surgeon should develop their own approach to managing these cases and observe the future literature for more validated decision-making processes.

Another method to treat intraoperative ulnar nerve subluxation after in situ decompression, is the use of a triceps sling reconstruction. With this technique, a small, distally-based strip of triceps tendon is harvested (Fig. 12.5a). The proximal end of the strip is then sutured to the posterior aspect of Osborne's ligament, thus creating a "sling" between the medial epicondyle and the olecranon (Fig. 12.5b). Any excess tendon is excised. At the completion, the ulnar nerve should be tension-free within the cubital tunnel without impingement from the triceps fascia.

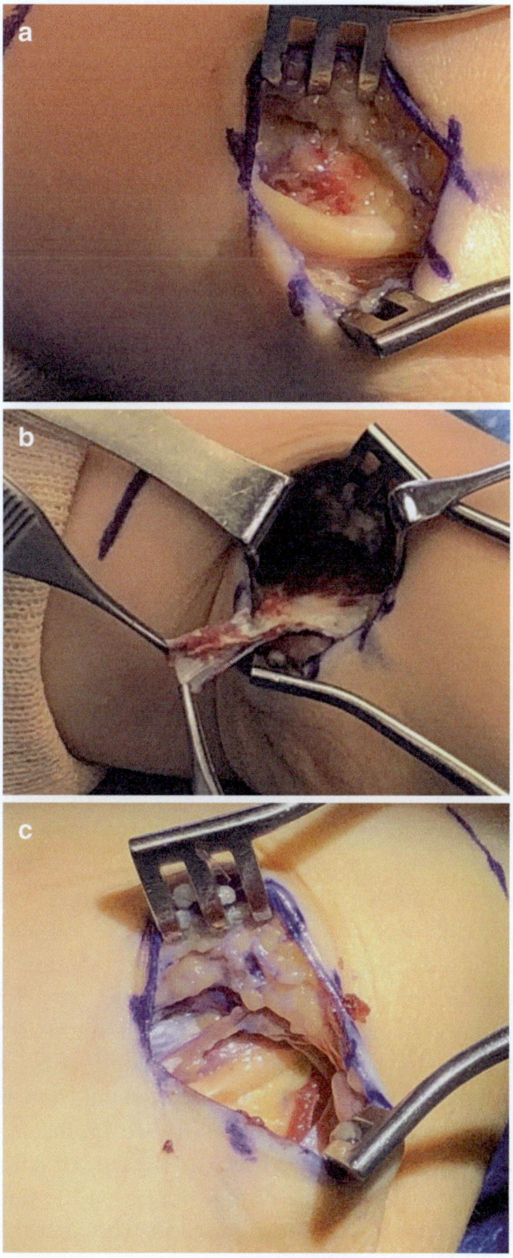

Fig. 12.4 After decompression of the ulnar nerve, the elbow is placed into maximum flexion. If the nerve is found to subluxate out of the groove, over the medial epicondyle (**a**), it is the author's recommendation to transpose the nerve. Through this same incision, the nerve can be mobilized, the medial intramuscular septum can be resected, and a fascial sling can be created (**b**). Particular care should be taken to the transition points between posterior and anterior, especially distally. Avoidance of a "Z" deformity by adequate release of the anterior FCU fascia is required to prevent post-transpositional impingement upon the nerve. After transposition, the nerve passes smoothly from proximal to distal (**c**)

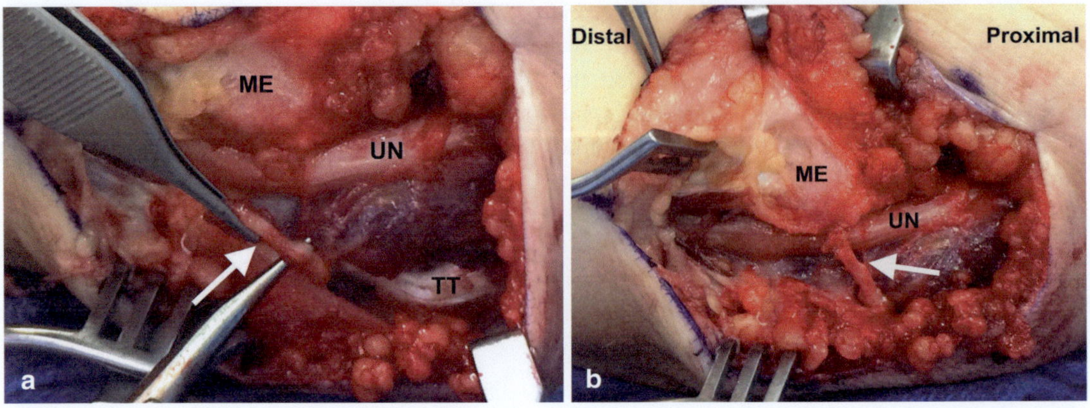

Fig. 12.5 (**a**) Harvesting of a small distally based strip of triceps tendon (white arrow) proximal end of tendon strip in forceps. (**b**) The proximal end of the triceps strip (white arrow) is sutured to the posterior aspect of Osborne's ligament. UN: ulnar nerve, ME: medial epicondyle, TT: triceps tendon. (Photo: courtesy of Dr. Dean Sotereanos)

There have been suggestions that because certain individuals in the population have an ulnar nerve that subluxates asymptomatically, that nerve transposition, in cases of subluxation after decompression, is not necessary [22]. The author does not agree with this conclusion for several reasons. Firstly, the asymptomatic ulnar nerve may be at risk for symptoms at a later time, and therefore there may be some benefit to transposition to avoid the potential need for additional surgery. Additionally, this author has had two patients develop symptomatic subluxation after in situ decompression earlier in his adoption of this technique. These patients required revision surgery which lead to symptom resolution after transposition. As mentioned previously, this is anecdotal and certainly decisions should not be made on such weak evidence. However, the second rational for transposition in the face of iatrogenic ulnar nerve instability hinges on the data supporting in situ decompression. The idea that the nerve "should not" be transposed suggest that the author in reference has concluded that in situ transposition is "better" than transposition when in fact it has only proved to be comparable. Therefore, the fact that in situ decompression and transposition have been found to have similar outcomes should not lead to the conclusion that in situ decompression is "better" because it is simpler. Rather, that data supports transposition for any reason, as it has shown the result of the two techniques to be equal. Therefore, it is reasonable and prudent for surgeons to judge the situation based on each individual situation and patient. As there is no objective downside to transposition, it may be considered for a variety of reasons [22].

When the nerve is determined to require transposition, this is done using the techniques detailed in the appropriate chapter on nerve transposition. The exact technique is up to the surgeon. It is possible, after some experience with the limited incision, to resect the medial intramuscular septum, transpose the nerve in a subcutaneous, intramuscular, or sub-muscular fashion, and achieve a straight course for the nerve across the elbow without extending the incision. When initially using this limited skin incision, it is likely best to extend it for a transposition. With experience, the incisional length can be progressively shortened, and the "window" technique used to affect the transposition effectively.

Following decompression, the wound is irrigated and closed with several deep absorbable sutures and then nylon sutures in the skin. The stresses on this incision with elbow flexion necessitate a layered closure and at least 10 days for maintenance of the nylon skin sutures. A soft dressing and compressive elastic bandage are applied and left in place. On post-operative day 4, the patient is allowed to remove the dressing, wash the wound, dry it well, and apply a clean adhesive bandage which is changed daily. Motion and activities are allowed to resume as tolerated. The patient is seen back in the office in 10–14 days. In most cases, formal therapy is unnecessary, as most patients have regained almost normal motion at this time. If they have not, they are instructed in a home passive motion program and instructed to call in 2 weeks if they have not regained full motion, at which time a formal therapy program is begun.

At the first post-operative visit, an assessment of symptoms should be gathered. Patients are expected to have post-operative incisional pain, as well as pain along the length of the decompression. It is valuable to assess between tenderness and pain, in contrast to dysesthesias consistent with MABC irritation, the latter of these taking longer to resolve. Resolution of the patients elbow pain due to ulnar nerve compression has frequently resolved by this visit, as have positional numbness and dysesthesias. Patients that only had positional symptoms pre-operatively are typically asymptomatic and are instructed to schedule a follow-up appointment at 3 months. If they remain asymptomatic and have no further complaints, they are instructed to cancel the appointment when they are called by the office to confirm it a few days prior. For patients that had constant numbness, weakness, or atrophy pre-operatively, they have typically seen a resolution of their dysesthesias, but little improvement in their other symptoms. If the surgeon has educated them well pre-operatively, this will be expected by the patient, although it is not uncommon for patients to forget this pre-operative education. The patients should be monitored post-operatively to make certain these symptoms resolve or until their recovery plateaus and the symptoms cease diminishing.

A valuable tool to assess the nerve dysfunction is a Semmes Weinstein test. This should be done pre-operatively for any patient that has subjective numbness without provocation pre-operatively. When it is done post-operatively and can give both the surgeon and the patient an idea of the progress of ulnar nerve recovery and potential for long-term improvements in function [5].

Simple decompression has been shown to be successful in treating cubital tunnel syndrome. Prospective randomized studies have shown results of simple decompression to be equal to anterior transposition [10, 12, 14, 23]. In one study, 152 patients were randomized to simple decompression (75 patients) and anterior ulnar nerve transposition (77 patients). In this study, the length of surgery was highly significantly longer for transposition. There was no significant difference in symptom resolution, reoperation, or failure between the groups. There was, however, a significantly lower complication rate in the simple decompression group (9.6%) compared to the transposition group (31.1%).

The severity of symptoms pre-operatively does not appear to affect the results of in situ decompression compared to anterior ulnar nerve transposition [12, 13].

Complications

In situ decompression has been shown to have a lower complication rate than submuscular transposition [11, 12, 15, 23], and therefore may be preferred over transposition. Biggs et al [23] showed a higher wound complication rate with transposition and, as mentioned previously, Bartels et al [12] showed nearly triple the complication rate for transposition. It should be noted that Bartels at al included peri-incisional numbness as a complication. If these patients were excluded, the complication rate was still much higher, but only double that of in situ decompression.

In situ decompression also appears to have a low failure rate. A study of 56 patients (69 extremities) who underwent in situ decompression of the ulnar nerve showed that five limbs (7%) had persistent symptoms postoperatively. These recurrent symptoms were relieved after anterior sub-muscular transposition. This data suggest in situ decompression is a reliable treatment with a low failure rate, and anterior transposition can be used to treat those patients with recurrent symptoms [24].

The posterior branch of the medial antebrachial cutaneous nerve is encountered in all surgical approaches to the ulnar nerve. Injury to the nerve can cause painful neuroma, hyperesthesia, hyperalgesia in the forearm and a painful scar [21]. Care must be taken throughout any ulnar nerve surgery to identify and protect any branches of the MABC that may be encountered. As mentioned previously, the author prefers the small incision for ulnar nerve surgery to minimize manipulation of these branches, but by no means is there any good data to suggest that injury to the MABC is less with this surgical technique.

Subluxation may occur with simple decompression alone. Intraoperative assessment of the nerve's stability is necessary to avoid this complication. If it is appreciated post-operatively, transposition, minimal medial epicondylectomy or triceps sling technique is required to eliminate the symptoms of a painful subluxating nerve. Persistent symptoms after cubital tunnel surgery are usually the result of incomplete decompression while recurrent symptoms are usually the result of perineural scarring [25]. The treatment of recurrent disease requires complete assessment of each potential site of compression. This includes the Arcade of Struthers, the medial intramuscular septum, the medial epicondyle, the cubital tunnel, Osbourne's ligament, and the aponeurosis of the flexor-pronator mass. Incomplete release of these structures can lead to persistent or recurrent symptoms. After transposition, attention should be focused on these areas as well as on the proximal and distal sites of transposition, where the nerve crosses from posterior to anterior and back again [26]. Surgical options for failed cubital tunnel syndrome include: anterior submuscular transposition, anterior intramuscular transposition, and anterior subcutaneous transposition [27, 28]. Medial epicondylectomy is another option, however, anterior transposition remains the preferred technique [29]. An adjunctive procedure for cubital tunnel revision is the addition of some form of soft-tissue coverage. These procedures are designed to provide a more hospitable bed for the nerve following transposition to limit perineural scarring. Options include vein-wrapping, triceps muscle flap, and pedicle fat flap [30, 31].

Conclusions

The surgical treatment of cubital tunnel syndrome can be helpful in minimizing symptoms and preventing functional loss in the hand. Several techniques for decompression have been described and have found through multiple studies to demonstrate comparable results. The use of in situ decompression should be considered as possibly the "simplest" (though by no means proven "best") option for treatment of cubital tunnel syndrome. There may be a slightly lower complication rate after simple decompression when compared against anterior ulnar nerve transposition. Following in situ decompression, the author recommends assessing the nerve for post-decompression instability. If this instability is present, transposition, triceps sling or medial epicondylectomy should be considered to prevent post-surgical symptoms. After ulnar nerve surgery using any of the common techniques, intermittent symptom resolution is common, while more advanced constant symptoms and weakness are less reliably resolved quickly. For these more advanced cases, patients should be educated that symptom resolution will be very slow and may be incomplete at final follow-up.

References

1. Bozentka DJ. Cubital tunnel syndrome pathophysiology. Clin Orthop Relat Res. 1998;351:90–4.
2. Boone S, Gelberman RH, Calfee RP. The management of cubital tunnel syndrome. J Hand Surg Am. 2015;40(9):1897–904; quiz 904.
3. Svernlöv B, Larsson M, Rehn K, Adolfsson L. Conservative treatment of the cubital tunnel syndrome. J Hand Surg Eur Vol. 2009;34(2):201–7.
4. Wang Y, Sunitha M, Chung KC. How to measure outcomes of peripheral nerve surgery. Hand Clin. 2013;29(3):349–61.
5. Bell-Krotoski J, Tomancik E. The repeatability of testing with Semmes-Weinstein monofilaments. J Hand Surg Am. 1987;12(1):155–61.
6. Geutjens GG, Langstaff RJ, Smith NJ, Jefferson D, Howell CJ, Barton NJ. Medial epicondylectomy or ulnar-nerve transposition for ulnar neuropathy at the elbow? J Bone Joint Surg Br. 1996;78(5):777–9.
7. Staples R, London DA, Dardas AZ, Goldfarb CA, Calfee RP. Comparative morbidity of cubital tunnel surgeries: a prospective cohort study. J Hand Surg Am. 2018;43(3):207–13.

8. Watts AC, Bain GI. Patient-rated outcome of ulnar nerve decompression: a comparison of endoscopic and open in situ decompression. J Hand Surg Am. 2009;34(8):1492–8.
9. Zhang D, Earp BE, Blazar P. Rates of complications and secondary surgeries after in situ cubital tunnel release compared with ulnar nerve transposition: a retrospective review. J Hand Surg Am. 2017;42(4):294.e1–5.
10. Gervasio O, Gambardella G, Zaccone C, Branca D. Simple decompression versus anterior submuscular transposition of the ulnar nerve in severe cubital tunnel syndrome: a prospective randomized study. Neurosurgery. 2005;56(1):108–17; discussion 17.
11. Caliandro P, La Torre G, Padua R, Giannini F, Padua L. Treatment for ulnar neuropathy at the elbow. Cochrane Database Syst Rev. 2012;(7):CD006839.
12. Bartels RH, Verhagen WI, van der Wilt GJ, Meulstee J, van Rossum LG, Grotenhuis JA. Prospective randomized controlled study comparing simple decompression versus anterior subcutaneous transposition for idiopathic neuropathy of the ulnar nerve at the elbow: part 1. Neurosurgery. 2005;56(3):522–30; discussion–30.
13. Izadpanah A, Gibbs C, Spinner RJ, Kakar S. Comparison of in situ versus subcutaneous versus submuscular transpositions in the management of McGowan stage III cubital tunnel syndrome. Hand (N Y). 2019; https://doi.org/10.1177/1558944719831387.
14. Nabhan A, Ahlhelm F, Kelm J, Reith W, Schwerdtfeger K, Steudel WI. Simple decompression or subcutaneous anterior transposition of the ulnar nerve for cubital tunnel syndrome. J Hand Surg Br. 2005;30(5):521–4.
15. Chen HW, Ou S, Liu GD, Fei J, Zhao GS, Wu LJ, et al. Clinical efficacy of simple decompression versus anterior transposition of the ulnar nerve for the treatment of cubital tunnel syndrome: a meta-analysis. Clin Neurol Neurosurg. 2014;126:150–5.
16. Osbourne G. The surgical treatment of tardy ulnar neuritis. J Bone Joint Surg Am. 1957;39:782.
17. Feindel W, Stratford J. The role of the cubital tunnel in tardy ulnar palsy. Can J Surg. 1958;1(4):287–300.
18. Chan RC, Paine KW, Varughese G. Ulnar neuropathy at the elbow: comparison of simple decompression and anterior transposition. Neurosurgery. 1980;7(6):545–50.
19. Foster RJ, Edshage S. Factors related to the outcome of surgically managed compressive ulnar neuropathy at the elbow level. J Hand Surg Am. 1981;6(2):181–92.
20. Manske PR, Johnston R, Pruitt DL, Strecker WB. Ulnar nerve decompression at the cubital tunnel. Clin Orthop Relat Res. 1992;274:231–7.
21. Lowe JB, Maggi SP, Mackinnon SE. The position of crossing branches of the medial antebrachial cutaneous nerve during cubital tunnel surgery in humans. Plast Reconstr Surg. 2004;114(3):692–6.
22. Heithoff SJ. Cubital tunnel syndrome: ulnar nerve subluxation. J Hand Surg Am. 2010;35(9):1556; author reply –7.
23. Biggs M, Curtis JA. Randomized, prospective study comparing ulnar neurolysis in situ with submuscular transposition. Neurosurgery. 2006;58(2):296–304; discussion 296–304.
24. Goldfarb CA, Sutter MM, Martens EJ, Manske PR. Incidence of re-operation and subjective outcome following in situ decompression of the ulnar nerve at the cubital tunnel. J Hand Surg Eur Vol. 2009;34(3):379–83.
25. Rogers MR, Bergfield TG, Aulicino PL. The failed ulnar nerve transposition. Etiology and treatment. Clin Orthop Relat Res. 1991;269:193–200.
26. Lowe JB, Mackinnon SE. Management of secondary cubital tunnel syndrome. Plast Reconstr Surg. 2004;113:1e–16e.
27. Gabel GT, Amadio PC. Reoperation for failed decompression of the ulnar nerve in the region of the elbow. J Bone Joint Surg Am. 1990;72(2):213–9.
28. Caputo AE, Watson HK. Subcutaneous anterior transposition of the ulnar nerve for failed decompression of cubital tunnel syndrome. J Hand Surg Am. 2000;25(3):544–51.
29. Kleinman WB. Cubital tunnel syndrome: anterior transposition as a logical approach to complete nerve decompression. J Hand Surg Am. 1999; 24(5):886–97.
30. Varitimidis SE, Riano F, Sotereanos DG. Recalcitrant post-surgical neuropathy of the ulnar nerve at the elbow: treatment with autogenous saphenous vein wrapping. J Reconstr Microsurg. 2000;16(4):273–7.
31. Godette GA, Rayan GM. Medial triceps flap coverage for an ulnar neuroma. Orthop Rev. 1993; 22(5):603–6.

Endoscopic Ulnar Nerve Release

13

Margaret Woon Man Fok, Tyson Cobb, and Greg Bain

Introduction

Cubital tunnel syndrome, after carpal tunnel syndrome, is the second most common compressive nerve entrapments in the upper limb. It is defined as ulnar nerve compression around the elbow region. Apart from the cubital tunnel retinaculum (also known as the Osborne's ligament), compressive sites of the entrapment may involve: Arcade of Struthers, the fasciae of the medial triceps, medial intermuscular septum, medial epicondyle, aponeurosis of the two heads of the flexor carpi ulnaris (FCU) and anomalous anconeous epitrochlerais muscle (Fig. 13.1).

Patients suffering from cubital tunnel syndrome usually complain of intermittent numbness and paresthesia of their ulnar ½ of ring finger and little finger. This is usually aggravated by elbow flexion. They may notice weakness in grip strength and difficulty in buttoning or holding small objects. In severe cases, intrinsic muscle wasting, easily notable at the 1st web space and hypothenar area, and ulnar claw hand deformity (i.e. hyperextension of the metacarpal-phalangeal joint and flexion of the interphalangeal joints of the ring and little finger) can be observed. Tinel sign can be demonstrated along the route of ulnar nerve, posterior to the medial epicondyle.

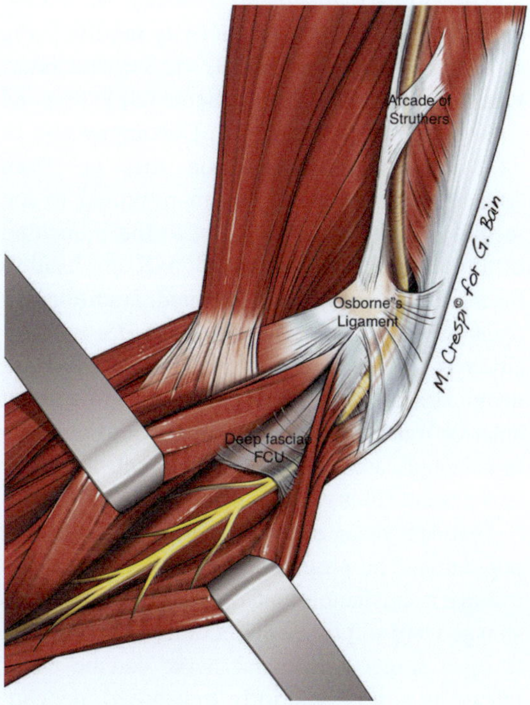

Fig. 13.1 Illustration of the extent of release in cubital tunnel syndrome

M. W. M. Fok
Department of Orthopaedics and Traumatology, Queen Mary Hospital, The University of Hong Kong, Hong Kong, China

T. Cobb
Shoulder Elbow wrist and Hand Center of Excellent, Davenport, IA, USA

G. Bain (✉)
Department of Orthopaedic Surgery, Flinders University, Adelaide, South Australia

D. G. Sotereanos, L. K. Papatheodorou (eds.), *Compressive Neuropathies of the Upper Extremity*,
https://doi.org/10.1007/978-3-030-37289-7_13

The cause of cubital tunnel is usually idiopathic. Nevertheless, elbow osteoarthritis, joint malalignment secondary to malunion of childhood elbow fracture, post-traumatic scarring, inflammatory arthropathy and ulnar nerve subluxation are some of the common predisposing factors. Cubital tunnel syndrome is a clinical diagnosis, based on history and physical examination. Yet, in cases of uncertainty or of medical – legal concerns, nerve conduction study can be used to confirm the diagnosis and to document the severity of the neuropathy. Radiographs and ultrasound are used if structural compression is suspected [1, 2].

The primary treatment modality of cubital tunnel is conservative with activity modification, splints and physiotherapy [3, 4]. Surgical intervention is indicated when patients fail to respond with conservative modalities. Decompression of all the potential compression sites i.e. from Arcade of Struthers, 8–10 cm proximal to the medial epicondyle proximally, to the branching of motor branches of the FCU, 5–8 cm distal to the medial epicondyle, is warranted. Traditionally, open cubital tunnel release with anterior transposition is the gold standard. Yet recent literature demonstrates that simple decompression without anterior transposition has comparable outcomes in selected cases, e.g. in cases which the ulnar nerve is not subluxable [5–8].

In recent years, endoscopic surgery has gained popularity. The proposed benefits are that it can achieve a satisfactory outcome with smaller incision and less soft tissue dissection [9, 10]. Similar to open surgery, the ulnar nerve can be either release in situ or anteriorly transposed, depending on the stability of the ulnar nerve and its surrounding environment.

Endoscopic Cubital Tunnel Release (Decompression of Ulnar Nerve In-Situ)

Indications

- Idiopathic cubital tunnel syndrome, preferably confirmed by nerve conduction study.

Contra-indications

- Unstable ulnar nerve, i.e. subluxation or dislocation of nerve during elbow flexion.
- Mass or space occupying lesion compressing onto the ulnar nerve.
- Hostile ulnar nerve bed, such as scarring from previous elbow surgery or trauma.
- Severe elbow contracture.
- Concomitant conditions necessitating anterior transposition (e.g. cubitus valgus or humeral malunion or non-union).
- Recurrent cubital tunnel syndrome.
- Limited external rotation of the shoulder (relative contra-indication).
  - Depends on surgeons' expertise in performing this surgery.

Surgical Techniques

Different techniques have been described for endoscopic cubital tunnel release. It can be classified into two types, the use of specialized dissection equipment, Storz instruments (Karl Storz, Tuttlingen, Germany) [11, 12], and Agee device (3M, Orthopaedic Products, St Pauls, MN, USA) [13] and the use of cannula. (Integra LifeSciences, Plainsboro, NJ, USA) [14, 15]. Each technique has its benefits and drawbacks. The choice depends on the surgeons' preference and the availability of the instruments.

Surgical Technique Using Storz Equipment (Karl Storz, Tuttlingen, Germany) [12, 16]

The patient is in supine position, under general or regional anesthesia, with the affected arm in 90° abduction and supination on a standard hand table. Pneumatic tourniquet is applied. The ulnar nerve is palpated and a 2 cm skin incision is made over the retro-condylar groove. Once the ulnar nerve is identified, tunneling forceps is introduced distally about 10–12 cm and proximally 8–10 cm from the medial epicondyle into the space between the fasciae and the subcutaneous tissue. An illuminated speculum is then inserted into this prepared space. Under direct vision, the fascial roof of the retrocondylar groove and the Osborne's ligament can be divided under direct vision.

A 4 mm 30° endoscope with a blunt dissector on its tip is introduced and advanced distally. The dissector is used to lift up the soft tissue, creating a space for better visualization of the nerve and its surrounding tissue. Under endoscopic guidance, a blunt-tipped scissors is used to release the forearm fasciae, followed by the fibrous raphe between the two muscular heads of the FCU and the fibrous bands over the ulnar nerve (Fig. 13.2). All the soft tissue overlying the ulnar nerve is released until the motor branches of the FCU come into view i.e. about 8 cm distal to the medial condyle.

Proximally, the endoscope is used to decompress the ulnar nerve in a similar fashion. The deep fascia and the arcade of Struthers above the ulnar nerve are divided, up to 10 cm proximal to the medial epicondyle. The intermuscular septum can be left alone if no impingement to the ulnar nerve is observed. Hemostasis can be achieved with long bipolar forceps or special bipolar micro-forceps (Fig. 13.3).

Post release, the ulnar nerve is checked for stability, by taking the elbow in full range of motion. If subluxation or dislocation of the nerve is noted, anterior transposition of the nerve is warranted. If the nerve remains stable, the wound is closed in layers. A suction drain may be inserted prior to closure.

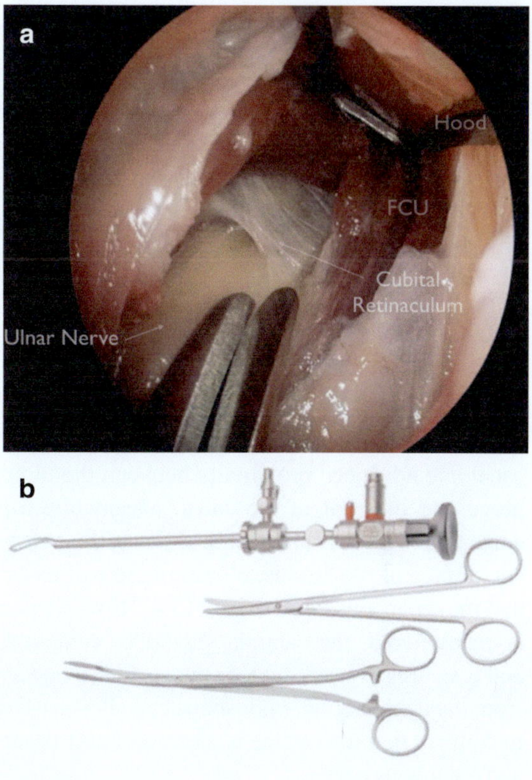

Fig. 13.2 (**a**) Endoscopic view of distal release using endoscope and specialized dissection equipment (Copyright Dr Gregory Bain). (**b**) illustration of the equipment used

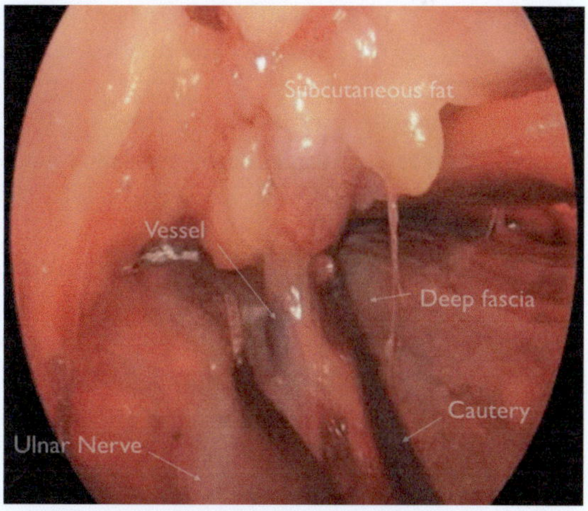

Fig. 13.3 Endoscopic view of cautery in order to achieve hemostasis. (Copyright Dr Gregory Bain)

Cannula Technique (Integra LifeSciences, Plainsboro, NJ, USA) [14, 15]

The patient is being prepared in a similar fashion, with arm board and anesthesia. A 2 cm incision is made over the retrocondylar groove, and the ulnar nerve is identified after incising the roof of the cubital tunnel. The spatula is inserted into the potential space between the ulnar nerve and the roof of the tunnel. The spatula should advance both proximally and distally without resistance to create a canal for the cannula.

A cannula specifically designed for cubital tunnel release is used. The cannula has a flat undersurface, which helps to hold the nerve under the cannula, and slots on the inferior surface, which allows visualization of the ulnar nerve during the release. The cannula has an attached retractor,

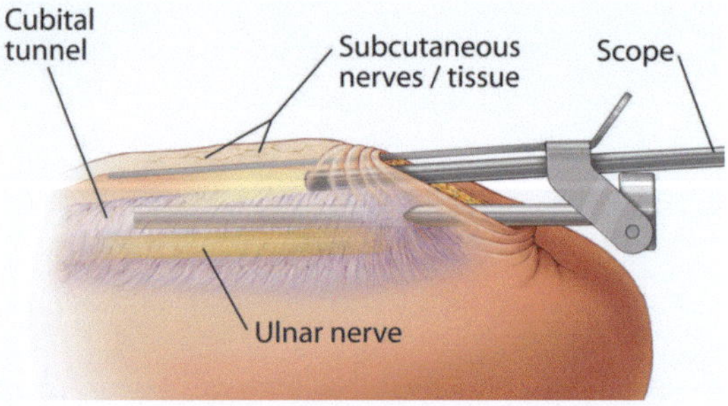

Fig. 13.4 Illustration of endoscope and cannula in place

which holds the soft tissue and the cutaneous nerve. The cannula with trocar is inserted into the canal and advanced proximally between the ulnar nerve and the roof of the canal. Meanwhile the attached retractor is allowed to slide on the extensor surface of the fasciae, elevating the soft tissue and the cutaneous nerves (Fig. 13.4). If resistance is encountered, the cannula should be removed, and a spatula is used to clear the soft tissue away from the deep fasciae. Endoscope can also be used to confirm that the fasciae is cleared of soft tissue and cutaneous nerves.

Once the cannula/trocar has been placed into the canal, the trocar is removed. A 4 mm 30° endoscope is inserted into the cannula. The inferior slot of the cannula is viewed, confirming that the ulnar nerve is protected by the cannula. The fasciae (roof of the canal) is then divided with a blade, along the superior slot of the cannula. Following the release of the fascia, the completeness of the release is checked by gradually pulling the cannula back on the scope and out of the canal.

A similar procedure is performed for the distal release. Prior to closure, the endoscope is inserted again at the space where the retractor is placed, to check the completeness of the release both proximally and distally. After confirmation of the stability of the ulnar nerve, the wound is closed in layers.

Surgical Technique Using Agee Device (3M, Orthopaedic Products, St Pauls, MN, USA) [13, 17]

This is the most economical techniques especially if one uses the Agee device for endoscopic carpal tunnel release. Its technical details are similar to the Cobbs cannula technique. The patient is put under anaesthetia with the inflation of the tornqiuet. Similar incision is made over the retro-condylar groove and the unar nerve is identified. A spatula is used to free the nerve from the surrounding soft tissue and fasciae. Then, instead of the inserting the cannula, the Agee endoscope is inserted into the prepared canal. The Agee device has 30° endoscope optic and a pistol-grip hand piece with a trigger mechanism that activates a retractable blade immediately distal to the window. After obtaining a clear and safe view of the cubital retinaculum, and confirming that the ulnar nerve and its branches are not at risk, the trigger mechanism is activated and the entire device is withdrawn, incising the retinaculum. If any at-risk structures are seen in the visual view, the knife is retracted by releasing the trigger. This procedure can be done both distally and proximally in a repeated manner until the ulnar nerve is completely released. Prior to closure, the ulnar nerve is checked for stability by taking the elbow in full range of motion.

Tips and Tricks

- This is an advanced technique. It is recommended that surgeons are familiarized with all the instruments, preferable in a cadaveric setting
- For the first few cases, the surgeon is advised to perform endoscopic release in thin patients as their anatomy can be more easily identified and the ulnar nerve more easily localized.
- A 3–4 cm longitudinal incision instead of 2 cm incision is recommended for the initial few cases, until surgeon is familiarized with the techniques. Larger incision may be needed for patients who are overweight or have a large build.
- Cutaneous nerves may be encountered in the incision. While surgeons do not need to look for them, if seen, they should be protected to avoid injury and neuroma.
- All instruments including endoscope/spatula/cannula should advance without resistance.

In cases which resistance is encountered, surgeons should withdraw the instruments from the canal and proceed with the following checklist:
- Ensure the incision in the cubital tunnel retinaculum is large enough so that the instrument does not bend as it is placed into the canal.
- Ensure the elbow is not overly flexed to create impingement.
- Wet the instruments to minimize friction.
- Use a spatula to ensure the appropriate plane is well developed and the angle of advancement is identified.

- The ulnar nerve must be well visualized before the dissection of the soft tissue with dissecting forceps.
- Adipose tissue may interfere with the endoscope view. Endoscope has to be cleaned often with the adipose tissue removed.
- Protection of the vascular supply of the ulnar nerve is mandatory.
- The motor branches of the FCU needs to be well visualized and should be protected during dissection.
- Good hemostasis is needed to prevent postoperative hematoma. Deflation of tourniquet is recommended prior to wound closure. Alternatively, a drain may be inserted for 1–2 days.
- After release, stability of the nerve should be checked by taking elbow in full range of motion. If subluxation of the ulnar nerve is noted, proceed to anterior transposition (see below section "Endoscopic Cubital Tunnel Release and Anterior Transposition").
- If there is any difficulty while performing this procedure e.g. if the ulnar nerve cannot be well visualized or if hemostasis cannot be achieved, the surgeon should convert to an open procedure.

Postoperative Protocol

A bulky compression dressing is applied for 2–3 days. It is then changed to simple dressing. Motion is allowed within the limits of patient's comfort. Patients can expect to return back to office activity on the first post-operative day. Full range of motion is expected in 1 week. For patients who need to return to sports or return to moderate to heavy duty, they are typically restricted for 1 week and then advanced to full duty over the subsequent 2–3 weeks.

Complications

- One of the most common complications following endoscopic cubital tunnel release is hematoma formation. It is minimized by:
  - Handling soft tissue with care, especially during dissection of soft tissue away from the fasciae.
  - Deflating the tourniquet prior to wound closure followed by good hemostasis,
  - Using local anesthesia with epinephrine at wound closure.
  - Placement of drain for 1–2 days.
- Medial antebrachial cutaneous nerves of the arm may be injured, resulting in neuroma or paresthesia of the medial forearm. This can be minimized by attention to details during dissection and the avoidance of multiple layer of soft tissue dissection.
- The main ulnar nerve or one of its branches can be injured during decompression. The nerve needs to be well visualized at all times.
- Unrecognized subluxation of the ulnar nerve can be minimized by checking the stability of the ulnar nerve in full range of elbow motion post nerve release.
- Wound dehiscence can be minimized by ensuring a tight closure, with wound closed in layers.

Results

Satisfactory and comparable results were noted by using different techniques of endoscopic cubital tunnel release.

Seventy-five patients with seventy-six ulnar nerves underwent endoscopic cubital tunnel release in situ using the Storz instruments [11].

Sensory improvement was noted in 96% of patients and grip strength was noted to be significantly improved (30.5%) as compared with preoperatively. Even patients with preoperative severe symptoms (based on Dellon's classification [18]) had 89% good to excellent results based on the modified Bishop rating [19]. Four patients suffered from hematomas and nine patients had sensory loss over the medial antebrachial cutaneous nerve of the arm. There was no recurrence at a mean follow-up of 11 months.

Cobb et al reported the use of cannula for endoscopic cubital tunnel release in 172 cases [20]. At a mean follow-up of 30 months, 96% had good to excellent results based on the modified Bishop rating [19]. The average return to normal work was 8 days following endoscopic cubital tunnel release compared with 71 days following anterior transposition of the ulnar nerve. Seven patients had complications including wound dehiscence, postoperative hematoma and superficial infection. There were four patients requiring revision surgery due to persistent symptoms or recurrence.

With the use of Agee endoscope, 27 cases of cubital tunnel were studied [17]. With a mean follow up of 112 weeks, 81% of patients showed a clinical improvement of the McGowan grade [13]. Two patients suffered from wound dehiscence, with one requiring revision surgery. No subluxation of the ulnar nerve nor iatrogenic ulnar nerve injury was noted.

Current Literature

Endoscopic cubital tunnel release is a minimally invasive technique which is postulated to have theoretical benefits of a small incision, less soft tissue dissection and low complication rate as compared with the conventional open cubital tunnel release. In a cadaveric study, Said et al demonstrated that the visualization of the ulnar nerve around the elbow region can be accomplished by a 2 cm incision instead of a 4 cm open incision [21]. In addition, authors using different endoscopic techniques have shown that it can lead to an adequate ulnar nerve decompression and a satisfactory outcome in both cadaveric studies and clinical settings [11, 13, 17, 20].

In spite of these promising results, studies comparing open and endoscopic cubital tunnel release in situ are mixed and not conclusive. In a prospective randomized double-blind study of 56 cubital tunnel syndrome cases, Schmidt et al demonstrated that there was no difference with respect to clinical improvement between the two techniques in both early or late follow-up [9]. Hematoma was significantly more frequent in the endoscopic group (i.e. seven cases versus one case). Meanwhile, in a retrospective cohort study of 114 patients with cubital tunnel syndrome [22], the endoscopic group had better short term results and comparable long term outcomes when compared with the open release group. Seventy-six percent of patients after endoscopic surgery returned to their full functionality within 1 week as opposed to 19% patients after open surgery. Nineteen patients in the open group suffered from complications of loss of sensation over the medial antebrachial cutaneous nerve of the arm, scar pain and superficial wound infection while six patients in the open group suffered from complications of ulnar nerve subluxation and hematoma formation. Four patients, two with hematoma and two with nerve subluxation, required additional surgeries. Similarly, the conclusion of two recent systematic reviews comparing the two techniques are mixed. Toirac et al [23], after reviewing eight articles, suggested that the clinical outcomes of endoscopic technique were more superior than open technique in regards to both complication rates and patients satisfaction. The rate of excellent/good Bishop score was 92% for the endoscopic group as compared with 83% for open group. The breakdown of each complication was not stated. In contrast, Aldekhayel et al, reviewed 20 studies and concluded that there was similar effectiveness between the endoscopic and open techniques for treatment of cubital tunnel syndrome with similar outcomes, complication profiles and reoperation rates [24].

Endoscopic Cubital Tunnel Release and Anterior Transposition

This describes subcutaneous anterior transposition of the ulnar nerve performed under endoscopic guidance.

Indications

- Unstable ulnar nerve, either pre-operatively or post nerve release.
- Hostile ulnar nerve bed, such as scarring from previous trauma or elbow surgery.

Contraindications

- Previous trauma or surgery to the ulnar nerve and/or elbow.
- Severe elbow contracture.
- Concomitant conditions necessitating open surgery such as management of humeral malunion or non-union.
- Patients' particular conditions necessitating sub-muscular transposition, e.g. thin patient who is prone to have ulnar nerve irritation.
- Limited external rotation of the shoulder (relative contra-indication).
  - Depends on surgeons' expertise in performing this surgery.

Surgical Technique

Endoscopic ulnar nerve release is performed as described in the endoscopic cubital tunnel release in situ section, using either Storz instruments (Karl Storz, Tuttlingen, Germany) or specific designed cannula (Integra LifeSciences, Plainsboro, NJ, USA). In cases which subluxation of the ulnar nerve is observed either pre-operatively or post ulnar nerve decompression, anterior transposition of the nerve is recommended [25].

Starting proximally, the medial intermuscular septum (MIMS) identified during the decompression must be excised. The MIMS does not usually cause impingement of the ulnar nerve if the nerve is decompressed in situ. Yet. If the nerve is transposed, impingement of the nerve is likely. Excision of the MIMS is needed.

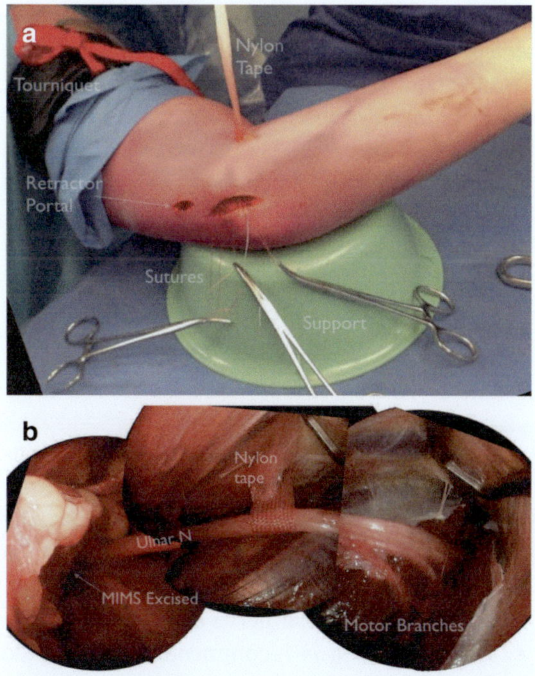

Fig. 13.5 (**a**) Additional portal for anterior transposition. (**b**) nylon tape. (Copyright Dr Gregory Bain)

The tunneling forceps or spatula is used to create an anterior subcutaneous space into which the nerve will be placed after transposition. In order to aid in the mobilization of the ulnar nerve into the anterior compartment, an additional subcutaneous portal is created at this space just distal to the medial epicondyle (Fig. 13.5). A nylon tape is then introduced into this portal for the manipulation of the nerve. The ulnar nerve, together with its accompanied vessels is mobilized from the loose areolar tissue under endoscopic guidance.

Once the ulnar nerve is freed and positioned anteriorly to the medial condyle, the entire "new" course of the nerve is checked to ascertain that there is no new site of compression or kinking of the nerve. The nerve is then secured to prevent subluxation back into its original position. First, the medial condyle is rasped, in order to promote adhesion to the adjacent soft tissue. The subcutaneous tissue is then sutured to the medial condyle to prevent the nerve from falling back behind the epicondyle. To ensure the stability of the nerve in its new course, the position of the ulnar nerve is checked, taking the elbow in its entire range of motion. Hemostasis is performed after the deflation of the tourniquet. The wound is closed in layers, taking care of not catching the nerve. An arm sling is given to keep the elbow in flexed position.

Tips and Tricks

- This is an advanced technique, with a significant learning curve. Surgeons are recommended to be familiarized with the technique of endoscopic release of ulnar nerve prior to his/her attempt in performing anterior transposition of the ulnar nerve endoscopically.
- Larger incision is recommended to be made for the initial few cases and for overweight patients.
- When using the nylon tape to retract the ulnar nerve during the mobilization from its native bed, it is important not to employ significant traction, as this may result in iatrogenic ulnar nerve palsy.
- The MIMS is to be excised in a generous manner prior to the transposition of the ulnar nerve. This is to prevent a new site of ulnar nerve impingement.
- During the creation of the subcutaneous tunnel, the medial antebrachial cutaneous nerve of the arm may be damaged. The surgeon is recommended to dissect just above the fasciae using forceps and spatula. Dissection in multiple planes should be avoided.
- Prior to closure, the surgeon should ensure that there is no new site of compression and the ulnar nerve is stable in its new route. The elbow should be taken over its entire course of motion for confirmation.
- Hemostasis should be achieved by using bipolar forceps under endoscopic guidance to prevent haematoma formation. Drain may be placed for 1–2 days. It is recommended to close the wound in layers to avoid wound dehiscence.

Postoperative Protocol

A longer rehabilitation period is needed after anterior transposition as compared with decompression in situ. An arm sling is used for 10 days. Gentle active elbow mobilization is allowed out of the sling, but the elbow should be not straightened. Full elbow mobilization exercise is only permitted after 10 days, allowing the soft tissue to heal around the nerve. Light duties can resume after 10 days. Patients should delay return to moderate to heavy duties or return to sports for 6–12 weeks.

Complications

- Iatrogenic injury to the ulnar nerve or its branches may occur. Patients usually complain of persistent or worsen symptoms and signs. Ulnar nerve must be well visualized under direct or endoscopic vision at all times. Significant traction should be avoided during the retraction of the ulnar nerve.
- Subluxation of the ulnar nerve back to its original route may be observed especially if patients undergo excessive movement of the elbow in the early post-operative period. A snapping sensation may be noted during elbow movement.
- New site of ulnar nerve compression may be noted if the MIMS is not excised or if the nerve is not completely mobilized and not completely seated in its new bed in a tension free manner.
- Paresthesia of medial forearm due to injury of the medial antebrachial cutaneous nerve of the arm.
- Wound dehiscence and hematoma formation may be encountered.

Results

Eleven patients with an average age of 52 years old underwent endoscopic cubital tunnel release and transposition over a 3 year period [25]. Satisfactory relief in symptoms was noted in most patients, though patients with significant preoperative nerve involvement (e.g. McGowen Grade 3) [26] had persistent paresthesia and muscle wasting post-operatively. Snapping of the ulnar nerve was resolved for patients with subluxable ulnar nerve. There was no major complication including reoperations, infections, nerve injures, or recurrent ulnar nerve instability.

Current Literature

There is limited literature on endoscopic cubital tunnel release with anterior transposition [25, 27]. Kirshnan et al described 11 patients with cubital tunnel syndrome irrespective of ulnar nerve stability undergoing endoscopic release and transposition. At a mean follow-up of 15.5 months, 91% showed good to excellent results, based on the modified Bishop rating [19], with no complications. Current literature supports that both simple cubital tunnel release in situ and cubital tunnel release with anterior transposition resulted in comparable outcomes [5, 6]. Yet most of these prospective randomized controlled trials exclude patients with ulnar nerve hypermobility. Bartels et al [8] randomized patients into simple release and anterior transposition irrespective of the ulnar nerve stability. It reported that just over 50% of patients had completely resolved symptoms in both groups with no statistical significance between groups. It is generally accepted that anterior transposition of ulnar nerve is indicated in patients with ulnar nerve hypermobility or hostile ulnar nerve bed or recurrent cubital tunnel syndrome [28, 29]. Higher complication rates of up to 31% as opposed to 9.1% has been reported with open nerve release with anterior transposition in a prospective randomized trial. The majority of complications were loss of sensation around the scar and superficial wound infection [8]. With the growing familiarity of performing cubital tunnel release under endoscopic guidance, concomitant anterior transposition appears to be a viable option. The preliminary result shows promising outcomes with minimal complication.

Learning New Techniques

As the interest of endoscopic ulnar nerve release is growing, a rise in complications is foreseeable if training of using endoscopic equipment is not adapted accordingly. To master this endoscopic technique, a detailed knowledge of the anatomy, pathology and necessary equipment is essential.

Surgeons should be equipped with general arthroscopic skills prior to the attempt of performing endoscopic procedure. As the decompression is under close proximity of the ulnar nerve and its accompanied vessels, good hand – eye coordination and triangulation techniques, acquired by mastering arthroscopic skills is essential. Surgeon must be familiarized with the anatomical environment around the ulnar nerve, so that they can avoid any potential injury to the surrounding area e.g. medial antebrachial cutaneous nerve of the arm. Soft tissue needs to be handled carefully in order to minimize iatrogenic nerve injury and hematoma formation.

In order to train specific psychomotor skills for the endoscopic nerve release, actual instruments handling on a regular basis is preferably performed in a simulated training setting away from the patients. This can be done through hands on cadaver courses, anatomic bench-top models or even virtual reality simulators. Unfortunately, high-fidelity virtual reality simulators include both passive and active haptic devices to perform a full-scale simulation are not yet commercially available for elbow region.

Authors recommended that interested surgeons should start endoscopic technique initially in uncomplicated patients requiring a simple ulnar nerve release. The surgeon should start with a larger Incision (i.e. >2 cm) until they are familiarized with the procedure. In cases which the visuality of the nerve is not good, one should convert to an open procedure without hesitation.

References

1. Doughty CT, Bowley MP. Entrapment neuropathies of the upper extremity. Med Clin North Am. 2019;103(2):357–70.

2. Beekman R, Schoemaker MC, Van Der Plas JPL, Van Den Berg LH, Franssen H, Wokke JHJ, et al. Diagnostic value of high-resolution sonography in ulnar neuropathy at the elbow. Neurology. 2004;62(5):767–73.
3. Dellon AL, Hament W, Gittelshon A. Nonoperative management of cubital tunnel syndrome: an 8-year prospective study. Neurology. 1993;43(9):1673–7.
4. Svernlöv B, Larsson M, Rehn K, Adolfsson L. Conservative treatment of the cubital tunnel syndrome. J Hand Surg Eur Vol. 2009;34(2):201–7.
5. Nabhan A, Shariat K, Steudel WI, Kelm J, Ahlhelm F. Two year outcome following surgical therapy for cubital tunnel syndrome. Simple decompression or subcutaneous anterior transposition? Aktuelle Neurol. 2006;33(S1):P485.
6. Gervasio O, Gambardella G, Zaccone C, Branca D. Simple decompression versus anterior submuscular transposition of the ulnar nerve in severe cubital tunnel syndrome: a prospective randomized study. Neurosurgery. 2005;56(1):108–17.
7. Biggs M, Curtis JA. Randomized, prospective study comparing ulnar neurolysis in situ with submuscular transposition. Neurosurgery. 2006;58(2):296–304.
8. Bartels RHMA, Verhagen WIM, van der Wilt GJ, Meulstee J, van Rossum LGM, Grotenhuis JA. Prospective randomized controlled study comparing simple decompression versus anterior subcutaneous transposition for idiopathic neuropathy of the ulnar nerve at the elbow: part 1. Neurosurgery. 2005;56(3):522–30.
9. Schmidt S, Kleist Welch-Guerra W, Matthes M, Baldauf J, Schminke U, Schroeder HWS. Endoscopic vs open decompression of the ulnar nerve in cubital tunnel syndrome: a prospective randomized double-blind study. Neurosurgery. 2015;77(6):960–70; discussion 970–1.
10. Heikenfeld R, Godolias G. Ulnar nerve decompression in cubital tunnel syndrome – open in situ decompression versus endoscopic decompression. Arthroscopy. 2013;29(10):e98.
11. Hoffmann R, Siemionow M. The endoscopic management of cubital tunnel syndrome. J Hand Surg Br. 2016;31(1):23–9.
12. Hoffmann R, Lubahn J. Endoscopic cubital tunnel release using the Hoffmann technique. J Hand Surg Am. 2013;38(6):1234–9.
13. Bain GI, Bajhau A. Endoscopic release of the ulnar nerve at the elbow using the Agee device: a cadaveric study. Arthroscopy. 2005;21(6):691–5.
14. Cobb T. Endoscopic cubital tunnel release. In: Operative techniques: shoulder and elbow surgery. Amsterdam: Elsevier; 2011. p. 891–903.
15. Cobb TK. Endoscopic cubital tunnel release. J Hand Surg Am. 2010;35(10):1690–7.
16. Hoffmann R, Siemionow M. Miniinvasive, endoscopic cubital tunnel release. J Hand Surg Am. 2003;28:72.
17. Stadie AT, Keiner D, Fischer G, Conrad J, Welschehold S, Oertel J. Simple endoscopic decompression of cubital tunnel syndrome with the Agee system. Oper Neurosurg. 2010;66(1):325–32.
18. Dellon AL. Techniques for successful management of ulnar nerve entrapment at the elbow. Neurosurg Clin N Am. 1991;2(1):57–73.
19. Kleinman WB, Bishop AT. Anterior intramuscular transposition of the ulnar nerve. J Hand Surg Am. 1989;14(6):972–9.
20. Cobb TK, Walden AL, Merrell PT, Lemke JH. Setting expectations following endoscopic cubital tunnel release. Hand (N Y). 2014;9(3):356–63.
21. Said J, Frizzell K, Heimur J, Kachooei A, Beredjiklian P, Rivlin M. Visualization during endoscopic versus open cubital tunnel decompression: a cadaveric study. J Hand Surg Am. 2019;44(8):697.e1–6.
22. Dützmann S, Martin KD, Sobottka S, Marquardt G, Schackert G, Seifert V, et al. Open vs retractor-endoscopic in situ decompression of the ulnar nerve in cubital tunnel syndrome: a retrospective cohort study. Neurosurgery. 2013;72(4):605–16; discussion 614–6.
23. Toirac A, Giugale JM, Fowler JR. Open versus endoscopic cubital tunnel in situ decompression: a systematic review of outcomes and complications. Hand (N Y). 2017;12(3):229–35.
24. Aldekhayel S, Govshievich A, Lee J, Tahiri Y, Luc M. Endoscopic versus open cubital tunnel release. Hand (N Y). SAGE Publications Sage CA: Los Angeles, CA. 2016;11(1):36–44.
25. Morse LP, McGuire DT, Bain GI. Endoscopic ulnar nerve release and transposition. Tech Hand Up Extrem Surg. 2014;18(1):10–4.
26. McGowan AJ. The results of transposition of the ulnar nerve for traumatic ulnar neuritis. J Bone Joint Surg Br. The British Editorial Society of Bone and Joint Surgery. 1950;32-B(3):293–301.
27. Krishnan KG, Pinzer T, Schackert G. A novel endoscopic technique in treating single nerve entrapment syndromes with special attention to ulnar nerve transposition and tarsal tunnel release: clinical application. Neurosurgery. 2006;59(1 Suppl 1):ONS89–100; discussion ONS89–100.
28. Boone S, Gelberman RH, Calfee RP. The management of cubital tunnel syndrome. J Hand Surg Am. 2015;40(9):1897–904; quiz 1904.
29. DeGeorge B Jr, Kakar S. Decision-making factors for ulnar nerve transposition in cubital tunnel surgery. J Wrist Surg. Thieme Medical Publishers. 2019;8(2):168–74.

14 Subcutaneous Transposition of the Ulnar Nerve

Natalie H. Vaughn, Brittany E. Homcha, and Alexander H. Payatakes

Introduction

Though ulnar neuropathy of the elbow is often attributed to intrinsic compression at the cubital tunnel, this is not always the only pathophysiological mechanism at play. The ulnar nerve undergoes multiple changes at the elbow, with the medial epicondyle acting as a fulcrum about which the nerve deforms and sustains traction. A patient may experience subluxation or frank instability of the ulnar nerve about the medial epicondyle, which may be further exacerbated by decompression of the ulnar nerve at the cubital tunnel with an *in situ* release. As such, the technique of anterior transposition was first proposed by Curtis in 1898 [1]. This technique moves the nerve to a position of lower tension and theoretically protects the nerve from dynamic instability that may cause further irritation. Additionally, it is thought to avoid some of the morbidity associated with a larger dissection necessary for deeper transposition (i.e. intramuscular or submuscular). Limited high-level evidence is available to compare *in situ* decompression, subcutaneous transposition, and intramuscular/submuscular transposition, but these techniques have been found to be comparable in several randomized trials and large outcomes series.

Pertinent Anatomical Considerations

The ulnar nerve has both an intrinsic and an extrinsic blood supply. The intrinsic blood supply is contained within the epineurial sheath. Regarding the extrinsic supply, there are three major vascular pedicles to the ulnar nerve at the level of the elbow: the superior ulnar collateral artery proximally, the inferior ulnar collateral artery (which may not be present in all patients), and the posterior ulnar recurrent artery distally [2, 3]. The superior ulnar collateral artery has an average length of 16–17 cm. It originates from the brachial artery 16–18 cm proximal to the medial epicondyle, then courses parallel to the ulnar nerve [2, 4]. The inferior ulnar collateral artery, which some authors describe as a minor pedicle to the nerve, originates 6–7 cm proximal to the medial epicondyle. This artery runs deep to the intermuscular septum and deep to the ulnar nerve [4]. The posterior ulnar recurrent artery has an average length of 7 cm and originates from the ulnar artery 6–7 cm distal to the medial epicondyle. It runs proximally towards the ulnar nerve,

N. H. Vaughn · B. E. Homcha
Department of Orthopaedics, Penn State Health Milton S. Hershey Medical Center, Hershey, PA, USA

A. H. Payatakes (✉)
Department of Orthopaedics, Bone and Joint Institute, Penn State Health Milton S. Hershey Medical Center, Hershey, PA, USA
e-mail: apayatakes@pennstatehealth.psu.edu

D. G. Sotereanos, L. K. Papatheodorou (eds.), *Compressive Neuropathies of the Upper Extremity*,
https://doi.org/10.1007/978-3-030-37289-7_14

deep and posterior [2, 4]. One of the stated concerns about anterior transposition is that the dissection necessary to mobilize the ulnar nerve anterior to the medial epicondyle may devascularize the nerve to the point of functional impairment. In a canine model, ulnar nerve perfusion after anterior transposition with extrinsic vessel ligation was found to be 45% of normal controls, as opposed to 80% of controls when the extrinsic vessels were preserved [5]. Multiple studies on monkeys have also been performed to investigate blood flow to the ulnar nerve. Ogata et al found that in Macaca monkeys at 3 days post-transposition, blood flow to the ulnar nerve was decreased compared to the expected baseline of 0.5 mL/min/mL tissue [6]. However, the blood flow was noted to improve to the level of baseline flow at 7 days post-operatively. The same research team subsequently assessed ulnar nerve vascular supply (using a hydrogen washout test) and nerve conduction velocity in the setting of nerve compression, devascularization, and short-duration ischemia followed by compression [7]. They found that the effects of nerve compression were potentiated by ischemia of the limb. Prolonged compression of the ulnar nerve significantly decreased blood flow and led to significantly decreased conduction velocity at 28 min post-compression. Disruption of the ulnar nerve blood supply over a short segment decreased the recorded blood flow to the nerve, but did not affect nerve conduction velocity, though it did diminish the amplitude significantly after 44 min. Whole-arm ischemia with the use of a tourniquet followed by nerve compression caused the nerve conduction amplitude to diminish during the compression phase only.

Clinical data has suggested that with preservation of the superior ulnar collateral artery and inferior ulnar collateral artery, satisfactory clinical results are obtained despite the theoretical risk of devascularization [4, 5]. Nakamura et al performed laser Doppler flow studies before and after anterior transposition in patients randomized to either vascular pedicle-sparing or ligation groups and compared their clinical results up to 12 months postoperatively [4]. The authors found that blood flow in the ligation group decreased to 28–52% from pre-transposition baseline values. At 6 months, there were no significant differences in clinical outcomes between the two groups (including Disabilities of the Arm, Shoulder and Hand [DASH] score, grip strength, pinch strength, 2-point discrimination, and McGowan classification). At 12 months, however, the vascular-sparing group was found to have a significantly lower average DASH score compared to the ligation group. No significant differences were noted in other outcomes measures.

Biomechanical Considerations

The ulnar nerve runs behind the medial epicondyle, which serves as a fulcrum when the elbow enters a flexed position. This changes the inherent forces placed on the nerve. Multiple authors have measured the pressures on the ulnar nerve at various degrees of elbow flexion and at various sites along the nerve, both in cadaveric models and intraoperatively. These series consistently noted an increase of intraneural pressure with elbow flexion [8–13]. The position of the surrounding joints of the arm has an impact on the ulnar nerve pressure as well. Shoulder abduction, elbow flexion, and wrist extension place the nerve under maximum pressure [11, 13]. The cross-sectional area of the ulnar nerve decreases 33–50% and the overall area of the cubital tunnel decreases 30–41% from elbow extension to flexion [9]. Intraneural pressure is relatively higher than extraneural pressure with terminal elbow flexion, suggesting that flexion and traction on the ulnar nerve associated with this motion contributes to the changes in pressures around the nerve [9]. Intraneural hypertension may disrupt vascular supply to the nerve nerve. Clinical interventions for cubital tunnel syndrome should thus relieve this pressure to alleviate symptoms. Cadaveric studies have demonstrated a decrease in the maximal pressure within the cubital tunnel by 50% with release of the cubital tunnel with the elbow in flexion [13]. In one intraoperative series measuring ulnar nerve pressures around the cubital tunnel in elbow flexion and extension, there was a positive correlation between the pressure and the stage of neuropathy and disease duration [12]. However, simple *in situ* release of the arcuate ligament over the ulnar nerve did not change pressure in the cubital tunnel at the common flexor aponeurosis, suggesting that multiple sites of compression must be addressed in order to adequately decompress the ulnar nerve and address all sites of pathology [10].

The nerve shape also changes with elbow motion. Flexion of the elbow elongates the ulnar nerve approximately 4–5 mm [14, 15]. *In situ* decompression of the ulnar nerve changes the location at which elongation occurs from the epicondylar groove to a more proximal level. Anterior subcutaneous transposition restores the site of elongation to the segment of the nerve previously within the epicondylar nerve groove or distal to the flexor carpi ulnaris (FCU) aponeurosis [15, 16]. Clinical intra-operative assessments of ulnar nerve strain before and after anterior subcutaneous transposition have demonstrated that the strain on the ulnar nerve is significantly reduced with the elbow in flexion, but is elevated with the elbow in extension when compared to *in situ* decompression [16].

Techniques of Anterior Subcutaneous Transposition

Surgical treatment for cubital tunnel syndrome is indicated when the patient fails nonoperative treatment (including activity modification, positional changes, avoiding prolonged flexion of the elbow, and nighttime splinting) with persistent hand numbness and/or weakness. Subcutaneous transposition of the ulnar nerve was first described by Curtis in 1898 [1]. Since that time, multiple descriptions of the surgical technique have been published [17–21]. Decompression of the ulnar nerve is performed in the same general fashion as an *in situ* decompression. However, the skin incision may need to be extended both proximally and distally relative to an *in situ* to improve visualization of potential sites of compression (Fig. 14.1a). In total an incision of approximately 8–10 cm centered just posterior to the medial epicondyle may be necessary to fully visualize all potential sites of compression. Full-thickness subcutaneous flaps are created. Care is taken to avoid injury to branches of the medial antebrachial cutaneous nerve (MABC) during subcutaneous dissection to the cubital tunnel and subsequent preparation for the transposition (Fig. 14.1b). The ulnar nerve is usually easiest to identify proximal to the cubital tunnel. The cubital tunnel is then released, addressing the arcade of Struthers, medial intermuscular septum, medial triceps, cubital retinaculum, Osborne's ligament, fascial bands within the FCU, and possibly the anconeus epitrochlearis, if present. The ulnar nerve is dissected out proximally to the arcade of Struthers. With transposition, the medial intermuscular septum creates a new potential location for compression (Fig. 14.2a). A portion of the septum should be excised, or alternatively the septum may be simply released from the humerus to relieve its tension. Care must be taken to maintain hemostasis during this release, as a vascular leash is typically present in close proximity to or piercing the septum (Fig. 14.2b) [22]. The ulnar nerve is then freed distally, releasing the aponeurosis between the two heads of the flexor carpi ulnaris and any deep transverse fascial bands identified distally. Once decompression is satisfactory, the elbow is taken through the arc of motion to assess for instability (perching or subluxation, Fig. 14.3a, b).

If a decision is made to proceed with anterior transposition, the ulnar nerve is then mobilized. The vascular supply to the nerve should be maintained, if possible (Fig. 14.1c). Articular branches to the ulnohumeral joint are sacrificed. The first two motor branches to the flexor carpi ulnaris arise on average 1.6 and 3.4 cm distal to the medial epicondyle [23]. In order to adequately mobilize the ulnar nerve anteriorly, these motor branches must be identified and dissected out, possibly with sacrifice of the first branch (Fig. 14.1d). Every effort should be made to preserve the distal motor branches, as inadvertent injury may cause weakness of the flexor carpi ulnaris and affect wrist flexion. Dissection of the motor fascicles from the ulnar nerve may increase transposition distance substantially [23].

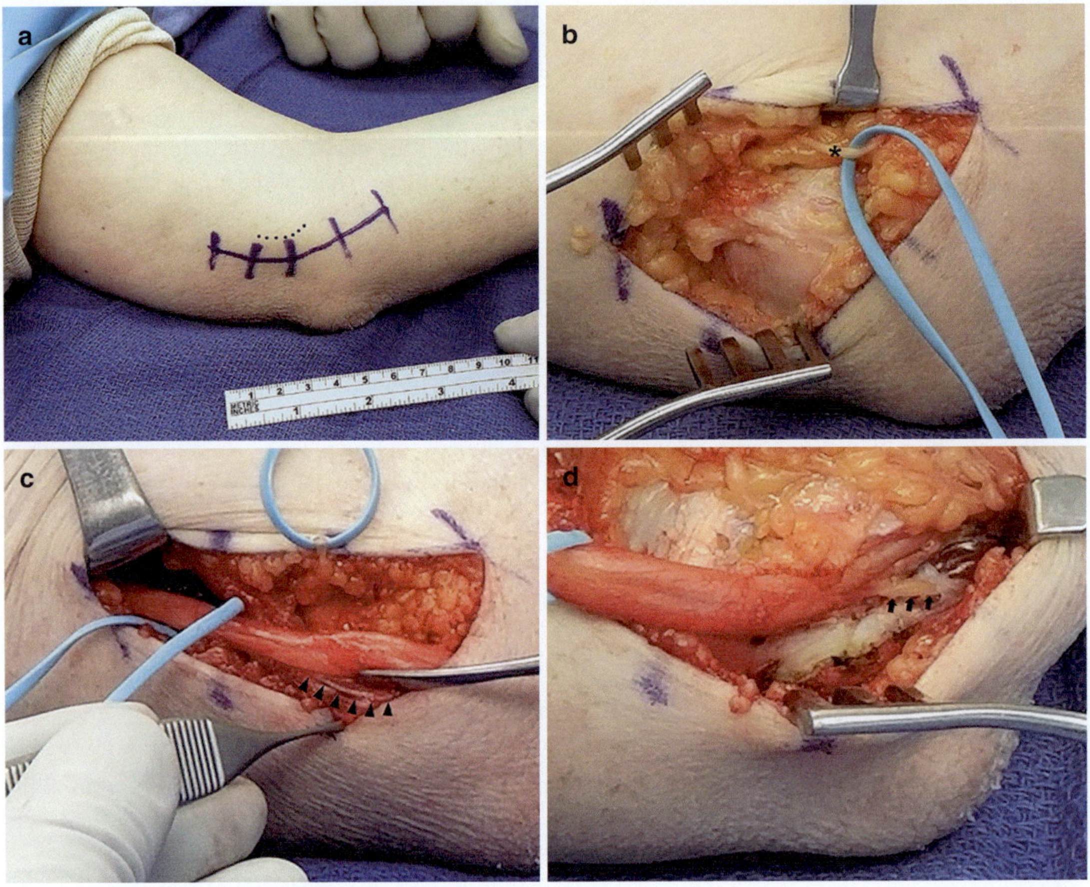

Fig. 14.1 Considerations for nerve decompression and transposition. **a**: The planned surgical incision is 8–10 cm in length (*dotted line:* medial epicondyle). **b**: The medial antebrachial cutaneous nerve branch(es) (*asterisk*) should be identified and protected. **c**: Care must be taken to maintain the extrinsic longitudinal bloody supply (*arrowheads*) to the ulnar nerve. **d**: Dissection of first motor branch of the ulnar nerve to the flexor carpi ulnaris (*arrows)* is often required for adequate mobilization

When the nerve has been adequately mobilized so that it can be repositioned anterior to the medial epicondyle without tension or kinking (proximal or distal), the nerve should be stabilized in its new course. This is achieved by utilizing one of several available anatomic features around the proximal and medial elbow. Described techniques include creation of a subcutaneous pocket, use of a fasciodermal sling, fascial sling, adipose flap, medial intermuscular septal sling, ligamentodermal sling or ligamentofascial sling.

Subcutaneous Pocket

The simplest form of transposition involves anterior transposition of the nerve followed by suturing of the fascia of the flexor-pronator mass (posterior to the desired position of the nerve) to the subcutaneous tissue overlying this spot on the skin flap. While technically straightforward, it does have the theoretical risk of failure of the fixation and of skin tethering. This technique provides only one to two single points of restraint against recurrent subluxation of the nerve at the site of the knots, and may serve as an additional point of kinking of the nerve if the force is not carefully distributed across its length.

Fasciodermal Sling

For additional stability, a fascial flap can be harvested from the fascia overlying the flexor-

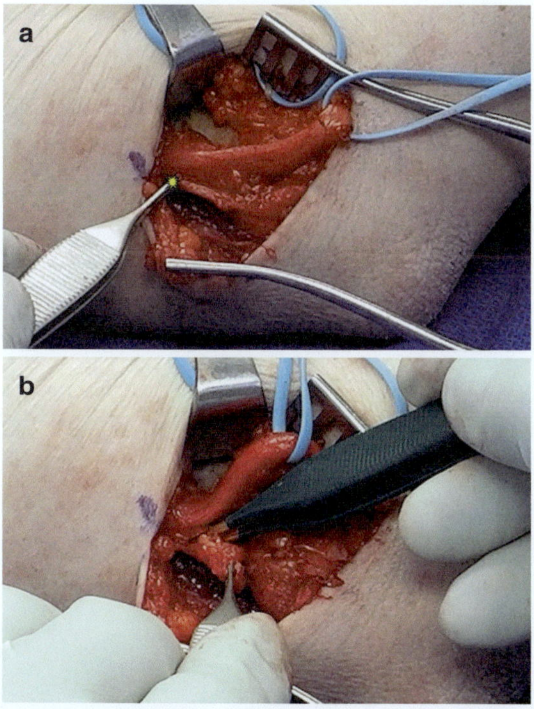

Fig. 14.2 Medial intermuscular septum. **a**: Failure to excise or release the intermuscular septum (*star*) may create kinking or compression of the anteriorly transposed nerve. **b**: Caution must be exercised when releasing the septum to prevent undue bleeding from the vascular leash just posterior to the septum

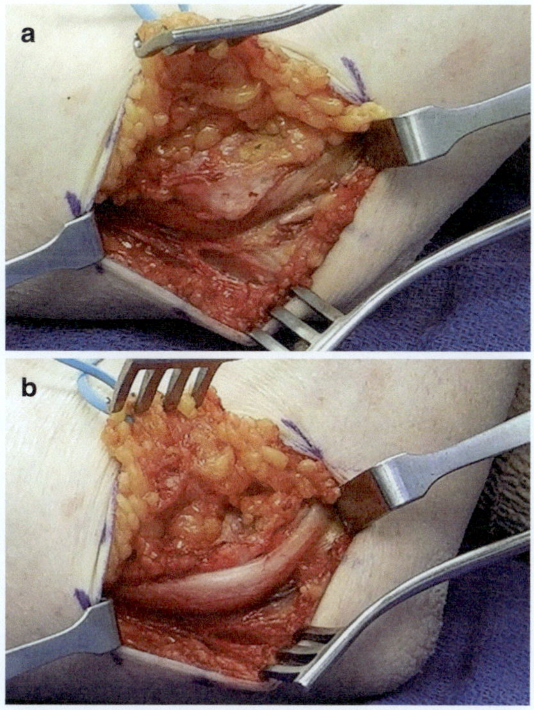

Fig. 14.3 Assessment for perching/subluxation of the nerve. **a**: The nerve should be assessed after decompression; here, the nerve sits posteriorly to the medial epicondyle in extension. **b**: With flexion of the elbow, the ulnar nerve is seen to subluxate anteriorly and perch over the medial epicondyle

pronator mass [17]. A marker is used to draw three sides of a square or rectangle at the desired flap site on the flexor-pronator mass (Fig. 14.4a). The flap should be designed 1–2 cm wide to distribute forces more widely across the nerve at this site. Three sides of the flap are sharply elevated with a scalpel, with a posteromedial base most commonly described (Fig. 14.4b). The appropriate anchoring location on the dermis of the anterior skin flap is identified. This is done by simulating wound closure and marking the position on the skin flap that corresponds to a location about 1 cm distal/lateral to the medial epicondyle (Fig. 14.4c). The superior and inferior corners of the free edge of the fascial flap are sutured to the dermis with absorbable suture, with the nerve transposed and held anterior to the medial epicondyle by this flap (Fig. 14.4d, e). Care must be taken to ensure there is sufficient space for the nerve after fixation of the sling. This may be assessed with use of a Freer elevator (Fig. 14.4f). If nerve compression or puckering of the skin is noted, the sling should be revised.

Fascial Sling

A variation of the aforementioned technique involves fixation of the fascial sling to the intact fascia, rather than to the overlying subcutaneous tissue. This technique provides the benefit of improved tissue quality for fixation (fascia rather than dermis). It does, however, run the risk of over-constraining the nerve and creating a new site of compression. If this technique is used, the surgeon must ensure sufficient length of the fascial flap by designing a more pronounced rectangular shape with longer superior and inferior limbs. This design prevents compression of the nerve and limitations in gliding.

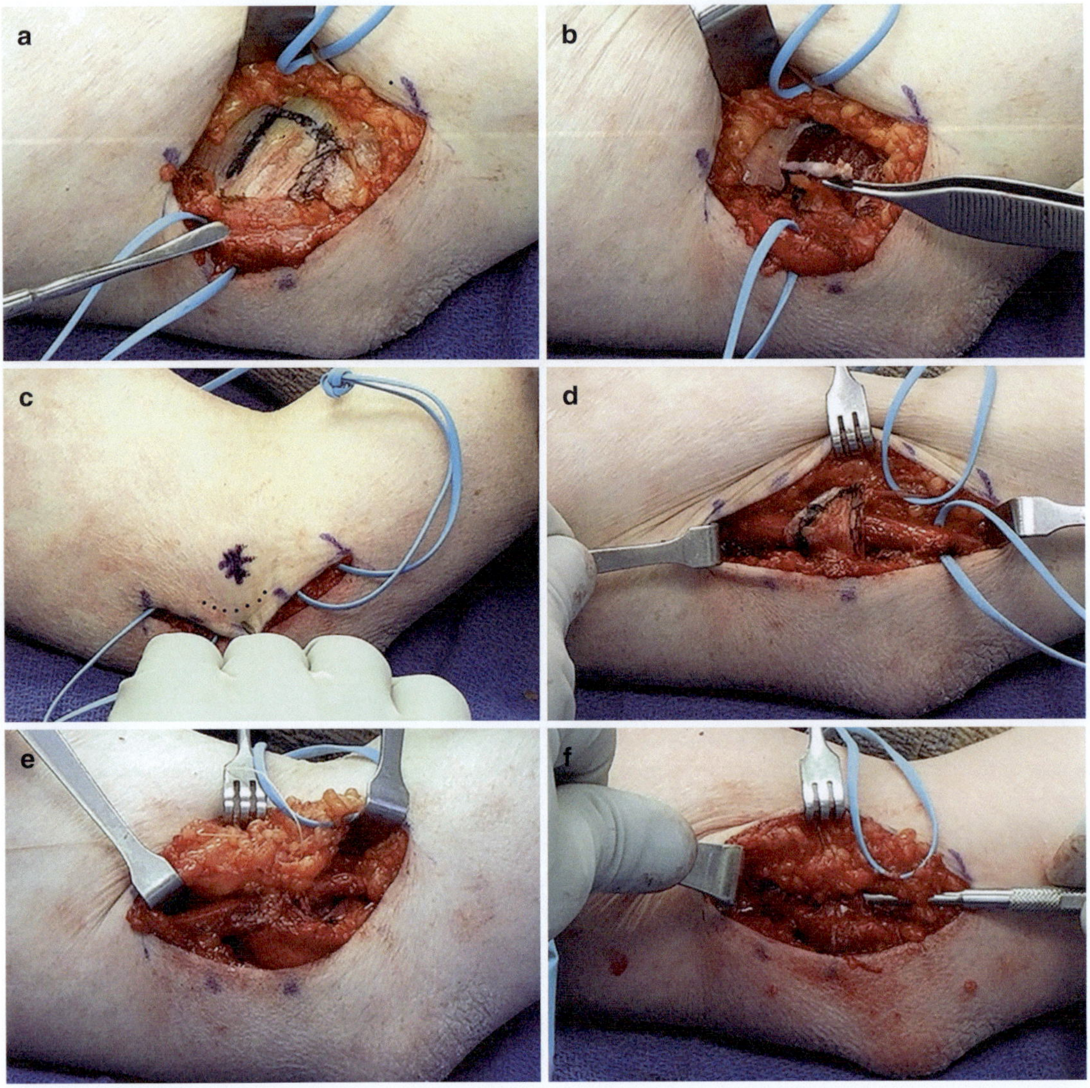

Fig. 14.4 Fasciodermal sling technique. **a**: A square or rectangular flap is drawn on the flexor-pronator fascia. **b**: The flap is sharply elevated, maintaining a posterior base. **c**: The appropriate anchoring site for the fascial sling is identified and marked (*asterisk*) by laying down the anterior skin flap over the medial epicondyle (*dotted line*) to simulate closure. **d**: The flap can be provisionally sutured to the dermis for assessment. **e**: The elbow should be gently ranged after flap suturing to rule out proximal or distal kinking or compression. **f**: A Freer elevator is used to rule out nerve compression by the sling

Adipose Flap

Use of an adipose flap has been described to minimize the scarring associated with the fascial sling method and to promote improved gliding of the nerve. In this technique, a subcutaneous adipose flap is elevated, maintaining its vascular pedicle to the skin. The anterior adipose flap is wrapped around the nerve and sutured to the anterior subcutaneous tissue [18, 21].

Medial Intermuscular Septal Sling

Use of the medial intermuscular septum has also been described as a potential restraint to prevent posterior subluxation of the ulnar nerve after transposition. In this technique, after release of the ulnar nerve from the cubital tunnel, the intermuscular septum is divided 3–4 cm proximal to its medial epicondyle insertion and dissected toward the medial epicondyle, leaving a 1 cm wide flap of fascial tissue attached only to the medial epicondyle. When the nerve is transposed anteriorly, the free end of the septum can be secured either to the dermis or to the fascia overlying flexor-pronator mass [19]. The flexor-pronator mass fascia should be palpated to ensure no sharp borders may kink or irritate the nerve; if present, the fascia at this location should be released. A modification of this technique has also been described [20], whereby a second limb of the septum sling is added to prevent kinking. This requires a more extensive release off the medial epicondyle, with an 8 cm strip of tissue required to create an inverted-V flap. The mid-portion of the septum is attached to the subcutaneous tissue or flexor-pronator mass as described above, forming the apex of the "V," while the most distal aspect of the septum is attached 1–1.5 cm distal to this, distributing the forces on the nerve.

Ligamentofascial/Ligamentodermal Sling

Finally, the tissue of Osborne's ligament can be used to create a ligamentofascial/ligamentodermal sling [24]. In this technique, Osborne's ligament is released posteriorly off the olecranon and preserved (rather than a release along the middle of the ligament, directly overlying the ulnar nerve, Fig. 14.5a). After transposition of the nerve, the free end of Osborne's ligament is sutured either to the dermis or the fascia overlying the flexor-pronator mass (Fig. 14.5b). This creates a relatively long ligamentous flap that theoretically avoids the risk of nerve kinking at the transposition fixation site.

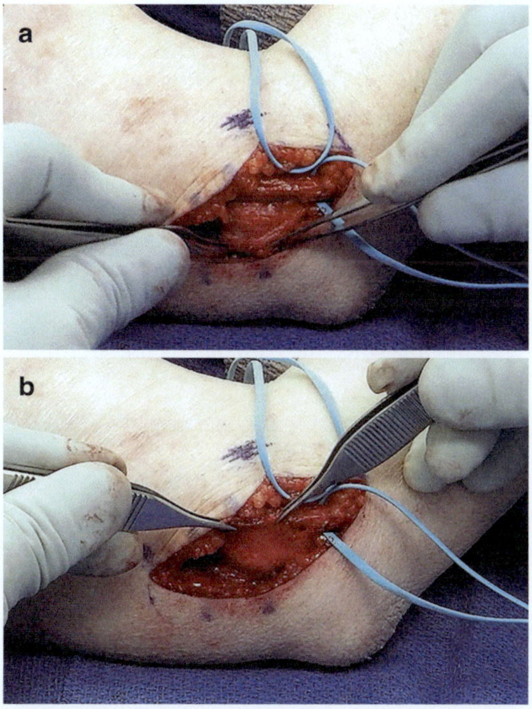

Fig. 14.5 Ligamentodermal sling. **a**: Osborne's ligament is released posteriorly and preserved as anteriorly based flap. **b**: The ligament is reversed anteriorly and sutured to the dermis, creating a stabilizing sling

Additional Considerations

Care must be taken to avoid creating new sites of compression with anterior transposition, especially the dreaded "omega (Ω) deformity." Ultrasound evaluation of patients with persistent symptoms after subcutaneous transposition have revealed "kinks" in the transposed nerves in the majority of cases [25]. These sites of fascial compression may prevent patients from achieving adequate symptomatic relief from their surgery. To avoid this, the surgeon should carefully palpate and visualize the entire course of the nerve after transposition to reveal any locations in which the nerve appears to deviate from a smooth, straight line. Any palpable sharp borders from remaining fascia should be released. Particular care should be taken proximally at the medial intermuscular septum.

The skin is then closed and dressings are applied. Some advocate immediate range of motion. Others recommend the use of a splint for 2 weeks for soft tissue rest prior to initiation of motion. A long-term outcome series revealed that at 2–14 years post-transposition, there were no differences in final range of motion in patients who had 2–3 weeks of immobilization versus those who had immediate range of motion. There were no differences in clinical outcomes between the groups. However, the patients who were immobilized missed more work, with an average return at 30 days versus 10 days in those who were not immobilized [26]. This is consistent with the findings of Weirich et al, who noted no differences in pain, functional improvements, or failure rates in patients permitted to undergo immediate elbow motion after transposition, compared with patients who were immobilized for 7–30 days [27]. The immediate mobilization group had the benefit of earlier return to work, at a median of 1 month post-operatively versus 2.75 months when the patient was immobilized.

Outcomes of Anterior Subcutaneous Transposition

A number of retrospective outcomes series have been published reporting clinical outcomes after anterior subcutaneous transposition. In general, patients tend to demonstrate good clinical improvement in symptoms, with 80–90% of patients reporting good or excellent results and over a 90% satisfaction rate [26, 28–33].

Simple decompression has been proposed as an effective alternative to transposition (Table 14.1; subcutaneous, intramuscular, submuscular). There has been a significant increase in the *in situ* decompression technique over time; in one registry review from 2005 to 2012, 80% of the procedures performed for cubital tunnel syndrome were *in situ* decompression, and only 16% involved anterior transposition [47]. Proponents of simple decompression cite similar clinical outcomes and higher morbidity of transposition techniques as reason to preferentially manage ulnar nerve compression at the elbow with simple decompression. These include higher postoperative narcotic use and patient-reported disability [32, 38, 39].

Table 14.1 Comparisons of *in situ* decompression to subcutaneous transposition of the ulnar nerve

Study	Study design	Patient population	Results
Bartels et al. (2005) [34]	Randomized Controlled Trial (RCT)	75 SD 77 SC	Higher complication rate in subcutaneous (31.1%) vs *in situ* (9.6%) No clinical differences regarding subluxation No significant differences in symptom outcomes
Nabhan et al. (2005) [35]	Randomized Controlled Trial	32 SD 34 SC	No significant differences in pain, motor or sensory deficits, or electrophysiological recordings at 3 and 9 months
Tawfik et al. (2017) [36]	Randomized Controlled Trial	10 SD 10 SC	No significant differences between groups for electrophysiological or clinical improvement at 6 months
Macadam et al. (2008) [37]	Meta-analysis of 10 studies	449 SD 342 SC 115 SM	Lower chance of improvement with simple *in situ* versus anterior transposition, odds ratio 0.751 (0.542–1.040) No significant differences on subgroup analysis
Zlowodzki et al. (2007) [38]	Meta-analysis of 4 RCTs	EMG scores: 49 SD 33 SC 18 SM Clinical scores: 130 SD 73 SC 58 SM	No significant differences in conduction velocity No clinical differences between groups
Chen et al. (2014) [39]	Meta-analysis of 13 studies	500 SD 381 SC 128 SM	No difference in clinical outcomes Higher rate of complications with transposition
Adelaar et al. (1984) [40]	Prospective Series	7 SD 22 SC 8 SM	Poor results correlated with symptoms longer than 36 months, presence of intrinsic muscle atrophy, presence of fibrillations on EMG, absence of ESP preoperatively, alcoholism No significant difference in outcomes between intervention groups

(continued)

Table 14.1 (continued)

Study	Study design	Patient population	Results
Staples et al. (2018) [32]	Prospective series	47 SD 35 SC 43 SM	Higher average narcotic consumption with transposition Higher patient-reported disability up to 8 weeks post-op with transposition At 8 weeks, only difference between groups was persistent olecranon paresthesias in transposition group At final follow-up, six revisions for failure (13%) after *in situ* vs. two after transposition (3%)
Paine et al. (1970) [41]	Retrospective review	50 SD 11 unspecified transpositions	Both groups showed improvement or complete resolution (90.9% transposition group vs 77.7%) Transposition less likely to make patients worse Favor transposition in setting of arthritis, cubitus valgus, or flexion deformity
Chan et al. (1980) [33]	Retrospective review	115 SD 71 SC 43 SM	Simple decompression had higher percentage of full nerve recovery Young men (age 50 or younger) with less than 12 months of symptoms had better results Both groups had symptom improvement in over 80% of cases
Foster et al. (1981) [42]	Retrospective review	29 SD 19 SC	Subcutaneous had higher percentage of complete symptom resolution ($p > 0.05$) Intraneural fibrosis at time of release related to poor outcome Better outcomes if symptoms present 12 months or less
Davies et al. (1991) [43]	Retrospective review	73 SD 105 SC	No significant difference in satisfaction; both groups improved postoperatively (60% SC vs 72% SD) Lower percentage with unsatisfactory results in the *in situ* group Age, preoperative symptom severity or duration, or intraneural fibrosis not related to poor outcome
Taha et al. (2004) [44]	Retrospective review	21 SD 17 SC	No statistical difference in improved sensory symptoms (48% SD group vs 59% SC group) Worse outcomes if symptoms were bilateral or if cervical disease present >1 year
Mitsionis et al. (2010) [45]	Retrospective review	31 SD 45 ME 37 SC	Subcutaneous transposition group had significantly inferior results (62% reporting good or excellent outcome) compared to *in situ* (84%) and medial epicondylectomy (80%)
Bacle et al. (2014) [29]	Retrospective review (4 centers)	44 SD 154 SC 82 SM 95 EN	Greater than 90% success rate (improvement or complete resolution of symptoms) regardless of method used
Zhang et al. (2017) [46]	Retrospective review	157 SD 29 SC 61 SM	Higher complications (3.8%) with *in situ* (infection, seroma, instability) versus transposition (2.2%) (MABC injury, infection) 11% of patients with initial transposition procedure required second surgery versus 2.5% for patients treated with *in situ* Prior trauma to elbow related to higher rate of second surgery

SD simple decompression, *SC* subcutaneous transposition, *SM* submuscular transposition, *ME* medial epicondylectomy, *EN* endoscopic, *MABC* medial antebrachial cutaneous

However, many of these differences are only temporary, resolving after 8 weeks [32]. In a cost analysis study, simple decompression was also favored based on similar outcome and lower cost of simple decompression, largely due to sick leave expenses [28]. In patients who fail initial decompression with simple decompression, anterior transposition is an effective treatment [32]. Few randomized controlled trials have been published directly comparing subcutaneous transposition and *in situ* decompression. Of these, patients have similar improvements in resolution of their symptoms at 6 months and 1 year post-operatively [34–36]. This has prompted some authors to recommend the *in situ* technique, as it tends to be less invasive. However, one meta-analysis identified a trend toward a lower chance of symptom improvement with simple decompression of the ulnar nerve compared to techniques which include anterior transposition, including subcutaneous technique, with an odds ratio of 0.75 [37].

Primary anterior transposition may be favored in patients who demonstrate subluxation or frank instability of the ulnar nerve preoperatively or intra-operatively. It should be noted that ulnar nerve subluxation occurs in 16% of healthy subjects [48]. In these patients, it is more common for the nerve to "perch" on the medial epicondyle without completely exiting the groove. This mobility is thought to exacerbate irritation of the ulnar nerve in the setting of cubital tunnel syndrome. However, Bartels et al found no clinical differences between patients treated with *in situ* decompression versus anterior transposition despite presence of luxation intra-operatively [34]. Unfortunately, no additional series have been published to date which specifically evaluate treatment techniques dependent upon the presence or absence of intraoperative nerve subluxation.

Subcutaneous transposition has been criticized for placing the ulnar nerve in a relatively vulnerable position. In thin patients, in whom there is little subcutaneous fat around the medial elbow, the nerve may be easily palpable below the skin. It may be susceptible to injury with blunt blows to the medial elbow, particularly in athletes such as basketball players who often sustain upper extremity injuries during play [49]. Performing a submuscular or intramuscular transposition, rather than subcutaneous, may better protect the nerve in such patients. In a rat model in which rats had paired transpositions (one submuscular, one subcutaneous), histology at 6 weeks post-transposition revealed a healthier appearance of the ulnar nerve axons and less perineural scar tissue associated with the submuscular technique [50]. Several series comparing subcutaneous and submuscular transposition found no differences between motor and sensory function after intervention (Table 14.2). Both groups were noted to have significant improvements at final follow-up [29, 38, 53]. In general,

Table 14.2 Comparisons of submuscular and subcutaneous transposition techniques

Study	Study design	Patient population	Results
Jaddue et al. (2009) [51]	Prospective series	26 consecutive patients, stratified by age and gender and placed into subcutaneous (13) or submuscular (13) groups; treated by two surgeons	92% good or excellent result in subcutaneous group versus 62% in submuscular Subcutaneous method required shorter incision, easier surgical technique, less operative time, less postoperative pain, earlier mobilization
Stuffer et al. (1992) [52]	Retrospective review	Compared 51 patients pre and post transposition., nonrandomized into submuscular (18) and subcutaneous (33)	18 cases had additional neurolysis Improved hand function, sensory nerve conduction, and two point discrimination with subcutaneous method
Charles et al. (2009) [53]	Retrospective review	49 patients with minimum 2 year follow up after transposition procedure, treated by a single surgeon; 25 submuscular, 24 subcutaneous	Poor outcome if symptoms present greater than 6 months Significant improvement in sensory and motor function after both transposition methods

a prolonged duration of symptoms (>6 months) tends to be predictive of a less favorable prognosis regardless of the technique used [31, 33, 53]. One group did note significantly better outcomes with a subcutaneous technique versus submuscular, with 92% good or excellent outcomes for the subcutaneous technique versus 62% for submuscular [51]. The authors listed easier surgical technique, shorter operative time (30 min versus 45 min), and less postoperative pain as additional reasons to choose a subcutaneous transposition technique rather than a submuscular.

Failures in patients initially treated with primary subcutaneous transposition has been attributed to recurrent subluxation over the medial epicondyle, perineural scarring, or incomplete release of proximal or distal sites of compression [54, 55]. Upon revision surgery for patients with failed subcutaneous transpositions, surgeons often note perineural scarring and fibrosis in the subcutaneous tunnel [54, 56]. However, development of fibrotic tissue encapsulating the ulnar nerve may also be found in failed submuscular transpositions and is not unique to subcutaneous transposition. Several risk factors have been identified for failed decompression in the setting of revision surgery for cubital tunnel syndrome, including age greater than 50 years, electromyography demonstrating denervation, previous treatment with submuscular transposition, and increasing number of previous procedures [56, 57]. Results after revision cubital tunnel surgery for failed subcutaneous transposition may not be as favorable as a successful primary surgery, with satisfaction rates of only 78% reported in one series after revision to submuscular transposition [55]. However, most patients do report some improvement in their pain and ability to return to daily functional activities.

Complications

The technique of subcutaneous anterior transposition of the ulnar nerve is not without complications. These can include peri-incisional numbness from injury to branches of the medial antebrachial cutaneous nerve, neuroma formation, infection, and elbow stiffness. The rate of complications is variable, with some authors reporting a higher rate with subcutaneous transposition as compared to *in situ* release (31% subcutaneous versus 10% *in situ*) while others report similar rates for the two techniques (3.4% subcutaneous versus 3.8% *in situ*) [34, 46]. A large meta-analysis comparing simple decompression versus anterior transposition of the ulnar nerve revealed similar improvement in ulnar neuritis symptoms in the two groups, but more complications associated with anterior transposition [39]. This study did not differentiate between transposition techniques.

Conclusions

Multiple treatment strategies have been described for cubital tunnel syndrome, all involving decompression of the ulnar nerve. Subcutaneous transposition was proposed to decrease pressure on the nerve during elbow flexion and to address potentially symptomatic nerve instability in certain susceptible individuals. Proponents of subcutaneous transposition cite its relative ease compared to other transposition techniques, while critics warn that perineural scarring may render it less effective than deeper transposition techniques. Outcomes following subcutaneous transposition are generally good or excellent, with high rates of symptom relief and patient satisfaction. No differences in outcomes have been reported when comparing subcutaneous transposition to *in situ* decompression or to submuscular and intramuscular techniques. In patients with ulnar nerve subluxation or frank instability, subcutaneous transposition is a relatively straightforward and reliable technique to prevent adverse effects of the medial epicondyle on the ulnar nerve.

Indications (for Anterior Transposition in general)

- *Absolute:* Symptomatic snapping of the ulnar nerve with elbow flexion necessitates anterior transposition (alternatively medial epicondylectomy)
- *Relative:*
  - Intraoperative subluxation of the ulnar nerve noted after *in situ* decompression
  - Failed *in situ* release

Contraindications (for Subcutaneous Technique)

- *Relative*: Very thin body habitus (consider intramuscular or submuscular technique)

Pearls

- The three vascular pedicles to the ulnar nerve should be preserved if possible when mobilizing the ulnar nerve.
- Perform careful dissection of the motor branches to the FCU. Sacrifice of first motor branch along with articular branches is often necessary for adequate anterior mobilization of the nerve.
- Plan fasciodermal (or ligamentodermal) sling by laying down the anterior skin flap over the medial epicondyle to simulate closure.

Pitfalls

- Use caution to protect the branches of the medial antebrachial cutaneous nerve while elevating the subcutaneous flaps for this approach.
- Avoid creating new sites of compression; a complete release should be performed to prevent kinking from the medial intermuscular septum, the flexor-pronator fascia, and the FCU fascia.
- Use caution not to over-constrain the nerve with stabilizing sling or flap.
- Consider patient habitus; very thin individuals may be susceptible to blunt injury to the ulnar nerve after subcutaneous transposition.
- If the dermis is felt to be tenuous, consider a fascial sling or intramuscular/submuscular technique.

References

1. Curtis B. Traumatic ulnar neuritis – transplantation of the nerve. J Nerv Ment Dis. 1898;25:480.
2. Prevel CD, Matloub HS, Ye Z, Sanger JR, John Yousif N. The extrinsic blood supply of the ulnar nerve at the elbow: an anatomic study. J Hand Surg Am. 1993;18:433–8.
3. Sunderland S. Blood supply of the nerve of the upper limb in man. Arch Neurol Psychiatry. 1945;53:91–115.
4. Nakamura K, Uchiyama S, Ido Y, Itsubo T, Hayashi M, Murakami H, et al. The effect of vascular pedicle preservation on blood flow and clinical outcome following ulnar nerve transposition. J Hand Surg Am. 2014;39:291–302.
5. Sugawara M. Experimental and clinical studies of the vascularized anterior transposition of the ulnar nerve for cubital tunnel syndrome. J Jpn Orthop Assoc. 1988;62:755–66.
6. Ogata K, Orthopaedic FT, Shimon S, Owen J, Manske PR. Effects of compression and devascularisation on ulnar nerve function: a quantitative study of regional blood flow and nerve conduction in monkeys. J Hand Surg. 1991;16B:104–8.
7. Ogata K, Manske PR, Lesker PA. The effect of surgical dissection on regional blood flow to the ulnar nerve in the cubital tunnel. Clin Orthop Relat Res. 1985;(193):195–8.
8. Dellon AL, Chang E, Henk Coert J, Campbell KR. Intraneural ulnar nerve pressure changes related to operative techniques for cubital tunnel decompression. J Hand Surg Am. 1994;19:923–30.
9. Gelberman RH, Yamaguchi K, Hollstien SB, Winn SS, Heidenreich FP, Bindra RR, et al. Changes in interstitial pressure and cross-sectional area of the cubital tunnel and of the ulnar nerve with flexion of the elbow: an experimental study in human cadavera. J Bone Joint Surg Am. 1998;80:492–501.
10. Green JR, Rayan GM. The cubital tunnel: anatomic, histologic, and biomechanical study. J Shoulder Elbow Surg. 1999;8:466–70.
11. Pechan J, Juliš I. The pressure measurement in the ulnar nerve. A contribution to the pathophysiology of the cubital tunnel syndrome. J Biomech. 1975;8:75–9.
12. Iba K, Wada T, Aoki M, Tsuji H, Oda T, Yamashita T. Intraoperative measurement of pressure adjacent to the ulnar nerve in patients with cubital tunnel syndrome. J Hand Surg Am. 2006;31:553–8.

13. Macnicol M. Extraneural pressures affecting the ulnar nerve at the elbow. Hand. 1982;14:5–11.
14. Apfelberg D, Larson S. Dynamic anatomy of the ulnar nerve at the elbow. Plast Reconstr Surg. 1973;51:79–81.
15. Grewal R, Varitimidis SE, Vardakas DG, Fu FH, Sotereanos DG. Ulnar nerve elongation and excursion in the cubital tunnel after decompression and anterior transposition. J Hand Surg Br. 2000; 25(5):457–60.
16. Foran I, Vaz K, Sikora-Klak J, Ward S, Hentzen E, Shah S. Regional ulnar nerve strain following decompression and anterior subcutaneous transposition in patients with cubital tunnel syndrome. J Hand Surg. 2016;41:e343–50.
17. Eaton RG, Crowe JF, Parkes JC. Anterior transposition of the ulnar nerve using a non-compressing fasciodermal sling. J Bone Joint Surg Am. 1980;62:820–5.
18. Danoff JR, Lombardi JM, Rosenwasser MP. Use of a pedicled adipose flap as a sling for anterior subcutaneous transposition of the ulnar nerve. J Hand Surg Am. 2014;39:552–5.
19. Pribyl CR, Robinson B. Use of the medial intermuscular septum as a fascial sling during anterior transposition of the ulnar nerve. J Hand Surg Am. 1998;23:500–4.
20. Tan V, Pope J, Daluiski A, Capo JT, Weiland AJ. The V-Sling: a modified medial intermuscular septal sling for anterior transposition of the ulnar nerve. J Hand Surg Am. 2004;29:325–7.
21. Verveld CJ, Danoff JR, Lombardi JM, Rosenwasser MP. Adipose flap versus fascial sling for anterior subcutaneous transposition of the ulnar nerve. Am J Orthop. 2016;45:53–7.
22. Glickel S, Gupta S, Catalano L. Decision making and operative tactics for ulnar nerve compression at the elbow. Tech Shoulder Elb Surg. 2006;7:52–60.
23. Watchmaker G, Lee G, Mackinnon S. Intraneural topography of the ulnar nerve in the cubital tunnel facilitates anterior transposition. J Hand Surg. 1994;19A:915–22.
24. Goldberg J, Burnham J, Dhawan V. Subcutaneous ulnar nerve transposition using Osborne's ligament as a ligamentodermal ligamentofascial sling. Am J Orthop. 2018;47:1–11.
25. Gruber H, Baur EM, Plaikner M, Loizides A. The ulnar nerve after surgical transposition: can sonography define the reason of persisting neuropathy? Fortschr Röntgenstr. 2015;187:998–1002.
26. Black B, Barron O, Townsend P, Glickel S, Eaton R. Stabilized subcutaneous ulnar nerve transposition with immediate range of motion. J Bone Joint Surg Am. 2000;82–A:1544–51.
27. Weirich SD, Gelberman RH, Best SA, Abrahamsson SO, Furcolo DC, Lins RE. Rehabilitation after subcutaneous transposition of the ulnar nerve: immediate versus delayed mobilization. J Shoulder Elbow Surg. 1998;7:244–9.
28. Bartels RHMA, Termeer EH, Van Der Wilt GJ, Van Rossum LGM, Meulstee J, Verhagen WIM, et al. Simple decompression or anterior subcutaneous transposition for ulnar neuropathy at the elbow: a costminimization analysis – part 2. Neurosurgery. 2005;56:531–5.
29. Bacle G, Marteau E, Freslon M, Desmoineaux P, Saint-Cast Y, Lancigu R, et al. Cubital tunnel syndrome: comparative results of a multicenter study of 4 surgical techniques with a mean follow-up of 92 months. Orthop Traumatol Surg Res. 2014;100:S205–8.
30. Gökay NS, Bagatur AE. Subcutaneous anterior transposition of the ulnar nerve in cubital tunnel syndrome. Acta Orthop Traumatol Turc. 2012;46:243–9.
31. Liu XH, Gong MQ, Wang Y, Liu C, Li SL, Jiang XY. Anterior subcutaneous transposition of the ulnar nerve affects elbow range of motion: a mean 13.5 years of follow-up. Chin Med J. 2018;131:282–8.
32. Staples R, London DA, Dardas AZ, Goldfarb CA, Calfee RP. Comparative morbidity of cubital tunnel surgeries: a prospective cohort study. J Hand Surg Am. 2018;43:207–13.
33. Chan R, Paine K, Varughese G. Ulnar neuropathy at the elbow: comparison of simple decompression and anterior transposition. Neurosurgery. 1980;7:545–50.
34. Bartels RHMA, Verhagen WIM, Van Der Wilt GJ, Meulstee J, Van Rossum LGM, Grotenhuis JA. Prospective randomized controlled study comparing simple decompression versus anterior subcutaneous transposition for idiopathic neuropathy of the ulnar nerve at the elbow: part 1. Neurosurgery. 2005;56:522–9.
35. Nabhan A, Ahlhelm F, Kelm J, Reith W, Schwerdtfeger K, Steudel WI. Simple decompression or subcutaneous anterior transposition of the ulnar nerve for cubital tunnel syndrome. J Hand Surg Am. 2005;30:521–4.
36. Tawfik MR, Khedr WM, Sakr MF, Farhoud AH, Fawzy W, Saadany E. Comparative study of outcome of simple decompression versus anterior transposition of ulnar nerve in the treatment of cubital tunnel syndrome. Natl J Health Sci. 2017;2:52–6.
37. Macadam SA, Gandhi R, Bezuhly M, Lefaivre KA. Simple decompression versus anterior subcutaneous and submuscular transposition of the ulnar nerve for cubital tunnel syndrome: a meta-analysis. J Hand Surg Am. 2008;33:1–12.
38. Zlowodzki M, Chan S, Bhandari M, Kalliainen L, Schubert W. Anterior transposition compared with simple decompression for treatment of cubital tunnel syndrome: a meta-analysis of randomized, controlled trials. J Bone Joint Surg Am. 2007;89(A):2591–8.
39. Chen HW, Ou S, Liu GD, Fei J, Zhao GS, Wu LJ, et al. Clinical efficacy of simple decompression versus anterior transposition of the ulnar nerve for the treatment of cubital tunnel syndrome: a meta-analysis. Clin Neurol Neurosurg. 2014;126:150–5.

15 Submuscular Transposition of the Ulnar Nerve

Maureen A. O'Shaughnessy and Marco Rizzo

Introduction

This chapter will delve into the surgical technique of submuscular transposition of the ulnar nerve. The chapter will cover the background of nerve transposition, the indications, described modifications of surgical technique, and outcomes. We will also cover in detail the authors' preferred surgical technique and postoperative care for submuscular transposition of the ulnar nerve.

Background

Ulnar neuropathy describes a spectrum of pathology. Ulnar pathology can masquerade in various ways, with compression coming from the spinal column, thoracic outlet, elbow, or wrist. The etiology may be from bony or muscular compression, vascular disorder, or even be physiologic.

The ulnar nerve receives its innervation from cervical roots C8–T1 which coalesce to form the medial cord of the brachial plexus. The primary function of the nerve is to supply the critical sensation and fine motor functions at the most distal hand and digits. Pathology leads to clawing of the hand and atrophy of the intrinsic muscles. Few options exist for the end-stage disease, with tendon transfers being much less successful than those for pathology of the radial or median nerves. Therefore, it is imperative to treat the disease early to avoid the dreaded late outcomes.

As previously described in other chapters, there are many ways to surgically manage cubital tunnel. The nerve may be released in situ (also known as simple decompression) or be mobilized to another position, called transposition. Various means to transpose the nerve have been described including subcutaneous, subfascial, sub- or intramuscular. Medial epicondylectomy has also been described. The surgical approach to nerve decompression has always had supporters of various anatomic approaches by master surgeons, signifying that no consensus has been reached.

Stability of the ulnar nerve at the elbow is a key element in discussion of what to do with the nerve. Patients with evidence of nerve subluxation on preoperative exam may worsen if the nerve is not stabilized with some type of transposition or epicondylectomy. The same can be said for a nerve which preoperatively is stable at the elbow in flexion and extension but becomes unstable intraoperatively after surgical decompression. Many surgeons argue that an unstable ulnar nerve (noted either pre- or intraoperatively) should be transposed.

M. A. O'Shaughnessy
Department of Orthopaedic Surgery, University of Kentucky, Lexington, KY, USA

M. Rizzo (✉)
Department of Orthopedic Surgery, Mayo Clinic, Rochester, MN, USA
e-mail: rizzo.marco@mayo.edu

D. G. Sotereanos, L. K. Papatheodorou (eds.), *Compressive Neuropathies of the Upper Extremity*,
https://doi.org/10.1007/978-3-030-37289-7_15

Revision cubital tunnel surgery is discussed in further detail in following chapters. However, it warrants mention in this section given that many of authors recommend submuscular anterior transposition for cases of revision surgery to help decrease the risk of perineural scarring and adhesions [1, 2].

History of Submuscular Transposition

The ulnar nerve courses posterior to the axis of rotation at the medial elbow putting it at risk of traction and compression with elbow flexion, potentially compromising its microcirculation; anterior transposition can eliminate these forces [3]. By moving the nerve to an anterior location, embedded within protective muscle, the local compressive and traction forces can theoretically be decreased. Advocates of transposition say that this addresses the dynamic compression of the nerve that occurs in elbow flexion [4, 5]. In submuscular transposition, the nerve is well protected and lies deep below substantial soft tissue [6]. Submuscular transposition lies close to the axis of motion and can eliminate iatrogenic-induced strain [7, 8]. The true submuscular pathway places the nerve directly over the elbow joint capsule which becomes the new bed in which the nerve lies [7].

The first description of the submuscular transposition was by Learmonth in 1942 [9]. This is what we now call anterior submuscular transposition (ASMT) of the ulnar nerve. Learmonth's technique was to detach the flexor-pronator mass from its insertion on the medial humeral epicondyle. The decompressed ulnar nerve was then transposed anteriorly and medially to the midline to lie next to the median nerve, coursing just over the smooth gliding surface of the anterior ulnohumeral joint capsule. The flexor-pronator mass was then reattached. Patients required postoperative splinting for several weeks with the elbow and the wrist flexed to ensure the musculotendinous insertion healed back to the epicondyle [10].

Dellon began using a modification of the Learmonth submuscular technique in 1980 and published his surgical technique several years later [10, 11]. This technique modification is referred to as a z-lengthening or V-Y advancement anterior submuscular transposition. Dellon's technique lengthens the flexor-pronator fascia to create space for the ulnar nerve in its transposed position while allowing repair of the flexor-pronator attachment without tension, all while allowing immediate flexion and extension of the elbow [10]. This modification is arguably the most common technique for ASMT currently. We refer the reader to a well-written surgical technique article by Dellon et al. in which they describe the V-Y submuscular lengthening in detail with clear intraoperative images and prudent surgical pearls [12].

A modification of the submuscular is intramuscular transposition, Adson is credited with first describing this in 1918 [13]. This modification consists of creating a trough in the flexor-pronator musculature in the projected line of pull of the nerve in its anterior transposed position [7, 14–17]. In this transposition, the flexor-pronator mass is *not* detached from the medial epicondyle. Proponents argue this allows earlier mobilization and less local trauma. Fascial flaps are raised, the muscular trough created, and the nerve is placed in its intramuscular position. Fascial flaps are repaired in a lengthened position to avoid undue tension on the nerve. This allows almost immediate mobilization of the wrist and elbow for early nerve gliding. A recent modification published by Henry merges the intramuscular and submuscular techniques and allows almost immediate motion for early nerve gliding [7].

Critics state that an intramuscular position may create a fibrotic scarring bed on the nerve that traps it and obstructs longitudinal nerve gliding [6]. However, work by Dellon et al. found no significant difference in nerve fibrosis, mean nerve fiber diameter, or percent of neural tissue when placing the ulnar nerve in a submuscular versus intramuscular position in a primate model [18].

In our review of the current literature, few current articles describe the intramuscular transposition which may hint that this technique has declined in popularity in relation to the modified submuscular transposition.

Several biomechanical and histologic studies have been published on ulnar nerve decompression and/or transposition. A biomechanical analysis using a micro-strain recording device found that 22 mm of ulnar nerve excursion is required at the elbow to prevent undue strain on the nerve [19]; any surgery aiming to mobilize the ulnar nerve at the elbow should aim to allow at least 2 cm of excursion.

Dellon et al. performed a cadaveric study to evaluate intraneural pressures following the common ulnar decompression techniques [20]. The authors found that ulnar nerve transposition and musculofascial lengthening reduced intraneural pressures both in elbow extension and flexion at 30°, 60°, and 90° by a minimum of 40% when compared to in situ decompression, medial epicondylectomy, subcutaneous transposition, and traditional Learmonth submuscular transposition.

A recent histologic study on a rat model showed healthier axons and less perineural scar tissue in rats treated with submuscular transposition compared to subcutaneous method [3].

Disadvantages of transposition include complexity of the procedure, extensive tissue dissection, risk of nerve devascularization, intraneural injury, perineural fibrosis, and chance of injury to the motor branch to the flexor carpi ulnaris (FCU) [21, 22]. Postoperative elbow immobilization may lead to contracture and prevent nerve gliding which can lead to adhesions.

Comparative Trials

In the early 2000s, studies emerged pitting head-to-head simple decompression and transposition. Gervasio et al. performed a prospective randomized trial of 70 patients with either in situ or submuscular transposition and found no statistically significant difference in clinical or electrophysiologic outcomes [6]. Charles et al. published a retrospective review comparing in situ and submuscular transposition and found no significant difference in sensory or motor recovery in McGowan II and III patients [23]. They did find that patients with symptoms lasting longer than 6 months had a worse prognosis regardless of technique. Biggs et al. conducted a prospective randomized trial of 54 patients comparing in situ decompression and submuscular transposition; they noted equally effective neurologic improvement but higher wound complications in the submuscular technique [24].

Following the publication of these and other high-quality studies, systematic reviews and meta-analyses were able to be performed. A 2007 meta-analysis of four randomized controlled trials of simple decompression and anterior transposition found no difference in motor nerve-conduction velocities or clinical outcomes [25]. Chung performed a literature review in 2008 which showed that no single procedure had shown to be best. He concluded that based on review of the best available evidence, he had changed practice of using subcutaneous anterior transposition in favor of in situ release [26]. Published in 2008, Macadam et al. performed a meta-analysis of comparative trials or randomized controlled trials comparing in situ and transposition release. The authors found no statistically significant difference but a trend towards improved clinical outcomes with transposition as opposed to simple decompression [27].

Based on large national databases, it appears that the pendulum has shifted to favor simple decompression for primary nerve release. A 2013 study of the United States national ambulatory surgery data from 1996 to 2006 showed that transposition dropped from 49% to 38% in 2006, with women more likely to have simple decompression (70%) [28]. A more recent state-wide Florida database retrospective cross-sectional analysis for 2005–2012 showed that of over 26,000 cubital tunnel releases performed, 80% underwent had situ decompression, 16% underwent transposition, and 4% underwent "other" [29]. During the study period, there was a statistically significant increase in in situ release and decrease in transposition. Females and patients treated by high-volume surgeons had a statistically higher rate of in situ release. The published data did not state whether the data set could determine if release was primary or revision.

In a letter to the editor in response to results of the Charles et al. [23] study, MacKinnon eloquently described what appears to be the current approach to the ulnar nerve. MacKinnon argued that technical details of ulnar nerve surgery such as kinking of the ulnar nerve, appropriate decompression of the tendinous leading edge of the FCU, and respect for the medial brachial and antebrachial cutaneous nerves are likely more important than which procedure is done [30]. She also argued that simple decompression is likely to relieve symptoms in the majority of patients unless there is resultant subluxation of the nerve [30]. Charles et al. agreed but also noted that patients with major sensory or motor deficits or anatomic abnormalities around the epicondyle should be considered for transposition [23].

Surgical Indications

Surgical decompression of the ulnar nerve at the elbow should only be performed after appropriate clinical workup.

A comprehensive physical exam is critical. The surgeon should document objective motor strength (grading M0–M5) and sensory discrimination with Semmes-Weinstein monofilament or two-point discrimination testing. Specific motor testing should include flexor digitorum profundus (FDP) to small finger, FCU, and first dorsal interossei. Specific sensory testing should document the palmar small and ring finger, dorsal ulnar hand (DSBUN) , and the medial distal arm (MBC) to rule out brachial plexus origin. The DSBUN and MBC can be graded using a 0–10 scale by the patient given that two-point and monofilament is difficult for the patient at these sites.

The absence or presence of ulnar pathologic signs should be described; these may include Wartenburg, Froment, Testut, first dorsal interosseous wasting, and clawing. The McGowan classification is unique for ulnar neuropathy and can be helpful to standardize the publication of results [31].

Appropriate workup with electromyography (EMG) and nerve conduction velocity (NCV) studies are usually indicated. This is helpful not only for staging the disease but also to monitor recovery or progression of pathology and is essential in the unfortunate event of medicolegal conditions.

The surgeon may want to send the patient through a dedicated course of physical and/or occupational therapy. Therapists work on scapular stabilization and nerve gliding for thoracic etiology [32, 33] and nerve gliding with dart throwers and FCU gliding for compression at the elbow [34, 35]. Nighttime splinting of the elbow in extension is also indicated in the nonoperative management of the disease [36, 37].

Once the appropriate workup and nonoperative course has been completed, surgery may be indicated. Surgical techniques vary widely and ultimately lie at the discretion of the treating surgeon. As described earlier, in situ decompression is usually sufficient for a primary cubital tunnel. For many surgeons, the current treatment algorithm begins with in situ release followed by subcutaneous or submuscular transposition if perching, subluxation, or dislocation is noted during surgery [38]; most surgeons regard ulnar nerve subluxation or dislocation as an indication for transposition [25]. Additionally, transposition may be indicated for a revision ulnar neurolysis at the elbow to help prevent scar formation [1, 2].

Submuscular Transposition of the Author's Preferred Surgical Technique

Our current indication for the submuscular transposition is a patient with symptomatic ulnar nerve compression at the elbow. We prefer to obtain preoperative EMG and NCVs for all patients, as well as exhaust nonoperative measures including rest, nighttime splinting, physical therapy to include nerve gliding, and postural retraining. When these have failed, surgery is discussed with the patient.

In our experience, the majority of patients with primary cubital tunnel syndrome can be treated with simple decompression. Patients in whom we prefer to treat with transposition include those with evidence of nerve instability either pre- or intraoperatively. Additionally, we prefer this technique for revision decompression.

13. Macnicol M. Extraneural pressures affecting the ulnar nerve at the elbow. Hand. 1982;14:5–11.
14. Apfelberg D, Larson S. Dynamic anatomy of the ulnar nerve at the elbow. Plast Reconstr Surg. 1973;51:79–81.
15. Grewal R, Varitimidis SE, Vardakas DG, Fu FH, Sotereanos DG. Ulnar nerve elongation and excursion in the cubital tunnel after decompression and anterior transposition. J Hand Surg Br. 2000; 25(5):457–60.
16. Foran I, Vaz K, Sikora-Klak J, Ward S, Hentzen E, Shah S. Regional ulnar nerve strain following decompression and anterior subcutaneous transposition in patients with cubital tunnel syndrome. J Hand Surg. 2016;41:e343–50.
17. Eaton RG, Crowe JF, Parkes JC. Anterior transposition of the ulnar nerve using a non-compressing fasciodermal sling. J Bone Joint Surg Am. 1980;62:820–5.
18. Danoff JR, Lombardi JM, Rosenwasser MP. Use of a pedicled adipose flap as a sling for anterior subcutaneous transposition of the ulnar nerve. J Hand Surg Am. 2014;39:552–5.
19. Pribyl CR, Robinson B. Use of the medial intermuscular septum as a fascial sling during anterior transposition of the ulnar nerve. J Hand Surg Am. 1998;23:500–4.
20. Tan V, Pope J, Daluiski A, Capo JT, Weiland AJ. The V-Sling: a modified medial intermuscular septal sling for anterior transposition of the ulnar nerve. J Hand Surg Am. 2004;29:325–7.
21. Verveld CJ, Danoff JR, Lombardi JM, Rosenwasser MP. Adipose flap versus fascial sling for anterior subcutaneous transposition of the ulnar nerve. Am J Orthop. 2016;45:53–7.
22. Glickel S, Gupta S, Catalano L. Decision making and operative tactics for ulnar nerve compression at the elbow. Tech Shoulder Elb Surg. 2006;7:52–60.
23. Watchmaker G, Lee G, Mackinnon S. Intraneural topography of the ulnar nerve in the cubital tunnel facilitates anterior transposition. J Hand Surg. 1994;19A:915–22.
24. Goldberg J, Burnham J, Dhawan V. Subcutaneous ulnar nerve transposition using Osborne's ligament as a ligamentodermal ligamentofascial sling. Am J Orthop. 2018;47:1–11.
25. Gruber H, Baur EM, Plaikner M, Loizides A. The ulnar nerve after surgical transposition: can sonography define the reason of persisting neuropathy? Fortschr Röntgenstr. 2015;187:998–1002.
26. Black B, Barron O, Townsend P, Glickel S, Eaton R. Stabilized subcutaneous ulnar nerve transposition with immediate range of motion. J Bone Joint Surg Am. 2000;82–A:1544–51.
27. Weirich SD, Gelberman RH, Best SA, Abrahamsson SO, Furcolo DC, Lins RE. Rehabilitation after subcutaneous transposition of the ulnar nerve: immediate versus delayed mobilization. J Shoulder Elbow Surg. 1998;7:244–9.
28. Bartels RHMA, Termeer EH, Van Der Wilt GJ, Van Rossum LGM, Meulstee J, Verhagen WIM, et al. Simple decompression or anterior subcutaneous transposition for ulnar neuropathy at the elbow: a costminimization analysis – part 2. Neurosurgery. 2005;56:531–5.
29. Bacle G, Marteau E, Freslon M, Desmoineaux P, Saint-Cast Y, Lancigu R, et al. Cubital tunnel syndrome: comparative results of a multicenter study of 4 surgical techniques with a mean follow-up of 92 months. Orthop Traumatol Surg Res. 2014;100:S205–8.
30. Gökay NS, Bagatur AE. Subcutaneous anterior transposition of the ulnar nerve in cubital tunnel syndrome. Acta Orthop Traumatol Turc. 2012;46:243–9.
31. Liu XH, Gong MQ, Wang Y, Liu C, Li SL, Jiang XY. Anterior subcutaneous transposition of the ulnar nerve affects elbow range of motion: a mean 13.5 years of follow-up. Chin Med J. 2018;131:282–8.
32. Staples R, London DA, Dardas AZ, Goldfarb CA, Calfee RP. Comparative morbidity of cubital tunnel surgeries: a prospective cohort study. J Hand Surg Am. 2018;43:207–13.
33. Chan R, Paine K, Varughese G. Ulnar neuropathy at the elbow: comparison of simple decompression and anterior transposition. Neurosurgery. 1980;7:545–50.
34. Bartels RHMA, Verhagen WIM, Van Der Wilt GJ, Meulstee J, Van Rossum LGM, Grotenhuis JA. Prospective randomized controlled study comparing simple decompression versus anterior subcutaneous transposition for idiopathic neuropathy of the ulnar nerve at the elbow: part 1. Neurosurgery. 2005;56:522–9.
35. Nabhan A, Ahlhelm F, Kelm J, Reith W, Schwerdtfeger K, Steudel WI. Simple decompression or subcutaneous anterior transposition of the ulnar nerve for cubital tunnel syndrome. J Hand Surg Am. 2005;30:521–4.
36. Tawfik MR, Khedr WM, Sakr MF, Farhoud AH, Fawzy W, Saadany E. Comparative study of outcome of simple decompression versus anterior transposition of ulnar nerve in the treatment of cubital tunnel syndrome. Natl J Health Sci. 2017;2:52–6.
37. Macadam SA, Gandhi R, Bezuhly M, Lefaivre KA. Simple decompression versus anterior subcutaneous and submuscular transposition of the ulnar nerve for cubital tunnel syndrome: a meta-analysis. J Hand Surg Am. 2008;33:1–12.
38. Zlowodzki M, Chan S, Bhandari M, Kalliainen L, Schubert W. Anterior transposition compared with simple decompression for treatment of cubital tunnel syndrome: a meta-analysis of randomized, controlled trials. J Bone Joint Surg Am. 2007;89(A):2591–8.
39. Chen HW, Ou S, Liu GD, Fei J, Zhao GS, Wu LJ, et al. Clinical efficacy of simple decompression versus anterior transposition of the ulnar nerve for the treatment of cubital tunnel syndrome: a meta-analysis. Clin Neurol Neurosurg. 2014;126:150–5.

40. Adelaar RS, Foster WC, McDowell C. The treatment of the cubital tunnel syndrome. J Hand Surg Am. 1984;9A:90–5.
41. Paine K. Tardy ulnar palsy. Can J Surg. 1970;13:255–61.
42. Foster R, Edshage S. Factors related to the outcome of surgically managed compressive ulnar neuropathy at the elbow level. J Hand Surg. 1981;6:181–92.
43. Davies M, Vonau M, Blum P, Kwok B, Matheson J, Stening W. Results of ulnar neuropathy at the elbow treated by decompression or anterior transposition. Aust N Z J Surg. 1991;61:929–34.
44. Taha A, Galarza M, Zuccarello M, Taha J, Huang JH, Feinberg DM, et al. Outcomes of cubital tunnel surgery among patients with absent sensory nerve conduction. Neurosurgery. 2004;54:891–6.
45. Mitsionis G, Manoudis G, Paschos N, Korompilias A, Beris A. Comparative study of surgical treatment of ulnar nerve compression at the elbow. J Shoulder Elbow Surg. 2010;19:513–9.
46. Zhang D, Earp BE, Blazar P. Rates of complications and secondary surgeries after in situ cubital tunnel release compared with ulnar nerve transposition: a retrospective review. J Hand Surg Am. 2017;42:294.e1–5.
47. Adkinson JM, Zhong L, Aliu O, Chung KC. Surgical treatment of cubital tunnel syndrome: trends and the influence of patient and surgeon characteristics. J Hand Surg Am. 2015;40:1824–31.
48. Childress H. Recurrent ulnar nerve dislocation at the elbow. J Bone Joint Surg Am. 1956;38–A:978–84.
49. Catalano L, Barron O. Anterior subcutaneous transposition of the ulnar nerve. Hand Clin. 2007;23:339–44.
50. Lee S, Sharma S, Silver B, Kleinman G, Hausman M. Submuscular versus subcutaneous anterior ulnar nerve transposition: a rat histologic study. J Hand Surg Am. 2009;34:1811–4.
51. Jaddue DA, Saloo SA, Sayed-Noor AS. Subcutaneous vs submuscular ulnar nerve transposition in moderate cubital tunnel syndrome. Open Orthop J. 2009;3:78–82.
52. Stuffer M, Jungwirth W, Hussl H, Schmutzhardt E. Subcutaneous or submuscular anterior transposition of the ulnar nerve? J Hand Surg Am. 1992;17:248–50.
53. Charles YP, Coulet B, Rouzaud JC, Daures JP, Chammas M. Comparative clinical outcomes of submuscular and subcutaneous transposition of the ulnar nerve for cubital tunnel syndrome. J Hand Surg Am. 2009;34:866–74.
54. Rogers M, Bergfield T, Aulicino P. The failed ulnar nerve transposition. Etiology and treatment. Clin Orthop Relat Res. 1991;269:193–200.
55. Vogel RB, Nossaman BC, Rayan GM. Revision anterior submuscular transposition of the ulnar nerve for failed subcutaneous transposition. Br J Plast Surg. 2004;57:311–6.
56. Gabel GT, Amadio PC. Reoperation for failed decompression of the ulnar nerve in the region of the elbow. J Bone Joint Surg Am. 1990;72:213–9.
57. Caputo A, Watson H. Subcutaneous anterior transposition of the ulnar nerve for failed decompression of cubital tunnel syndrome. J Hand Surg. 2000;25:544–51.

In a primary release, the surgical approach includes a curvilinear incision centered at the medial elbow in between the medial epicondyle and the olecranon (Fig. 15.1). Tourniquet is inflated and skin is incised. Dissection is taken down with the knife through skin only, followed by careful dissection with tenotomies paying close attention to identifying the MBC and MABC (Fig. 15.2). These are protected with vessiloops to prevent iatrogenic damage during surgery.

The nerve is then identified running posteriorly below Osborne's ligament (Fig. 15.3). The nerve is carefully decompressed proximally to the level of the triceps medial intramuscular septum at the middle to distal third of the humerus as the nerve crosses through the septum from anterior to posterior (Fig. 15.4). We prefer to excise the medial intermuscular septum at the distal third of the arm. Attention is taken to release the entire arcade of Struthers and carefully divide Osborne's arcuate ligament. Distally, the tendinous leading edge of the two heads of the FCU is divided (Fig. 15.5). Further, distal dissection ensures the nerve is released up to the fascial origin of the flexor digitorum superficialis to the ring finger.

Care is taken to perform external neurolysis so as not to unduly strip the nerve in order to preserve the vascular supply to the epineurium (Fig. 15.6). The above-described additional mobilization both proximal and distal is often required to allow the nerve to move anteriorly to its transposed position. The previous identification and protection of the MBC and MABC with vessiloops helps to speed this step. The nerve is then pulled anteriorly to check that appropriate mobilization has been completed.

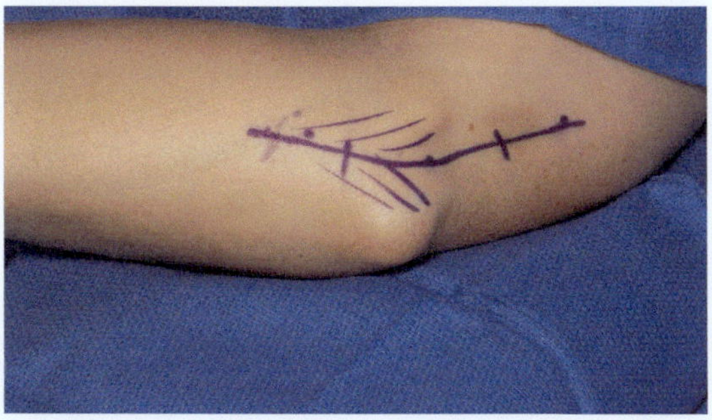

Fig. 15.1 Typical surgical incision for submuscular transposition centered at the medial elbow halfway between the olecranon and medial epicondyle

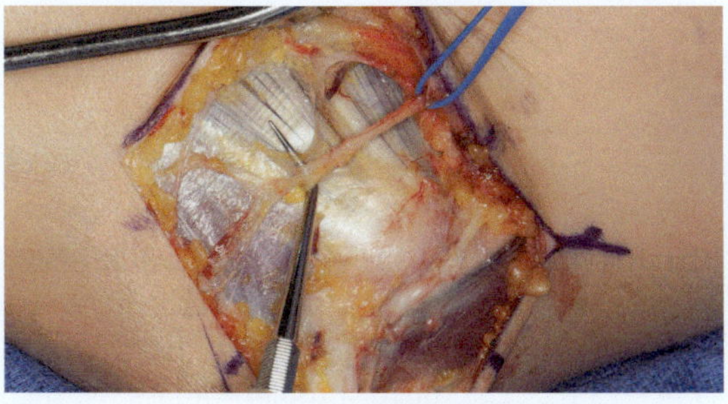

Fig. 15.2 After skin dissection, the medial brachial cutaneous nerve is identified and protected

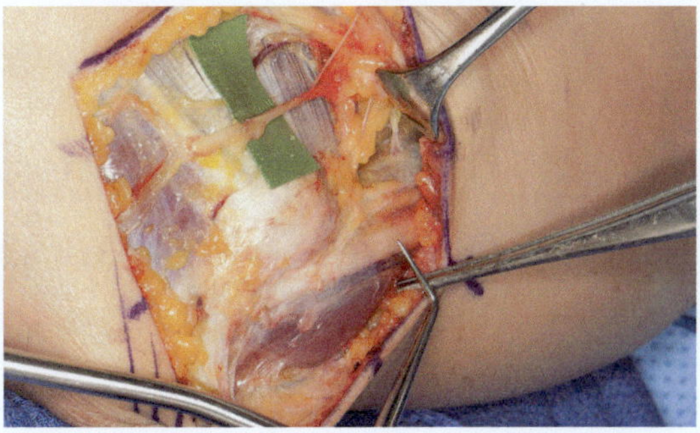

Fig. 15.3 Before decompression, the ulnar nerve is seen running posterior to the epicondyle, in the figure the probe is pointing to the nerve

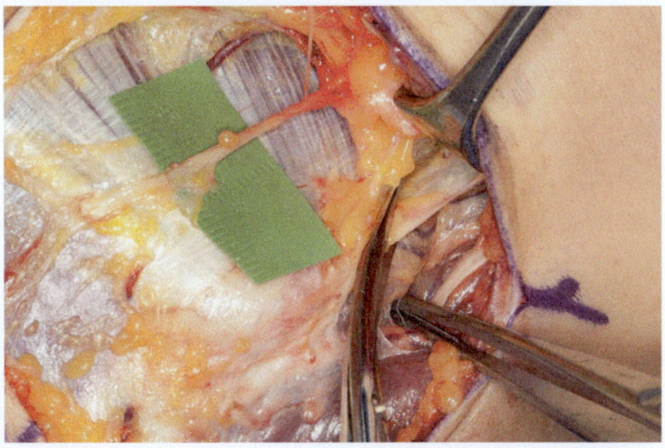

Fig. 15.4 The triceps intermuscular septum is carefully identified and excised to relief proximal sites of compression and to avoiding a site for kinking of the nerve after transposition

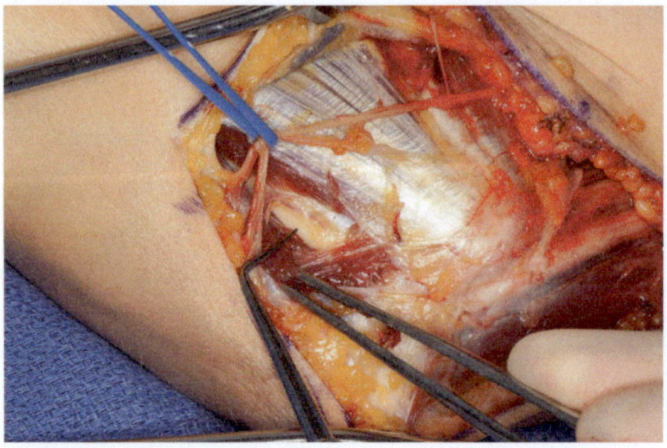

Fig. 15.5 The ulnar nerve is identified distally in the wound where the heads of the flexor carpi ulnaris are decompressed

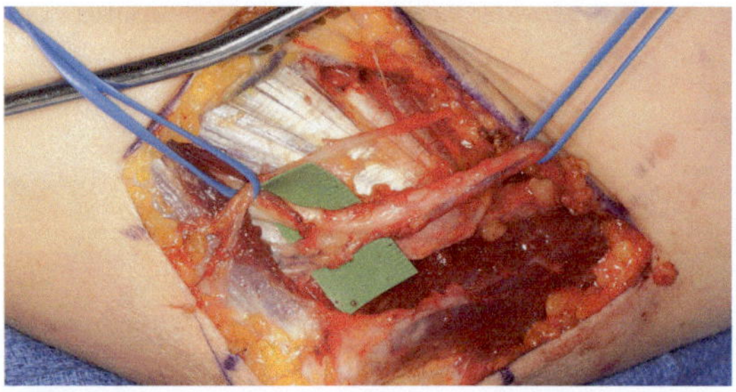

Fig. 15.6 The ulnar nerve is now decompressed and carefully lifted using vessiloops. The medial brachial cutaneous nerve is also seen anteriorly in the wound, protected by vessiloops

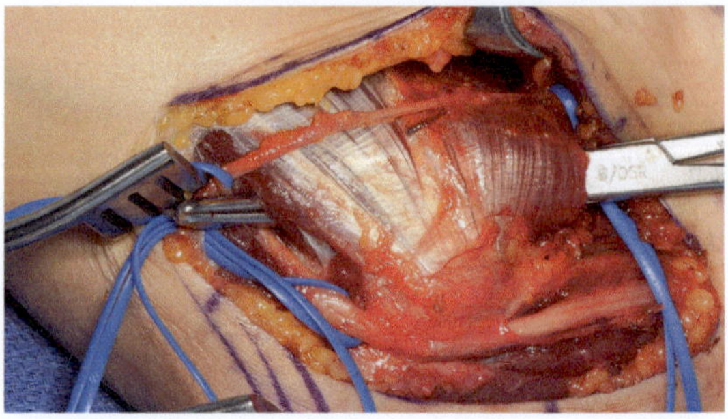

Fig. 15.7 Using gentle submuscular blunt dissection, the flexor-pronator mass is identified

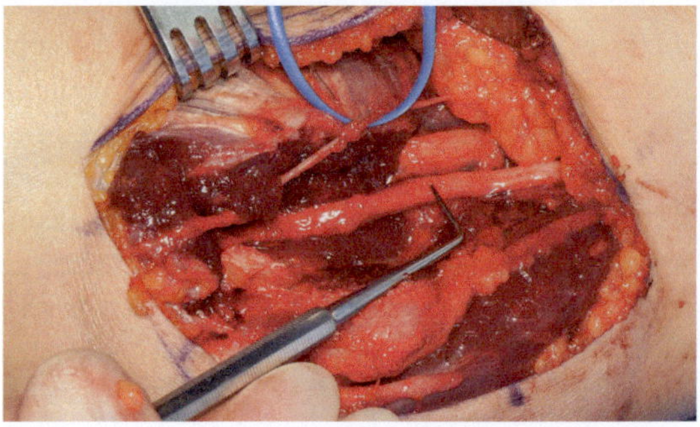

Fig. 15.8 After detachment of the flexor-pronator mass from its insertion, the ulnar nerve is placed into its transposed position

Once the nerve is sufficiently decompressed and mobilized, attention is turned to the submuscular transposition. Gentle dissection just below the flexor-pronator mass allows the muscular mass to be elevated with the least amount of intramuscular bleeding (Fig. 15.7). The flexor-pronator mass is then detached from the epicondyle en bloc, leaving a small cuff of facial attachment for later repair. Care is taken to mobilize the flexor-pronator mass medially to ensure no undue tension on the nerve.

Fractional lengthening is performed. The most superficial fascia is divided fully which allows several millimeters of increased muscular excursion. Several distinct longitudinal septa are present which are divided to allow fractional musculotendinous lengthening. The most important of these is the ring finger flexor digitorum superficialis origin. If not released at its origin, it creates a hard edge that the nerve winds around when it lies in its transposed position. The septa can be released in two stages, first when the nerve remains in situ and second during this second look.

The nerve bed is then chosen. We have noted that a natural plane can usually be found that runs parallel to the nerve's native course. The muscle fibers in this plane are carefully mobilized to create a trough the nerve will lie in. The bed is checked carefully for any remaining fascial fibers from previously divided septa that might create kinking and lead to adhesions.

The nerve is then moved anteriorly into its new submuscular position, sitting on top of the anterior elbow joint capsule and within the new muscular trough created to form its new bed (Fig. 15.8). The flexor-pronator mass is then pulled over the ulnar nerve and sutured down in a slightly loosened manner to prevent undue ten-

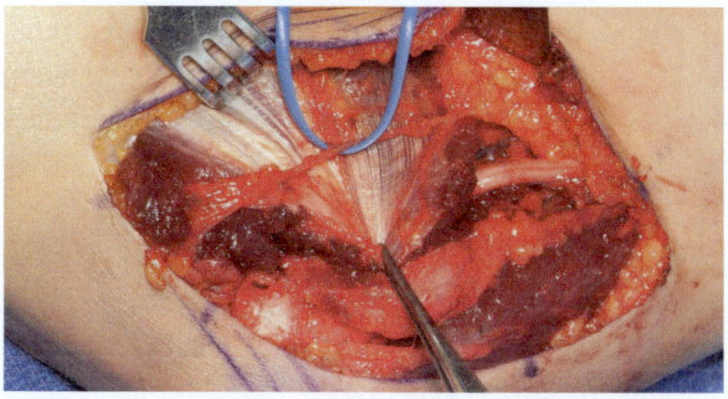

Fig. 15.9 The flexor-pronator mass is gently reapproximated and the nerve is checked to be free without any undue tension prior to approximation. If tension is noted, additional musculofascial lengthening should be performed

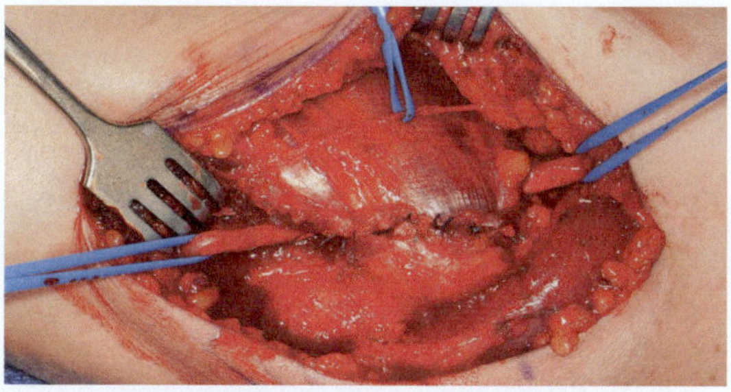

Fig. 15.10 Flexor-pronator mass is reattached using nonabsorbable suture to protect the repair

sion on the nerve in its transposed position (Fig. 15.9). We prefer to use non-absorbable suture such as 2-0 fiberwire. The elbow is then ranged through extension and flexion to ensure no kinking or excessive force on the nerve in the transposed position (Fig. 15.10).

Tourniquet is deflated and meticulous hemostasis obtained to help prevent postoperative hematoma. We prefer to leave a deep drain which is removed on postoperative day 1. Skin is closed in layers with deep dermal 3-0 absorbable monofilament, followed by either running 3-0 subcuticular absorbable monofilament or interrupted 3-0 nonabsorbable monofilament suture. A bulky compressive dressing is applied followed by a long arm splint with the arm at 70–90° of elbow flexion.

Depending on the stability of the repair, range of motion is usually begun at 10–14 days postoperatively and the patient is allowed early nerve gliding to decrease risk of adhesions and perineural scarring. The patient will work on motion for up to 6 weeks post-surgery and thereafter may initiate strengthening. They are typically released to unrestricted activity at 3 months postop.

Outcomes

Clinical outcomes are generally good for submuscular transposition. Dellon and Coert performed a prospective study of 161 extremities undergoing ASMT and found 88% good-excellent results at average follow-up of over 3.5 years [39]. Subgroup analysis found significant improvement among patient with diabetes, Workers' Compensation claim, and those with severe compression [39]. A study by Nouhan et al. found 97% good-excellent results [40], and Gervasio et al. noted 83% good-excellent outcomes [6]. Lee et al. performed a recent study of patients with severe disease undergoing V-Y lengthening ASMT; they noted 83% good-excellent results using a modified Bishop score [41]. Lee et al. noted a significant negative correlation between prolonged symptoms duration and modified Bishop score at final follow up, but age did not affect outcome [41].

Several studies have published objective results of nerve improvement. A prospective study of patients undergoing V-Y advancement ASMT found significant improvement in sensory and motor findings among all patients regardless of baseline nerve impairment [39]. A recent study of patients with severe disease (McGowan III) treated with submuscular transposition noted improvement of at least 1-McGowan grade in 94% of extremities [41]. Sixty-seven percent of patients had objective neurologic improvement in prospective randomized study in situ versus submuscular transposition [24].

The procedure is not without its complications. The incidence reported in the literature include symptomatic MABC neuroma requiring resection (1% [8] to 3% [39]), hematoma requiring drainage (0.5% [39]), reflex sympathetic dystrophy (1% [40]), and deep wound infection (1% [8] to 14% [24]).

Failure or recurrence rates with the submuscular technique vary. Dellon and Coert report 8% failure or recurrence [39] while Bacle et al. report a 7% recurrence rate [42]. A retrospective cohort study by Zhang et al. found secondary surgery rate of 11% for transposition compared to 2.5% for in situ release [8]. However, the results in Zhang et al.'s study may be skewed by selection bias given that patients undergoing transposition had higher McGowan grades and were more severe at baseline.

A recent systematic review by Macadam et al. showed that reliable, reproducible, and valid outcomes measures are lacking in the literature for cubital tunnel surgery [43]. The authors analyzed 42 studies and found 21 health outcomes measures, 2 generic instruments, 10 symptom-specific, author reported instruments; 3 symptom-specific, patient-reported instruments; and 6 patient questionnaires. Available data showed consistently high patient satisfaction after both simple decompression and submuscular transposition ranging from 65 to 92%, with no obvious association between author-reported and patient-reported results.

A multicenter group prospectively evaluated several outcome measures in patients undergoing simple decompression and found that the MHQ (Michigan Hand Questionnaire) and CTQ (Carpal Tunnel Questionnaire) are more responsive than DASH (Disabilities of the Arm, Shoulder and Hand) for ulnar neuropathy undergoing decompression [44]. These MHQ and CTQ questionnaires may be useful for detecting subtle outcomes differences in future studies of cubital tunnel decompression.

Summary

Submuscular transposition of the ulnar nerve can be technically demanding but, when indicated, can provide satisfactory outcomes for patients. Our preferred indication is a patient with nerve subluxation or in the revision setting. A short course of postoperative immobilization followed by early guided therapy can help improve nerve gliding and decrease risk of adhesions.

Our current body of evidence does not support the use of transposition over in situ release for primary surgery. Many authors argue that submuscular or intramuscular transposition is warranted in patients with instability or subluxation of the ulnar nerve, anatomic variants precluding in situ release, or in the revision setting [1, 2, 23, 30]. Regardless of specific technique, it is essential to fully decompress the nerve in an extra-neural fashion, preserve extrinsic vasculature, pay careful attention to protecting crossing cutaneous nerves, and ensure after mobilization that no undue tension or mechanical block precludes effortless, tension-free nerve gliding for optimal ulnar nerve recovery.

References

1. Vogel RB, Nossaman BC, Rayan GM. Revision anterior submuscular transposition of the ulnar nerve for failed subcutaneous transposition. Br J Plast Surg. 2004;57(4):311–6.
2. Ruchelsman DE, Lee SK, Posner MA. Failed surgery for ulnar nerve compression at the elbow. Hand Clin. 2007;23(3):359–71, vi–vii.
3. Lee SK, Sharma S, Silver BA, Kleinman G, Hausman MR. Submuscular versus subcutaneous anterior ulnar nerve transposition: a rat histologic study. J Hand Surg Am. 2009;34(10):1811–4.
4. Kleinman WB. Cubital tunnel syndrome: anterior transposition as a logical approach to complete nerve decompression. J Hand Surg Am. 1999;24(5):886–97.
5. Macnicol MF. The results of operation for ulnar neuritis. J Bone Joint Surg Br. 1979;61–B(2):159–64.
6. Gervasio O, Gambardella G, Zaccone C, Branca D. Simple decompression versus anterior submuscular transposition of the ulnar nerve in severe cubital tunnel syndrome: a prospective randomized study. Neurosurgery. 2005;56(1):108–17.
7. Henry M. Modified intramuscular transposition of the ulnar nerve. J Hand Surg Am. 2006;31(9):1535–42.
8. Zhang D, Earp BE, Blazar P. Rates of complications and secondary surgeries after in situ cubital tunnel release compared with ulnar nerve transposition: a retrospective review. J Hand Surg Am. 2017;42(4):294.e1–5.
9. Learmonth J. Technique for transplantation of the ulnar nerve. Surg Gynecol Obstet. 1942;75:792–3.
10. Williams EH, Dellon AL. Anterior submuscular transposition. Hand Clin. 2007;23(3):345–58.
11. Dellon A. Operative technique for submuscular transposition of the ulnar nerve. Oper Orthop. 1988;16:17–24.
12. Dellon AL, Coert JH. Results of the musculofascial lengthening technique for submuscular transposition of the ulnar nerve at the elbow. J Bone Joint Surg Am. 2004;86–A(Suppl 1(Pt 2)):169–79.
13. Adson A. The surgical treatment of progressive ulnar nerve paralysis. Minn Med. 1918;1:455–60.

14. Leone J, Bhandari M, Thoma A. Anterior intramuscular transposition with ulnar nerve decompression at the elbow. Clinial Orthop Relat Res. 2001;387: 132–9.
15. Kleinman WB, Bishop AT. Anterior intramuscular transposition of the ulnar nerve. J Hand Surg Am. 1989;14(6):972–9.
16. Glowacki KA, Weiss APC. Anterior intramuscular transposition of the ulnar nerve for cubital tunnel syndrome. J Shoulder Elb Surg. 1997;6(2):89–96.
17. Emamhadi M, Emamhadi A, Andalib S. Intramuscular compared with subcutaneous transposition for surgery in cubital tunnel syndrome. Ann R Coll Surg Engl. 2017;99(8):653–7.
18. Dellon AL, MacKinnon SE, Hudson AR, Hunter DA. Effect of submuscular versus intramuscular placement of ulnar nerve: experimental model in the primate. J Hand Surg Br. 1986;11(1):117–9.
19. Wright TW, Glowczewskie F, Cowin D, Wheeler DL. Ulnar nerve excursion and strain at the elbow and wrist associated with upper extremity motion. J Hand Surg Am. 2001;26(4):655–62.
20. Dellon AL, Chang E, Coert JH, Campbell KR. Intraneural ulnar nerve pressure changes related to operative techniques for cubital tunnel decompression. J Hand Surg Am. 1994;19(6):923–30.
21. Heithoff SJ. Cubital tunnel syndrome does not require transposition of the ulnar nerve. J Hand Surg Am. 1999;24(5):898–905.
22. Teoh LC, Yong FC, Tan SH, Andrew Chin YH. Anterior subfascial transposition of the ulnar nerve. J Hand Surg Br. 2003;28(1):73–6.
23. Charles YP, Coulet B, Rouzaud JC, Daures JP, Chammas M. Comparative clinical outcomes of submuscular and subcutaneous transposition of the ulnar nerve for cubital tunnel syndrome. J Hand Surg Am. 2009;34(5):866–74.
24. Biggs M, Curtis JA. Randomized, prospective study comparing ulnar neurolysis in situ with submuscular transposition. Neurosurgery. 2006;58(2):296–304; discussion 296–304.
25. Zlowodzki M, Chan S, Bhandari M, Kalliainen L, Schubert W. Anterior transposition compared with simple decompression for treatment of cubital tunnel syndrome. J Bone Joint Surg Am Vol. 2007;89(12):2591–8.
26. Chung KC. Treatment of ulnar nerve compression at the elbow. J Hand Surg Am. 2008;33(9):1625–7.
27. Macadam SA, Gandhi R, Bezuhly M, Lefaivre KA. Simple decompression versus anterior subcutaneous and submuscular transposition of the ulnar nerve for cubital tunnel syndrome: a meta-analysis. J Hand Surg Am. 2008;33(8):1314–24.
28. Soltani AM, Best MJ, Francis CS, Allan BJ, Panthaki ZJ. Trends in the surgical treatment of cubital tunnel syndrome: an analysis of the national survey of ambulatory surgery database. J Hand Surg Am. 2013;38(8):1551–6.
29. Adkinson JM, Zhong L, Aliu O, Chung KC. Surgical treatment of cubital tunnel syndrome: trends and the influence of patient and surgeon characteristics. J Hand Surg Am. 2015;40(9):1824–31.
30. Mackinnon SE. Comparative clinical outcomes of submuscular and subcutaneous transposition of the ulnar nerve for cubital tunnel syndrome. J Hand Surg Am. 2009;34(8):1574–5; author reply 1575.
31. McGowan AJ. The results of transposition of the ulnar nerve for traumatic ulnar neuritis. J Bone Joint Surg Br. 1950;32–B(3):293–301.
32. Gambhir RPS, Valenti D, Rashid H. Compliance with physical therapy is a key determinant of success of thoracic outlet surgical decompression. J Am Coll Surg. 2015;221(3):778.
33. Novak CB, Collins ED, Mackinnon SE. Outcome following conservative management of thoracic outlet syndrome. J Hand Surg Am. 1995;20(4):542–8.
34. Coppieters MW, Bartholomeeusen KE, Stappaerts KH. Incorporating nerve-gliding techniques in the conservative treatment of cubital tunnel syndrome. J Manip Physiol Ther. 2004;27(9):560–8.
35. Lund AT, Amadio PC. Treatment of cubital tunnel syndrome: perspectives for the therapist. J Hand Ther. 2006;19(2):170–9.
36. Szabo RM, Kwak C. Natural history and conservative management of cubital tunnel syndrome. Hand Clin. 2007;23:311–8.
37. Andrews K, Rowland A, Pranjal A, Ebraheim N. Cubital tunnel syndrome: anatomy, clinical presentation, and management. J Orthop. 2018;15:832–6.
38. Eberlin KR, Marjoua Y, Jupiter JB. Compressive neuropathy of the ulnar nerve: a perspective on history and current controversies. J Hand Surg. 2017;42:464–9.
39. Dellon AL, Coert JH. Results of the musculofascial lengthening technique for submuscular transposition of the ulnar nerve at the elbow. J Bone Joint Surg Am. 2003;85–A(7):1314–20.
40. Nouhan R, Kleinert JM. Ulnar nerve decompression by transposing the nerve and Z-lengthening the flexor-pronator mass: clinical outcome. J Hand Surg Am. 1997;22(1):127–31.
41. Lee SK, Lee GS, Choy WS. V-Y lengthening technique of the flexor-pronator mass for anterior submuscular transposition of the ulnar nerve in severe cubital tunnel syndrome. Ann Plast Surg. 2018;80(5):533–8.
42. Bacle G, Marteau E, Freslon M, Desmoineaux P, Saint-Cast Y, Lancigu R, et al. Cubital tunnel syndrome: comparative results of a multicenter study of 4 surgical techniques with a mean follow-up of 92 months. Orthop Traumatol Surg Res. 2014;100(4 Suppl):S205–8.
43. Macadam SA, Bezuhly M, Lefaivre KA. Outcomes measures used to assess results after surgery for cubital tunnel syndrome: a systematic review of the literature. J Hand Surg Am. 2009;34(8):1482–91.
44. Song JW, Waljee JF, Burns PB, Chung KC, Gaston RG, Haase SC, et al. An outcome study for ulnar neuropathy at the elbow: a multicenter study by the surgery for ulnar nerve (SUN) study group. Neurosurgery. 2013;72(6):971–81.

Minimal Medial Epicondylectomy

16

Loukia K. Papatheodorou, Dimitrios G. Vardakas, and Dean G. Sotereanos

Introduction

There are several accepted techniques for the surgical treatment of cubital tunnel syndrome [1]. Medial epicondylectomy combined with ulnar nerve decompression is one of them and its primary advantage is the preservation of the ulnar nerve's intraneural and extraneural blood supply, as compared to other ulnar nerve transposition techniques [2]. However, complications after conventional medial epicondylectomy, such as medial elbow instability and weakness related to detachment of the flexor pronator origin, have been reported [3–5].

To prevent these potential complications, investigators have advocated further modifications of the conventional medial epicondylectomy. The partial medial epicondylectomy is a modified technique in which approximately 40% of total width of medial epicondyle in the coronal plane is excised [6–9]. Despite the good outcomes that have been reported with the partial medial epicondylectomy, valgus instability of the elbow may occur postoperatively [8].

L. K. Papatheodorou · D. G. Sotereanos
Orthopaedic Specialists - UPMC,
University of Pittsburgh, Pittsburgh, PA, USA

D. G. Vardakas (✉)
General Hospital of Ioannina "G. Hatzikosta",
Department of Orthopaedic Surgery,
Ioannina, Greece

In an anatomic study of the medial ulnar collateral ligament in 10 cadaver elbows, O'Driscoll et al observed that only 19% of the width of the medial epicondyle in the coronal plane could be resected without potentially violating the anterior band of the medial collateral ligament [10]. Subsequently, authors have described modifications of the minimal medial epicondylectomy. With this modified technique, less than 20% of medial epicondyle in the coronal plane is excised, preserving the medial collateral ligament [11–15]. Thus the potential disadvantage of elbow instability can be minimized with the minimal medial epicondylectomy [11–14].

Indications

The minimal medial epicondylectomy combined with in situ ulnar nerve decompression is indicated for surgical treatment of primary cubital tunnel syndrome. This technique is particularly useful for cases of concomitant ulnar nerve subluxation, allowing smooth gliding of the ulnar nerve during the elbow range of motion.

In addition, the minimal medial epicondylectomy is indicated in cases of recurrent cubital tunnel syndrome after failed anterior, submuscular or subcutaneous, ulnar nerve transposition. In these cases, the posterior aspect of the ulnar nerve is compressed against the anterior aspect of the medial epicondyle, resulting in a z-deformity of

D. G. Sotereanos, L. K. Papatheodorou (eds.), *Compressive Neuropathies of the Upper Extremity*,
https://doi.org/10.1007/978-3-030-37289-7_16

the ulnar nerve [16, 17]. The minimal medial epicondylectomy, along with the revision decompression of the ulnar nerve, can eliminate the anterior tether by the medial epicondyle and allow the ulnar nerve to travel in a straight course throughout the elbow range of motion.

Surgical Technique

The minimal medial epicondylectomy combined with ulnar nerve decompression can be performed under general or regional anesthesia. The patient is positioned supine with the arm extended on a hand table. Under tourniquet control and loupe magnification, a medial incision 5 cm proximally and 5 cm distally to the medial epicondyle is made (Fig. 16.1). Dissection is carried down through the skin and subcutaneous tissue with attention being paid to identifying and protecting the medial antebrachial cutaneous nerve (Fig. 16.2).

The ulnar nerve is identified under the medial intermuscular septum, which is released and resected to avoid impingement on the nerve. The arcade of Struthers is released proximally and then the ulnar nerve is released through Osborne's ligament and the cubital tunnel (Fig. 16.3). Care is taken to release the Osborne ligament as posterior as possible to avoid subluxation of the ulnar nerve. Then the ulnar nerve is decompressed distally releasing the aponeurosis and deep fascia of

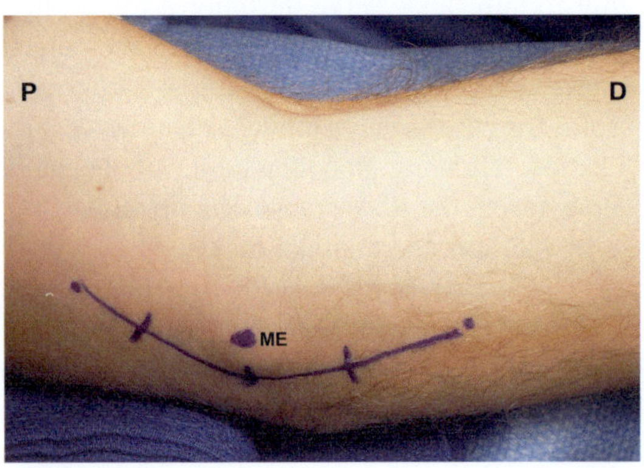

Fig. 16.1 Skin incision for minimal medial epicondylectomy centered over medial epicondyle. D: distal, P: proximal, ME: medial epicondyle

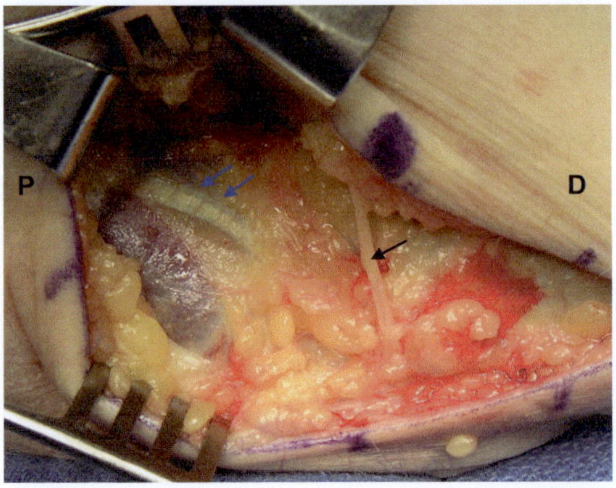

Fig. 16.2 Intra-operative photograph demonstrates identification of the medial antebrachial cutaneous nerve (black arrow) and the medial intermuscular septum (blue arrows). D: distal, P: proximal

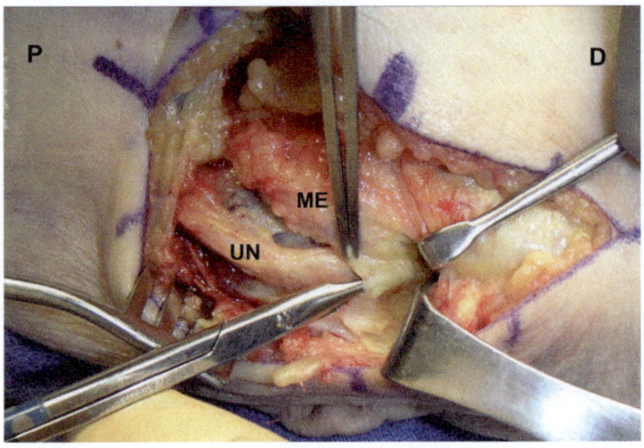

Fig. 16.3 Intra-operative photograph demonstrates release of the ulna nerve through Osborne's ligament and the cubital tunnel. UN: ulnar nerve, ME: medial epicondyle, D: distal, P: proximal

the flexor carpi ulnaris. Attention is paid to preserve the perineural bloody supply throughout the ulnar nerve decompression.

Upon completion of the ulnar nerve decompression, the medial epicondyle is exposed with a sharp subperiosteal dissection of the flexor-pronator origin. Care is taken to preserve good flaps anteriorly and posteriorly to facilitate closure (Fig. 16.4). Under visualization of the medial collateral ligament, a minimal, less than 20%, bony resection of the medial epicondyle is performed. The osteotomy is performed with the use of a small 12 mm osteotome, from distal to proximal, removing more bone posteriorly than

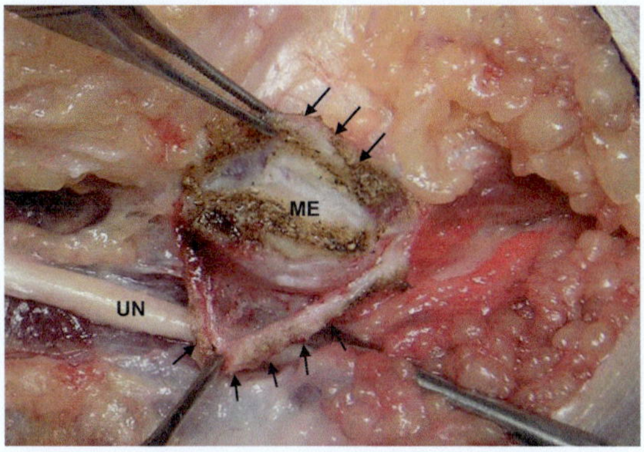

Fig. 16.4 Intra-operative photograph demonstrates the exposure of the medial epicondyle with subperiosteal dissection preserving good flaps anteriorly and posteriorly (black arrows). UN: ulnar nerve, ME: medial epicondyle

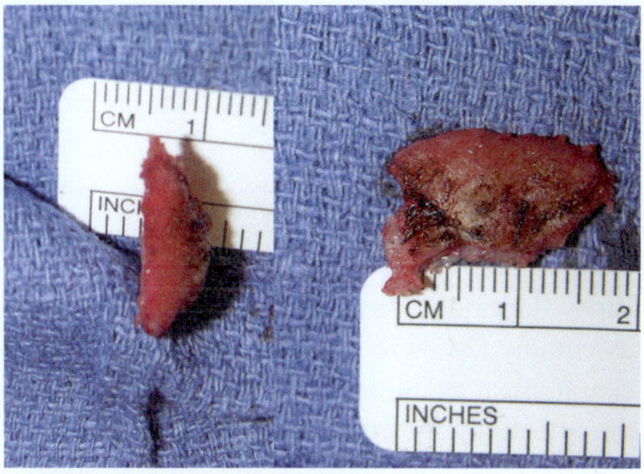

Fig. 16.6 Measurement of the size of the osteotomy fragment, less than 20% of the medial epicondyle was resected

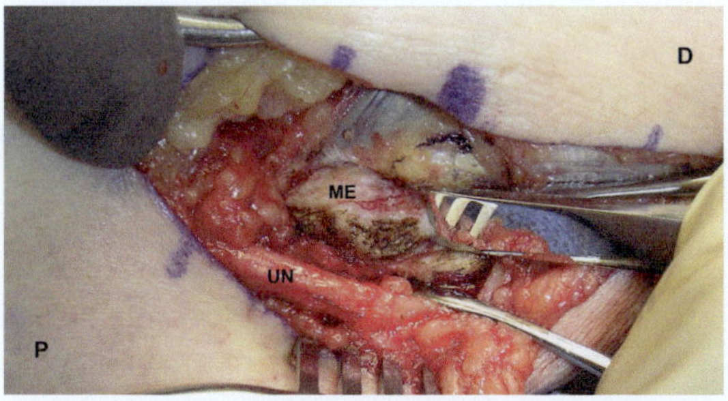

Fig. 16.5 Intra-operative photograph demonstrates the use of a small osteotome to perform a minimal medial epicondylectomy form distal to proximal. UN: ulnar nerve, ME: medial epicondyle, D: distal, P: proximal

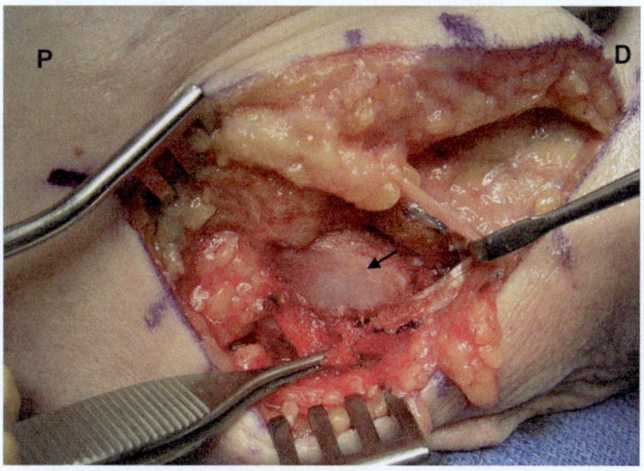

Fig. 16.7 Intra-operative photograph demonstrates the application of bone wax at the osteotomy site (black arrow). D: distal, P: proximal

anteriorly while protecting the anterior band of the medial collateral ligament (Figs. 16.5 and 16.6). After smoothing all sharp edges with a rongeur, bone wax is applied at the osteotomy site (Fig. 16.7) and the elbow is flexed and extended to ensure that the nerve is gliding over a smooth surface with elbow motion. Then, subperiosteal flap closure is performed with sutures buried (Fig. 16.8). Care is taken to ensure that the ulnar nerve is not subluxated anteriorly over the medial epicondyle with a dynamic flexion test of the elbow. After deflation of the tourniquet and proper hemostatsis, the wound is irrigated and the incision is closed in layers. At the conclusion of the procedure, the arm is placed in a bulky soft dressing. Early mobilization is suggested with gentle active range of motion exercises of the

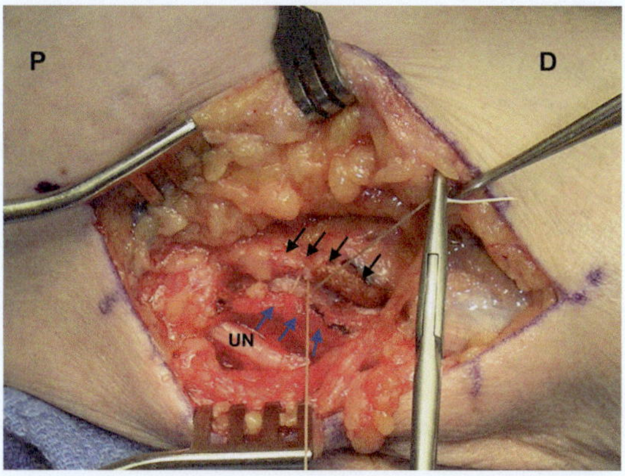

Fig. 16.8 Intra-operative photograph demonstrates subperiosteal flap closure (black arrows: anterior flap and blue arrows: posterior flap) with sutures buried. UN: ulnar nerve

elbow on the first postoperative day. Normal elbow motion is encouraged at the beginning of the second postoperative week.

Complications

Elbow instability can occur after medial epicondylectomy [3–5]. To avoid this potential complication, great attention must be paid to the size of the osteotomy. When less than 20% of the width of the medial epicondyle in the coronal plane is resected the risk of injury of the anterior band of the medial collateral ligament is minimized preventing valgus instability of the elbow.

Additional reported complications after medial epicondylectomy include grip weakness, tenderness at the osteotomy site and ulna nerve subluxation [3–8, 14, 16]. Grip weakness related to detachment of the flexor pronator origin can be avoided with careful dissection. Transient medial elbow pain at the site of osteotomy may occur up to 6–12 months after minimal medial epicondylectomy [3–8, 11–14]. To avoid ulna nerve subluxation over the remaining medial epicondyle, correct surgical technique must be used to create smooth surface allowing the ulnar nerve to freely glide throughout the elbow motion. The risk of damage to the medial antebrachial cutaneous nerve can be lessened by careful dissection.

Outcomes

In general, the clinical outcomes of minimal epicondylectomy were reported as 79–94% good to excellent based on the Wilson and Krout criteria [6–9, 11–14]. These results compare favorably to those of the other surgical treatment options for cubital tunnel syndrome. However, it is difficult to compare the outcomes between surgical techniques due to the lack of randomized prospective studies and the heterogeneity in reports.

Based on the Wilson and Krout grading system [18], excellent means minimal sensory and motor deficit and no tenderness at the incision site; good means mild deficit but occasional ache or tenderness at the incision or osteotomy site; fair means an improvement but persistent deficit; and poor means no improvement or a worsened condition.

Gobel et al reviewed 64 patients (66 elbows) with cubital tunnel syndrome that were treated with minimal medial epicondylectomy [11]. Excellent outcomes were reported in 44%, good in 35%, fair in 10% and poor in 6% of patients [11]. The authors noted no clinical signs of elbow instability, ulnar nerve subluxation or ulnar nerve palsy during the follow up period [11]. Similar results were reported by Kim et al in 25 patients after minimal medial epicondylectomy [12]. The authors reported excellent results in 64%, good in 20%, fair in 8% and poor in 8% of patients [12]. None of the patients showed clinical evidence of ulnar nerve subluxation or medial elbow instability after the minimal medial epicondylectomy [12].

In another clinical study, Osei et al evaluated 27 patients treated with a modified oblique minimal medial epicondylectomy for cubital tunnel syndrome [13]. The authors achieved good to excellent results in 25 of 27 patients (93%) according to the Wilson and Krout criteria [13]. No symptomatic ulnar nerve subluxation or elbow instability with valgus stress testing was noted postoperatively [13].

Beak et al performed a retrospective study of 56 patients with cubital tunnel syndrome, comparing the outcomes between minimal medial epicondylectomy and the anterior subcutaneous transposition [19]. In the 22 patients who were treated with minimal medial epicondylectomy, excellent results were reported in 41%, good in 45%, fair in 9% and poor in 5% of patients [19]. In the 34 patients who were treated with anterior subcutaneous transposition, excellent results were reported in 41%, good in 38%, fair in 6% and poor in 3% of patients [19]. The authors found no significant difference between the two surgical techniques [19].

In the senior author's (D.G.S.) personal series, since the original clinical study [11], consistently good to excellent results with the minimal medial epicondylectomy have been noted in more than three hundred patients with primary or recurrent cubital tunnel syndome.

Conclusion

The minimal medial epicondylectomy is an effective alternative technique for the surgical treatment of primary or recurrent cubital tunnel syndrome. This technique can address the compressive and tensile forces on the ulnar nerve while minimizing injury to the blood supply to the ulnar nerve. However, great attention must be paid to the size of the osteotomy to avoid potential complications. Resection less than 20% of the width of the medial epicondyle in the coronal plane can minimize the risk of damage of the anterior band of the medial collateral ligament preventing valgus instability of the elbow.

References

1. Adkinson JM, Zhong L, Aliu O, Chung KC. Surgical treatment of cubital tunnel syndrome: trends and the influence of patient and surgeon characteristics. J Hand Surg Am. 2015;40(9):1824–31.
2. Ogata K, Manske PR, Lesker PA. The effect of surgical dissection on regional blood flow to the ulnar nerve in the cubital tunnel. Clin Orthop Relat Res. 1985;193:195–8.
3. Heithoff SJ, Millender LH, Nalebuff EA, Petruska AJ Jr. Medial epicondylectomy for the treatment of ulnar nerve compression at the elbow. J Hand Surg Am. 1990;15(1):22–9.
4. Bednar MS, Blair SJ, Light TR. Complications of the treatment of cubital tunnel syndrome. Hand Clin. 1994;10(1):83–92.
5. King T, Morgan FP. Late results of removing the medial humeral epicondyle for traumatic ulnar neuritis. J Bone Joint Surg Br. 1959;41(1):51–5.
6. Popa M, Dubert T. Treatment of cubital tunnel syndrome by frontal partial medial epicondylectomy: a retrospective series of 55 cases. J Hand Surg Br. 2004;29(6):563–7.
7. Kaempffe FA, Farbach J. A modified surgical procedure for cubital tunnel syndrome: partial medial epicondylectomy. J Hand Surg Am. 1998;23(3):492–9.
8. Muermans S, De Smet L. Partial medial epicondylectomy for cubital tunnel syndrome: outcome and complications. J Shoulder Elbow Surg. 2002;11(3):248–52.
9. Amako M, Nemoto K, Kawaguchi M, Kato N, Arino H, Fujikawa K. Comparison between partial and minimal medial epicondylectomy combined with decompression for the treatment of cubital tunnel syndrome. J Hand Surg Am. 2000;25(6):1043–50.
10. O'Driscoll SW, Jaloszynski R, Morrey BF, An KN. Origin of the medial ulnar collateral ligament. J Hand Surg Am. 1992;17(1):164–8.
11. Gobel F, Musgrave DS, Vardakas DG, Vogt MT, Sotereanos DG. Minimal medial epicondylectomy and decompression for cubital tunnel syndrome. Clin Orthop Relat Res. 2001;(393):228–36.
12. Kim KW, Lee HJ, Rhee SH, Baek GH. Minimal epicondylectomy improves neurologic deficits in moderate to severe cubital tunnel syndrome. Clin Orthop Relat Res. 2012;470(5):1405–13.
13. Osei DA, Padegimas EM, Calfee RP, Gelberman RH. Outcomes following modified oblique medial epicondylectomy for treatment of cubital tunnel syndrome. J Hand Surg Am. 2013;38(2):336–43.
14. Erol B, Tetik C, Sirin E. The mid-term results of minimal medial epicondylectomy and decompression for cubital tunnel syndrome. Acta Orthop Traumatol Turc. 2004;38(5):330–6.
15. Jarrett CD, Papatheodorou LK, Sotereanos DG. Cubital tunnel syndrome. Instr Course Lect. 2017;15(66):91–101.
16. Rogers MR, Bergfield TG, Aulicino PL. The failed ulnar nerve transposition. Etiology and treatment. Clin Orthop Relat Res. 1991;269:193–200.
17. Dellon AL. Techniques for successful management of ulnar nerve entrapment at the elbow. Neurosurg Clin N Am. 1991;2(1):57–73.
18. Wilson DH, Krout R. Surgery of ulnar neuropathy at the elbow: 16 cases treated by decompression without transposition. J Neurosurg. 1973;38(6):780–5.
19. Baek GH, Kwon BC, Chung MS. Comparative study between minimal medial epicondylectomy and anterior subcutaneous transposition of the ulnar nerve for cubital tunnel syndrome. J Shoulder Elbow Surg. 2006;15(5):609–13.

Revision Cubital Tunnel: Surgical Options

17

Aikaterini G. Bavelou, Efstratios G. Papanikos, Panayotis N. Soucacos, and Zinon T. Kokkalis

Introduction

Cubital tunnel syndrome is the second most common upper extremity compressive neuropathy [1, 2], with an increased incidence in men [3]. Different procedures have been described for the release of the ulnar nerve at the elbow ranging from simple decompression to medial epicondylectomy, as well as anterior transposition (subcutaneous, intramuscular, or submuscular). There is still no clear consensus regarding the best operation [4]. The rate of surgical management has increased during the last decades, with a preference for simple decompression [1], and failure rates ranging from 3% to 35% have been reported in the literature, depending on the severity of symptoms before surgery [5–11].

Etiology

We can categorize patients who have failed a primary cubital tunnel release procedure into three groups: those with persistent symptoms, recurrent symptoms, or new symptoms. Patients with persistent symptoms, who have no relief or incomplete relief after the primary surgery, are likely to have had an incorrect diagnosis or a missed concomitant diagnosis, an inadequate release, or an irreversible intraneural pathology. Recurrent symptoms may result from scar and perineural fibrosis after surgery, and new symptoms may occur after iatrogenic creation of a new compression site or iatrogenic nerve injury, such as a medial brachial and antebrachial cutaneous nerve (MABCN) injury [12].

We can also categorize the reasons to failure as diagnostic, biologic, or technical. Biologic reasons can be perineural fibrosis formed after the primary surgery, or severe preoperative ulnar nerve damage from long-standing compression. Diagnostic causes can be an incorrent diagnosis or even a missed concomitant diagnosis, such as a C8 radiculopathy. Finally the technical causes may be incomplete decompression, iatrogenic creation of a new site of compression, nerve injury and instability of the ulnar nerve after the primary surgery [13].

There are also factors associated with increased rates of revision surgery. Krogue et al. [10] found that prior elbow fracture or dislocation and McGowan stage I disease were associated with revision surgery and that concurrent surgical procedures were protective against revision surgery. Increased risk for recurrence may also exist for patients with

A. G. Bavelou · E. G. Papanikos · Z. T. Kokkalis (✉)
Department of Orthopaedics,
University Hospital of Patras, Patras, Greece

P. N. Soucacos
Orthopaedic Research and Education Center (OREC), Attikon University Hospital, University of Athens, School of Medicine, Department of Orthopaedics, Athens, Greece

D. G. Sotereanos, L. K. Papatheodorou (eds.), *Compressive Neuropathies of the Upper Extremity*,
https://doi.org/10.1007/978-3-030-37289-7_17

hypercoagulable disorder, tobacco use, chronic anemia, chronic liver disease, age <65 years, diabetes mellitus, obesity and morbid obesity, and hyperlipidemia [14]. In addition, it is found that patients with chronic kidney disease are at higher risk for complications after cubital tunnel surgery and that the secondary surgery rate is higher for patients who have undergone transposition than for patients who have undergone in situ decompression [15]. This may be due to devascularization of the nerve, entrapment in scar, or a combination.

Evaluation

History

The patients who visit us after a failed primary cubital tunnel surgery deserve time in order to fully understand their symptoms and how they evolved. After a thorough history we should be able to recognize the difference between the preoperative and postoperative symptoms, the possible improvement and the period of it before the recurrence or the worsening of the symptoms. There are also pain evaluation forms that can be completed by the patients and help us determine the cause of their complaints [4].

Physical Examination

The physical examination should address all the possible causes, beginning from the cervical spine in order to assess for evidence of cervical radiculopathy, which can mimic or contribute to cubital tunnel syndrome symptoms with double crush lesion. Other conditions, such as thoracic outlet syndrome, a Pancoast lung tumor or brachial plexus injury should also be ruled out. We should examine all the possible sites of compression of the ulnar nerve, inspect the patient for possible clawing, atrophy or elbow deformity that can cause elbow stiffness and contribute to ulnar neuritis. In addition, evaluation of the sensory function, as well as palpation of the ulnar nerve for assessment of possible instability are also necessary. Lastly, examination of the scar can help us understand if all possible sites of compression were released.

Testing

We should repeat the nerve conduction and electromyography (EMG) studies and compare their results with the preoperative ones. A completely released ulnar nerve cannot be easily distinguished from an incompletely released ulnar nerve because the studies often show no improvement, but worse result may indicate need for reexplorationbecause of possible perineural fibrosis or ulnar nerve injury. If radiculopathy or Guyon canal compression is suspected, magnetic resonance imaging (MRI) may be helpful. Ultrasound could also be useful in order to assess for changes in the ulnar nerve diameter, perineural scarring, the position of the nerve or even MABCN neuromas.

Management

If symptoms do not alleviate after the primary surgery and other causes have been excluded, then the goal of revision surgery must be to completely decompress the ulnar nerve. Similar to the situation for primary cubital tunnel surgery, there is no widely accepted superior technique for revision surgery. Submuscular transposition seems to be the most commonly recommended revision technique [8, 16–20]. Other options include simple neurolysis [21], subcutaneous transposition [19, 22] and intramuscular transposition [23]. Revision surgery should be performed after thorough diagnosis by a highly experienced surgeon [24]. The results are generally not as good as for primary techniques [5, 18]. In general the surgical management of persistent or recurrent peripheral nerve compression needs a more aggressive surgical approach [25]. Complete visualization and release of all potential sites compression is critical and neuromas of superficial sensory nerves need also to be addressed. According to Sarris et al. [26] great care must be taken in identifying and preserving the branches of the medial cutaneous nerves during both primary and revision cubital tunnel surgery, as an injury to these branches can compromise the overall results following revision cubital tunnel surgery.

The literature is still limited in studies evaluating outcomes after revision cubital tunnel surgery, but till now most of the existing studies recommend external neurolysis and submuscular transposition as the method of choice.

Gabel and Amadio performed a retrospective review of 30 patients who were followed for a minimum of 2 years postoperatively. They suggested that for a reoperation to be successful all potential levels of compression must be released. They also found that an age of more than 50 years, electromyographic evidence of denervation and previous submuscular transposition were associated with poor outcomes [19].

Rogers et al. [17] reported their results or revision with external neurolysis and anterior submuscular transposition. All patients with McGowan grades I-II improved in almost all parameters, 3 (from 14) patients, who had McGowan grade III, had no improvement in sensation or motor weakness, and all patients returned to work.

Caputo and Watson [22] reported their results on 20 patients treated with neurolysis and anterior subcutaneous transposition and had 75% excellent or good results. They also suggested that increasing age and procedures were associated with fair or poor results.

Dagregorio and Saint-Cast [21] described external neurolysis in situ of the previously submuscularly transposed ulnar nerve in nine patients and reported 89% good or fair Wilson-Krout grade.

Vogel et al. [18] described submuscular transposition in 18 patients with persisted cubital tunnel syndrome after failed surgery. They concluded that most patients had partial relief of their pain and the satisfaction rate was 78%.

Bartels and Grotenhuis [27] reported their results on external neurolysis with anterior submuscular transposition in 40 patients and found that 20% had an excellent result whereas only one patient self-reported a complete cure.

There is also literature suggesting the use of adjunctive techniques. Varitimidis et al. [28] described neurolysis and autogenous saphenous vein wrapping in four patients with recurrent cubital tunnel syndrome. All patients reported significant pain relief and improvement in sensation. Two-point discrimination and EMG findings also improved.

Kokkalis et al. [29] also used autologous vein wrapping in 17 patients with recurrent cubital tunnel syndrome. All patients reported significant pain relief, and improvements in grip strength and 2-point discrimination were observed. Vein grafts are found to improve the recovery of nerve function by protecting the nerve from surrounding scar and so they are proven to be an effective and feasible technique for the surgical treatment of recurrent compressive neuropathy [30, 31].

Papatheodorou et al. [32] described the use of porcine extracellular matrix wrap in addition to decompression and minimal medial epicondylectomy in 12 patients and reported a significant improvement in postoperative pain levels, grip strength and pinch strength, as well as 2-point discrimination.

Other techniques such as amniotic membrane nerve wrapping [33] and ulnar nerve wrapping with a tissue engineered bioscaffold [34] have also been described and reported good results but the indication for all types of adjunctive techniques is still debatable and their efficacy is still to be studied (Fig. 17.1).

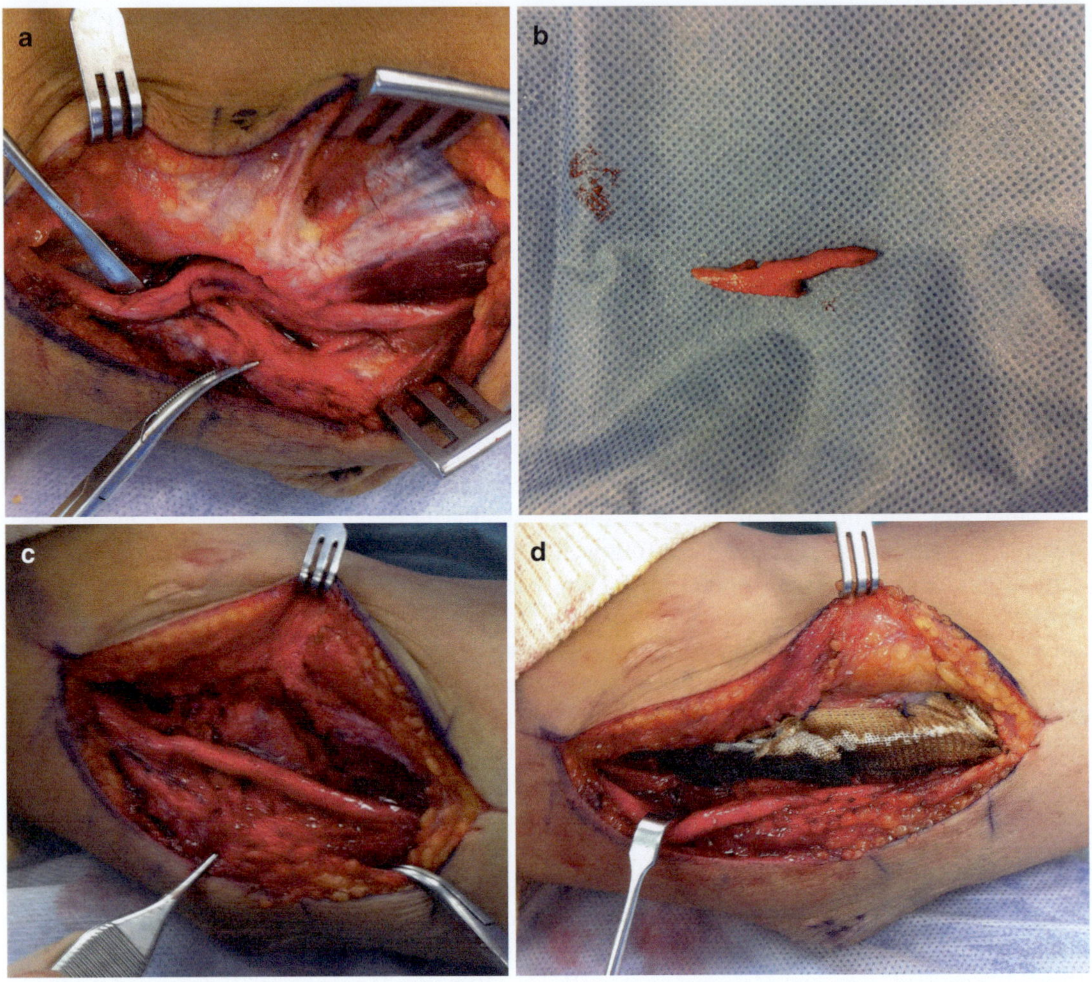

Fig. 17.1 A 40-year-old male patient after previous simple decompression of the ulnar nerve undergoing revision surgery. (**a**) Compressed ulnar nerve by a bony spur at the site of the medial epicondyle. (**b**) The bony spur compressing the ulnar nerve excised. (**c**) The completely decompressed ulnar nerve. (**d**) Dural allograft positioned at the medial epicondyle for protection of the ulnar nerve during gliding and avoidance of the formation of new adhesions

Surgical Techniques

As we have previously analyzed, there is not enough evidence to suggest a superior technique for revision cubital tunnel surgery. There is also literature suggesting the repositioning of the ulnar nerve in the cubital tunnel if possible, in order to regain its regular function [35], but most surgeons agree that the surgical technique tailored according to the intraoperative findings [36]. So, over the last decades, the most accepted techniques for revision surgery are the subcutaneous and submuscular anterior transposition with complete decompression and external neurolysis when needed. In order to achieve complete decompression one must be familiar with all five basic potential sites of compression encountered in primary surgery: the arcade of Struther's, the medial intermuscular septum, the medial epicondyle, the cubital tunnel with the arcuate ligament of Osborne as its roof, and the aponeurosis of the flexor carpi ulnaris [37], or any other possible fascial bands overlying the ulnar nerve [38, 39]. As for preserving the vascular supply to the ulnar nerve, it is found that the appropriate distance that the vascularized ulnar nerve can be moved into the subcutaneous tissue under tension-free conditions is 1.8 ± 0.6 cm (1.1–2.5 cm) [40].

Subcutaneous Transposition

The incision for the revision surgery incorporates the scar when possible, but extends proximal and distal. The most difficult part is to isolate the nerve from the surrounding scar tissue. This may need a nerve stimulator especially for cases with prior multiple surgeries. External neurolysis then is always necessary, but internal neurolysis may not be required. We should also excise any neuromata of the MACN and transpose them in soft tissues away from the surgical wound. Afterwards, all possible areas of entrapment must be released. A large strip of the medial intermuscular septum is excised, protecting the vessels to the ulnar nerve, and a large fascial window is created in the fascial origin of the flexor carpi ulnaris with excision of the superficial to deep fascial septae within muscle mass. The nerve then lies anteriorly without tension (Fig. 17.2). One 3-0 suture is used to approximate the adipose tissue from the anterior flap to the medial epicondyle and to prevent return of the nerve into the epicondylar groove. Complete proximal and distal decompression is confirmed and the surgical wound is closed. The patient is immobilized for 2 weeks in 90° flexion and then subsequently allowed to progressively begin full active range of motion.

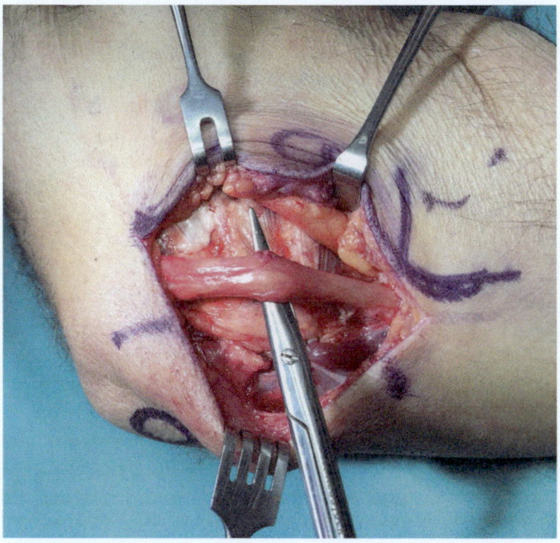

Fig. 17.2 Ulnar nerve after complete decompression lying anteriorly without any tension

Submuscular Transposition

After following the same steps as in the subsutaneous transposition till the stage of the complete decompression, as described above, we lengthen the medial epicondylar muscles by first developing a flap with distal pedicle on the lateral half of the medial epicondylar muscles, and then on the medial half. Next a fascial and tendon flap pedicled to the epicondyle is developed. The ulnar nerve is then transposed and then we oppose and suture the various fascial and tendinous flaps of the medial epicondylar muscles. Postoperatively the patient is immobilized with the arm in 90° flexion, allowing minimal forearm pronation. Subsequently, the patient undergoes 2 weeks of passive mobilization in a sling, followed by 3 weeks of active mobilization without lifting objects weighing more than 1 kg.

Conclusion

As discussed before, the rates of primary cubital tunnel surgery are continuously increasing. As a result of that we may also anticipate an increased need for revision surgeries in the future. We should be ready to face the difficulties of one or multiple revision cubital tunnel surgeries and most of all respect the anatomy of the area and keep a strong adherence to surgical principles in order to avoid ulnar nerve injury, that could worsen patient outcomes [41]. It is found that anterior transposition results in lower ulnar nerve strains than simple decompression during elbow flexion, but in higher nerve strains during elbow extension [42]. So, complete and careful decompression as well as external neurolysis must always accompany an anterior transposition.

Further research comparing different techniques is needed, in order to provide stong evidence-based information about the technique that could provide better outcomes for the patients with recurrent cubital tunnel syndrome.

References

1. Soltani AM, Best MJ, Francis CS, Allan BJ, Panthaki ZJ. Trends in the surgical treatment of cubital tunnel syndrome: an analysis of the National Survey of Ambulatory Surgery database. J Hand Surg Am. 2013;38(8):1551–6.
2. Bebbington E, Furniss D. Linear regression analysis of Hospital Episode Statistics predicts a large increase in demand for elective hand surgery in England. J Plast Reconstr Aesthet Surg. 2015;68(2):243–51.
3. Latinovic R, Gulliford MC, Hughes RAC. Incidence of common compressive neuropathies in primary care. J Neurol Neurosurg Psychiatry. 2006;77(2):263–5.
4. Tang DT, Barbour JR, Davidge KM, Yee A, Mackinnon SE. Nerve entrapment: update. Plast Reconstr Surg. 2015;135(1):199e–215e.
5. Aleem AW, Krogue JD, Calfee RP. Outcomes of revision surgery for cubital tunnel syndrome. J Hand Surg Am. 2014;39(11):2141–9.
6. Bartels RH. History of the surgical treatment of ulnar nerve compression at the elbow. Neurosurgery. 2001;49(2):391–9; discussion 399–400.
7. Lancigu R, Saint Cast Y, Raimbeau G, Rabarin F. Dellon's anterior submuscular transposition of the ulnar nerve: retrospective study of 82 operated patients with 11.5 years' follow-up. Chir Main. 2015;34(5):234–9.
8. Dellon AL. Review of treatment results for ulnar nerve entrapment at the elbow. J Hand Surg Am. 1989;14(4):688–700.
9. Gaspar MP, Kane PM, Putthiwara D, Jacoby SM, Osterman AL. Predicting revision following in situ ulnar nerve decompression for patients with idiopathic cubital tunnel syndrome. J Hand Surg Am. 2016;41(3):427–35.
10. Krogue JD, Aleem AW, Osei DA, Goldfarb CA, Calfee RP. Predictors of surgical revision after in situ decompression of the ulnar nerve. J Shoulder Elbow Surg. 2015;24(4):634–9.
11. Mowlavi A, Andrews K, Lille S, Verhulst S, Zook EG, Milner S. The management of cubital tunnel syndrome: a meta-analysis of clinical studies. Plast Reconstr Surg. 2000;106(2):327–34.
12. Grandizio LC, Maschke S, Evans PJ. The management of persistent and recurrent cubital tunnel syndrome. J Hand Surg Am. 2018;43(10):933–40.
13. Tang P, Hoellwarth JS, Chauhan A. Recurrent cubital tunnel syndrome. JBJS Rev. 2016;4(3):e31–7.
14. Camp CL, Ryan CB, Degen RM, Dines JS, Altchek DW, Werner BC. Risk factors for revision surgery following isolated ulnar nerve release at the cubital tunnel: a study of 25,977 cases. J Shoulder Elbow Surg. 2017;26(4):710–5.
15. Zhang D, Earp BE, Blazar P. Rates of complications and secondary surgeries after in situ cubital tunnel release compared with ulnar nerve transposition: a retrospective review. J Hand Surg Am. 2017;42(4):294.e1–5.
16. Goldfarb CA, Sutter MM, Martens EJ, Manske PR. Incidence of re-operation and subjective outcome following in situ decompression of the ulnar nerve at the cubital tunnel. J Hand Surg Eur Vol. 2009;34(3):379–83.
17. Rogers MR, Bergfield TG, Aulicino PL. The failed ulnar nerve transposition. Etiology and treatment. Clin Orthop Relat Res. 1991;269:193–200.
18. Vogel RB, Nossaman BC, Rayan GM. Revision anterior submuscular transposition of the ulnar nerve for failed subcutaneous transposition. Br J Plast Surg. 2004;57(4):311–6.
19. Gabel GT, Amadio PC. Reoperation for failed decompression of the ulnar nerve in the region of the elbow. J Bone Joint Surg Am. 1990;72(2):213–9.
20. Wever N, de Ruiter GCW, Coert JH. Submuscular transposition with musculofascial lengthening for persistent or recurrent cubital tunnel syndrome in 34 patients. J Hand Surg Eur Vol. 2018;43(3):310–5.
21. Dagregorio G, Saint-Cast Y. Simple neurolysis for failed anterior submuscular transposition of the ulnar nerve at the elbow. Int Orthop. 2004;28(6):342–6.
22. Caputo AE, Watson HK. Subcutaneous anterior transposition of the ulnar nerve for failed decompression of cubital tunnel syndrome. J Hand Surg Am. 2000;25(3):544–51.
23. Kleinman WB. Cubital tunnel syndrome: anterior transposition as a logical approach to complete nerve decompression. J Hand Surg Am. 1999;24(5):886–97.
24. Davis GA, Bulluss KJ. Submuscular transposition of the ulnar nerve: review of safety, efficacy and correlation with neurophysiological outcome. J Clin Neurosci. 2005;12(5):524–8.
25. Mackinnon SE, Novak CB. Operative findings in reoperation of patients with cubital tunnel syndrome. Hand. 2007;2(3):137–43.
26. Sarris I, Göbel F, Gainer M, Vardakas DG, Vogt MT, Sotereanos DG. Medial brachial and antebrachial cutaneous nerve injuries: effect on outcome in revision cubital tunnel surgery. J Reconstr Microsurg. 2002;18(8):665–70.
27. Bartels RH, Grotenhuis JA. Anterior submuscular transposition of the ulnar nerve. For post-operative focal neuropathy at the elbow. J Bone Joint Surg Br. 2004;86(7):998–1001.
28. Varitimidis SE, Riano F, Sotereanos DG. Recalcitrant post-surgical neuropathy of the ulnar nerve at the

elbow: treatment with autogenous saphenous vein wrapping. J Reconstr Microsurg. 2000;16(4):273–8.
29. Kokkalis ZT, Jain S, Sotereanos DG. Vein wrapping at cubital tunnel for ulnar nerve problems. J Shoulder Elbow Surg. 2010;19(2):91–7.
30. Xu J, Varitimidis SE, Fisher KJ, Tomaino MM, Sotereanos DG. The effect of wrapping scarred nerves with autogenous vein graft to treat recurrent chronic nerve compression. J Hand Surg Am. 2000;25(1):93–103.
31. Varitimidis SE, Vardakas DG, Goebel F, Sotereanos DG. Treatment of recurrent compressive neuropathy of peripheral nerves in the upper extremity with an autologous vein insulator. J Hand Surg Am. 2001;26(2):296–302.
32. Papatheodorou LK, Williams BG, Sotereanos DG. Preliminary results of recurrent cubital tunnel syndrome treated with neurolysis and porcine extracellular matrix nerve wrap. J Hand Surg Am. 2015;40(5):987–92.
33. Gaspar MP, Abdelfattah HM, Welch IW, Vosbikian MM, Kane PM, Rekant MS. Recurrent cubital tunnel syndrome treated with revision neurolysis and amniotic membrane nerve wrapping. J Shoulder Elbow Surg. 2016;25(12):2057–65.
34. Puckett BN, Gaston RG, Lourie GM. A novel technique for the treatment of recurrent cubital tunnel syndrome: ulnar nerve wrapping with a tissue engineered bioscaffold. J Hand Surg Eur Vol. 2011;36(2):130–4.
35. Filippi R, Charalampaki P, Reisch R, Koch D, Grunert P. Recurrent cubital tunnel syndrome. Etiology and treatment. Minim Invasive Neurosurg. 2001;44(4):197–201.
36. Antoniadis G, Richter HP. Pain after surgery for ulnar neuropathy at the elbow: a continuing challenge. Neurosurgery. 1997;41(3):585–9; discussion 589–91.
37. Amadio PC. Anatomical basis for a technique of ulnar nerve transposition. Surg Radiol Anat. 1986;8(3):155–61.
38. Siemionow M, Agaoglu G, Hoffmann R. Anatomic characteristics of a fascia and its bands overlying the ulnar nerve in the proximal forearm: a cadaver study. J Hand Surg Eur Vol. 2007;32(3):302–7.
39. Karatas A, Apaydin N, Uz A, Tubbs SR, Loukas M, Gezen F, et al. Regional anatomic structures of the elbow that may potentially compress the ulnar nerve. J Shoulder Elbow Surg. 2009;18(4):627–31.
40. Li M, He Q, Hu Z, Chen S, Lv Y, Liu Z, et al. Applied anatomical study of the vascularized ulnar nerve and its blood supply for cubital tunnel syndrome at the elbow region. Neural Regen Res. 2015;10(1):141.
41. Davidge KM, Ebersole GC, Mackinnon SE. Pain and function following revision cubital tunnel surgery. Hand. 2017;28:155894471774359.
42. Foran I, Vaz K, Sikora-Klak J, Ward SR, Hentzen ER, Shah SB. Regional ulnar nerve strain following decompression and anterior subcutaneous transposition in patients with cubital tunnel syndrome. J Hand Surg Am. 2016;41(10):e343–50.

18 Nerve Transfers for Neuropathies of the Median and Ulnar Nerve

Joshua Allan Gillis and Steven L. Moran

Introduction

Nerve transfers involve the division of an expendable motor or sensory nerve and anastomosing it to the distal intact portion of an injured nerve. Nerve coaptation can be performed in an end to end (ETE), or end to side (ETS) fashion beyond the zone of injury. The nerve transfer is ideally performed close to the end organ (muscle or skin); thus minimizing the time required for innervation from the donor transferred nerve. Historically, nerve transfers have been utilized for the treatment of traumatic proximal motor nerve injuries, particularly those involving the brachial plexus. Nerve transfers are most commonly used as an alternative to direct nerve repair and nerve grafting when the site of nerve damage is very proximal, precluding re-innervation of distal target muscles or when the area of injury is extensive, necessitating long intercalated nerve grafts with low potentials for meaningful recovery [1].

The use of nerve transfers, while rare in the majority of compressive neuropathies, can be considered in cases of severe proximal compression leading to axonal loss or in cases of iatrogenic injury following surgery. While most nerve transfers have classically been performed as ETE repairs, in this chapter we will advocate for the use of ETS transfers. ETS transfer allows for the preservation of recovering native nerve fibers while also allowing for the benefits of a distal ETS transfer. Recent data suggests that the benefits of ETS transfers can include preservation of motor end plates, improved native nerve recovery and additional axonal fiber ingrowth from the donor nerve [2, 3]. Such ETS transfers have been referred to as "supercharged" end to side transfers (SETS) and can help to preserve muscle function, restore protective sensation and potentially accelerate the recovery of native ingrowing nerve fibers [2, 4, 5]. Here we describe the principles and strategies for nerve transfers to restore sensation and muscle function in cases of severe median and ulnar compressive neuropathies.

Nerve Transfer Principles

Nerve transfers are performed as an alternative to direct nerve repair and nerve grafting. The procedure involves transfer a local, uninjured and expendable nerve or fascicle to the injured nerve close to the recipient end organ (muscle or skin). It effectively converts a proximal nerve injury into a distal injury. The classic example is that of the

J. A. Gillis
Maine General Medical Center, Department of Plastic Surgery, Augusta, ME, USA

S. L. Moran (✉)
Division of Plastic Surgery & Department of Orthopedic Surgery, Mayo Clinic, Rochester, MN, USA
e-mail: moran.steven@mayo.edu

D. G. Sotereanos, L. K. Papatheodorou (eds.), *Compressive Neuropathies of the Upper Extremity*,
https://doi.org/10.1007/978-3-030-37289-7_18

Oberlin transfer where a motor fascicle of the ulnar nerve is transferred to the biceps for restoration of elbow flexion following an upper trunk brachial plexus injury [6, 7]. The Oberlin procedure is illustrative of the potential advantages of nerve transfer procedures as the donor nerve is attached close to the biceps muscle, thus minimizing the time for innervation. Decreasing the time to innervation will theoretically decreasing the loss of motor end plates and fatty replacement of the denervated muscle [8]. The second major benefit is that the transfer can be performed out of the zone of injury. Theoretically one transferred nerve can innervate multiple muscle groups, such as the anterior interosseous nerve transferred to the motor branch of the ulnar nerve. Finally, nerve transfers, (if successful), can reestablish the native tendon muscle interaction which can restore independent finger motion, in comparison to tendon transfers which link muscle groups together.

More recent evidence has suggested that end to side motor transfers provide the added benefit of releasing neurotropic factors to the proximal and distal ends of the injured nerve which can stimulate the recovery of proximal native nerve fibers [2]. MacKinnon and colleagues have developed the term *supercharging* or *SETS* transfer, as a way to describe an ETS nerve transfers, which augment native nerve healing. The SETS transfer has been shown to add regenerating motor axons across the ETS coaptation to reinnervate the neuromuscular junction. Farber and colleagues looked at nerve recovery in an incomplete sciatic nerve injury model in mice, in which the tibial nerve was cut and a nerve allograft was interposed [2]. This was compared to those mice where the peroneal nerve was sutured in a SETS fashion in addition to the tibial nerve isograft. During nerve regeneration, they found axonal contribution from both the partially injured tibial nerve and axonal sprouting from the SETS peroneal nerve [2]. This correlated to increased function and a higher muscle specific force during sciatic nerve stimulation of the gastrocnemius muscle compared to the mice without the SETS transfer. When the peroneal nerve contribution was removed by cutting the coaptation, the increased force was no longer significant [2]. The authors believe that the SETS transfer acts to "babysit" the muscle and protect it from atrophy by providing axons at an earlier time point in addition to donating additional motoneurons to achieve target muscle reinnervation [2].

Nerve transfers are contraindicated when there is end-organ unresponsiveness, motor denervation for greater than 12 months, or loss of the musculotendinous unit due to trauma or fibrosis. A healthy donor nerve, as evident by a strong donor muscle, is required for a successful nerve transfer, typically greater than a Modified British Medical Research Council (BMRC) graded 4. In addition, there should be a large proportion of the type of axons required for the function you wish to restore (i.e.: large number of purely motor axons for motor reconstruction). Thus, one should strive for a pure motor or sensory nerve with greater than M4 or S4 at the time of transfer.

Joint releases, if necessary, should be performed prior to nerve transfer and passive motion of all effected joints maximized. If tendon transfers have been performed in addition to nerve transfers, then the tendon transfer rehabilitation will dictate the post-operative protocol [9]. The time required for functional recovery following nerve transfer can vary from 6 to 12 months or longer [6, 10].

Diagnosis

Nerve transfer for median or ulnar nerve compression should be reserved for cases exhibiting signs of pre-operative axonal injury. Compressive neuropathies progress in severity and early cases will present with intermittent symptoms and this is often a sign of dynamic reversible nerve ischemia. If compression is persistent, nerve ischemia can progress to demyelination; in these cases, the nerve conduction studies will show slowing conduction velocities. If compression is severe or long standing, nerve injury progresses from demyelination to axonal injury. These patients classically have signs of motor weakness on physical exam and evidence of muscle atrophy. For cases of severe ulnar nerve compression, we would expect to see intrinsic wasting, inability to cross the fingers, a positive Froment sign and clawing. For cases of severe median nerve compression at the level of the wrist one should see thenar atrophy and loss of palmar abduction of the thumb. These physical findings can be cooperated with the use of nerve conduction studies where one will see decrease amplitude. The EMG will show signs of fibrillations during the resting phase which is a definitive sign for denervation. If motor unit action potentials are seen during the recruitment phase of the EMG, this indicates collateral sprouting and evidence of attempted recovery.

In regard to chronic ulnar neuropathy, recent findings from Power and colleagues show that a reduction in compound muscle action potentials (CMAP) in the first dorsal interosseous muscle is a reliable indicator of axonal loss and substantial nerve compression [11]. In these cases, the nerve will recover at 1 mm per day in an ideal environment. This means that if the compression has occurred at the level of the elbow it may be over a year until the intrinsic muscles in the hand will receive re-innervation. Based on the time line of injury this may result in poor recovery of motor function without the aid of a SETS transfer.

SETS transfer should be reserved for patients with electro diagnostic evidence of denervation. Fibrillation in the intrinsic muscles in the hand points to recent denervation and the potential for re-innervation. CMAPs should be of low amplitude reflecting the severity of axonal involvement; however absence of CMAPs suggests that the amount of nerve injury has been present too long to allow for meaningful recovery [11]. Davidge and colleagues have shown that patients who showed little improvement following SETS transfer had absence of fibrillation and CMAPs preoperatively [12]. As a corollary, CMAPs of good amplitude suggest that recovery of function may occur with simple decompression and SETS may not be required. To summarize, the best patients for transfer will:

1. Have signs of ulnar atrophy/ or median nerve atrophy.
2. Have evidence of fibrillations on EMG.
3. Decreased, *but not absent*, CMAPs.

We will now examine the details of specific transfers for both ulnar and median nerve compression.

Ulnar Nerve Compression

Ulnar Nerve Compression Below the Elbow

In a low ulnar nerve palsy, the flexor carpi ulnaris (FCU) and flexor digitorum profundus (FDP) to the ring and little finger are spared. Thus, the deep motor branch to the intrinsic hand muscles is affected, in addition to the volar sensation to the little finger, half of the ring finger and the palm. Intrinsic motor loss can lead to a claw deformity. Coordinated flexion is lost as the lumbrical muscles first flex the metacarpophalangeal joints (MCPJ) when making a fist, followed by activation of the extrinsic flexor tendons. With intrinsic loss, the extrinsic flexors will initiate movement and finger flexion will begin at the interphalangeal joints (IPJs), which results in a rolling motion where the fingers prematurely close before they reach the palm [13]. Additionally, with the loss of the adductor pollicus, 1st dorsal interosseous, and deep head of the flexor pollicis brevis (FPB) key pinch is weakened. Due to loss of finger adduction from the interossei muscles, the little finger can develop an abducted posture due to the unopposed pull of the extensor digiti minimi, producing the Wartenberg's sign [13]. While most cases of compression do not display all of these signs we would advocate for SETS transfers for those with evidence of 1st dorsal interosseous atrophy and decreased CMAPs.

Motor SETS Transfer in Cases of Severe Lower Ulnar Compression

The target nerve for motor reconstruction of low ulnar nerve palsy is the deep motor branch of the ulnar nerve. This is usually found between the dorsal cutaneous branch of the ulnar nerve (DCBUN) and the sensory branch of the ulnar nerve [14]. The common donor nerve transfers are the anterior interosseous nerve (AIN) from the median nerve [4, 12, 15], and end to side from the thenar motor branch using a bridging nerve graft [16] (See Table 18.1 for list of possible nerve donors and recipients).

The AIN transfer can be done as ETE transfer or an end-to-side SETS "supercharge" transfer into the ulnar motor branch. The ETE transfer is typically performed if there is no chance of recovery of the ulnar nerve from a proximal injury. If there is an incomplete or mixed injury, as in the case of severe compression, where some motor recovery is expected, then a SETS transfer may be beneficial. This can help to reinnervate the distal targets quicker and preserve motor plate function while the native ulnar nerve recovers [2, 12, 14].

The SETS AIN to deep motor transfer has been shown to improve recovery of intrinsic function with complete ulnar nerve injury. Davidge and colleagues in 2015, reported the outcomes of their SETS AIN to ulnar motor transfer in a mixed group of patients with severe motor and sensory ulnar nerve dysfunction [12]. At an average of 8 months following SETS transfer, 70% of patients had BMRC >M3, as opposed to 15% preoperatively. Motor improvement was seen in 50% of patients between 3 and 12 months, which was attributed to the SETS transfer [12]. Those with

Table 18.1 Nerve transfers for ulnar and median neuropathies

Nerve deficit	Donor nerves	Recipient nerves	Function restored
Ulnar nerve			
Motor	1. AIN (median) 2. Bridging graft to median nerve	Deep motor branch	Intrinsic hand function
Sensory	1. 3rd webspace (median) 2. DCBUN (ulnar)(not available in a high injury) 3. Median nerve (end-to-side) 4. LABC/MABC 5. PCB of median or ulnar (not available in a high injury) 6. Bridging graft to median 7. RDN long or ring finger (median) 8. Radial sensory (radial)	1. 4th webspace 2. Ulnar sensory 3. Ulnar digital nerve of little finger 4. Dorsal cutaneous branch (in high injuries and possibly low)	Ulnar hand sensation
Median nerve			
Low motor	1. AIN (median) 2. FDS/FCR/PL (median) 3. Abductor digiti minimi (ulnar) 4. 3rd lumbrical (ulnar)	Recurrent motor branch	Thumb opposition
High motor	1. Brachialis (MCN) 2. Supinator (radial) 3. ECRB (radial) 4. FDS/FCR/PL (median) – if available 5. Bridging graft to ulnar	AIN	Wrist finger and thumb flexion
	1. ECRB (radial) 2. Brachioradialis (radial) 3. Supinator (radial) 4. FCU (ulnar) 5. FDS (median) – if available	Pronator teres	Forearm pronation
	1. Abductor digiti minimi (ulnar) 2. 3rd lumbrical (ulnar)	Recurrent motor branch	Thumb opposition
Sensory	1. 4th webspace (ulnar) 2. DCBUN (ulnar) 3. Radial sensory (radial) 4. LABC 5. Ulnar nerve (end-to-side)	1. 1st webspace 2. 2nd/3rd webspace	1. Sensation to thumb and index 2. Sensation to 2nd/3rd webspace (non-critical)
Combined palsy			
Motor	1. EDM/ECU (radial) 2. EIP/EPB/APL (radial)	Deep motor branch of ulnar nerve	Intrinsic hand function
Sensory	1. Radial sensory (radial) 2. LABC	First webspace of median nerve	Sensation to thumb and index

AIN anterior interosseous nerve, *FDS* flexor digitorum profundus, *EDM* extensor digiti minimi, *ECU* extensor carpi ulnaris, *EIP* extensor indicis proprius, *EPB* extensor pollicis brevis, *APL* abductor pollicis longus, *DCBUN* dorsal cutaneous branch of ulnar nerve, *LABC* lateral antebrachial cutaneous, *MABC* medial antebrachial cutaneous, *PCB* palmar cutaneous branch, *RDN* radial digital nerve, *FCR* flexor carpi radialis, *PL* palmaris longus, *MCN* musculocutaneous nerve, *ECRB* extensor carpi radialis brevis, *FCU* flexor carpi ulnaris evidence of AIN injury or absent motor unit potentials on pre-operative EMG had worse recovery. Following sacrifice of the AIN they did not report any limitations in forearm pronation.

While the use of SETS transfers in chronic ulnar nerve compression is still controversial several studies have noted promising results. Barbour and colleagues suggest that the use of the SETS AIN transfer is an important adjunct in those patients with severe or failed cubital tunnel surgery [14]. In Davidge's study, there were 15 patients with a compression neuropathy at the elbow who underwent both SETS AIN to ulnar motor transfer in conjunction with an anterior transposition and Guyon's release; seven of these patients had a rapid recovery [12]. Unfortunately, they did not perform any subgroup analysis separating the compressive group from the other traumatic injuries. Baltzer and colleagues evaluated the use of the SETS AIN transfer in a matched cohort study comparing ulnar nerve repair alone with ulnar nerve repair and SETS AIN transfer, in addition to ulnar nerve release alone with ulnar nerve release and SETS AIN transfer. They found that the SETS AIN transfer improved intrinsic recovery, with 84% recovery with the transfer compared to 38% without. In this study, recovery of motor function was more rapid with SETS transfer occurring at an average of 3.4 months versus 12.0 months in those without the transfer [4]. It is important to note that the conventional group that received a cubital tunnel and Guyon's canal release and those with an added SETS transfer had a 67% chance long term of recovering intrinsic function [4]. While results with traumatic injuries are encouraging, more study will be needed to determine which patients with compressive neuropathies are the best candidates for SETS AIN transfer. Since the donor site morbidity is so low, we still recommend this procedure for patients with evidence of atrophy and low amplitude CMAP response in the first dorsal interosseous muscle (Fig. 18.1).

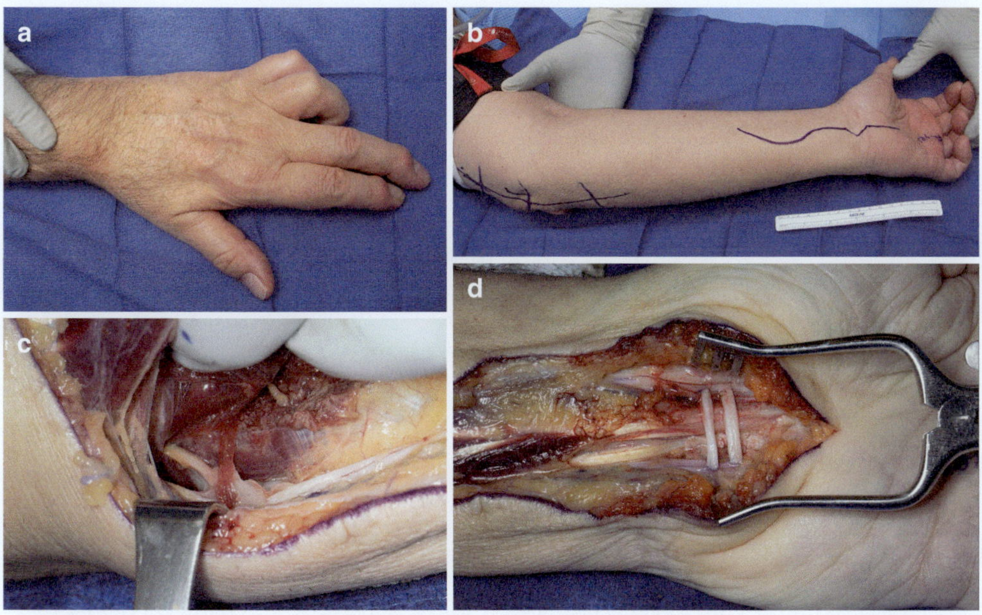

Fig. 18.1 A case of a 61 year old man with signs of severe ulnar nerve compression on EMG and nerve conduction studies. The site of compression is localized to the cubital tunnel. CMAPs were reduced in the ADM muscle and 1st dorsal interosseous muscle. (**a**) The patient's hand shows signs of clawing pre-operatively. (**b**) Incisions are planned for full ulnar nerve release with submuscular transposition, AIN distal SETS transfer, and cross bridging sensory graft from median to ulnar sensory nerve at the level of the wrist. (**c**) AIN transfer completed in an ETS fashion to ulnar motor branch. (**d**) Bridging allografts or "cross-cross grafts" were used to go from median sensory nerve to 3rd web space and long finger to both sensory fascicles of the ulnar nerve going to ring and small finger

As an alternative to the AIN SETS transfer, Sherif and Amr looked at using a nerve graft "bridge" sutured end to side into both the median and ulnar nerve in four patients with either a high median or ulnar nerve injury [16]. All cases were combined with grafting of the proximal injured nerve. The authors found early intrinsic hand muscle reinnervation with these high injuries, suggesting that reinnervation occurred through the bridge graft. In all patients, EMG studies had activation of the recipient nerve's intrinsic muscles through the donor nerve and bridge graft and not from the repaired ulnar nerve [16]. We find this a good option when severe compression has occurred at the level of Guyon's canal or in cases of severe proximal median nerve compression (Fig. 18.2).

Surgical Technique: AIN to Deep Ulnar Motor Branch SETS Technique

The ulnar nerve is exposed in the distal forearm through either a curvilinear or Bruner-style incision (Fig. 18.3). The flexor carpi ulnaris (FCU) tendon and muscle belly is retracted ulnarly to identify the ulnar artery and nerve. The branch point of the DCBUN is identified. *The most ulnar fascicle distal to this level will represent the deep motor branch, while the radial fascicle is the sensory nerve.* If needed, the ulnar nerve and deep motor branch can be identified distally with a Guyon's canal release and traced proximally to determine the correct ulnar nerve topography. The ulnar motor branch can be stimulated to

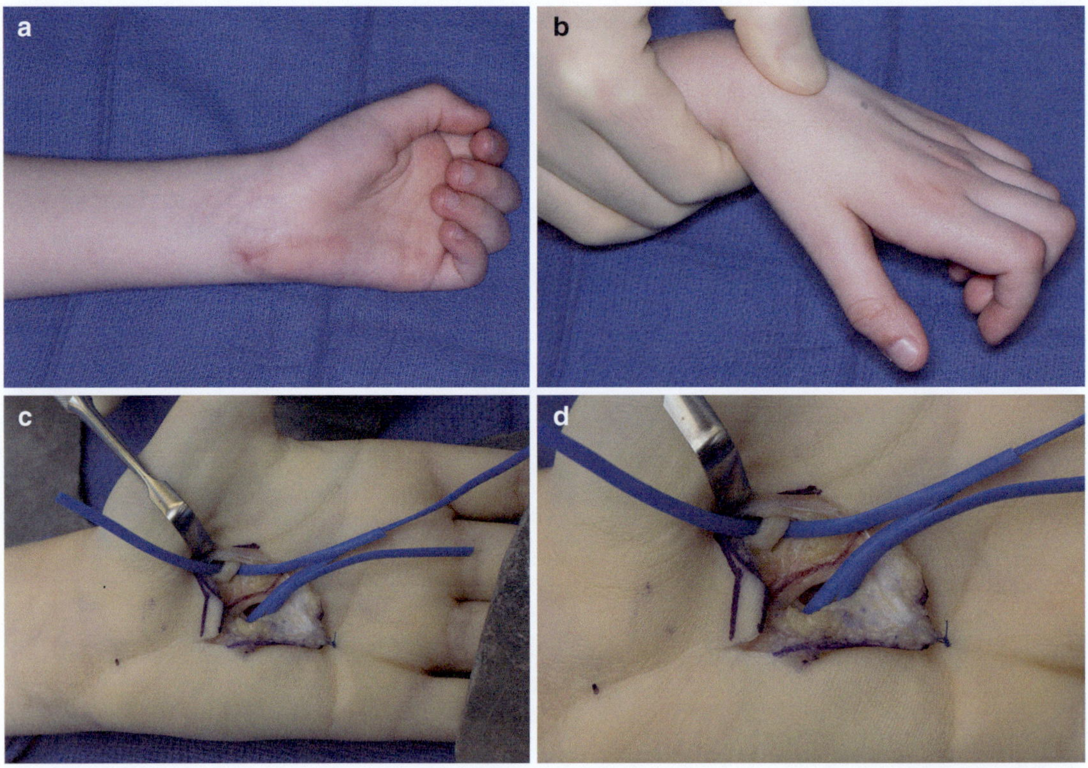

Fig. 18.2 An alternative to AIN SETS transfer in patients with pre-existing injury to AIN or injury distal to Guyon's canal is a bridge graft performed from in an ETS fashion from the median motor branch to the deep motor branch of the ulnar nerve. (**a–f**) A case of a 12 year old boy with an injury to the ulnar nerve at the level of Guyon's canal and inadequate motor recover despite nerve grafting at the site of injury. Image (**a**) shows scar over Guyon's canal and (**b**) shows persistent evidence of clawing and intrinsic weakness. Images (**c, d**) show palmar incision with isolation of recurrent thenar motor branch beneath superior blue vessel loop. Lower vessel loop surrounds ulnar motor branch. Image (**e**) shows nerve graft sew ETS into thenar motor branch. Image (**f**) shows completed graft going from median motor to ulnar motor branch. Figure (**g**) shows another case utilizing allograft for bridge grafting

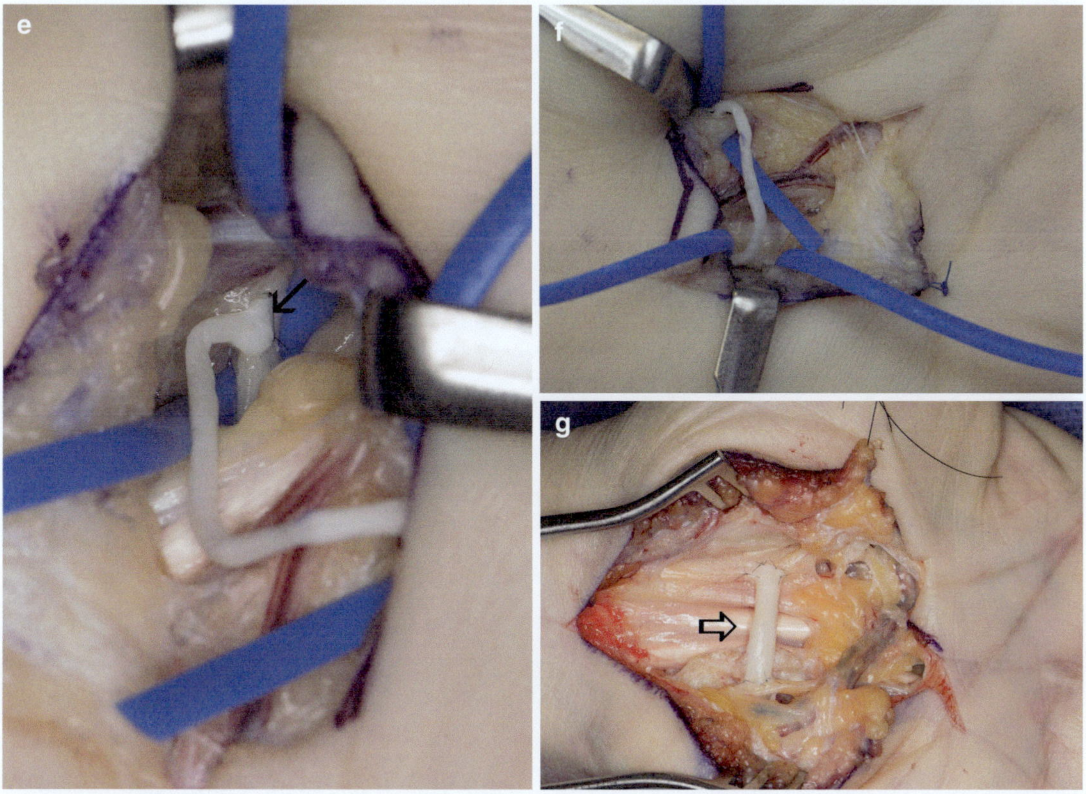

Fig. 18.2 (continued)

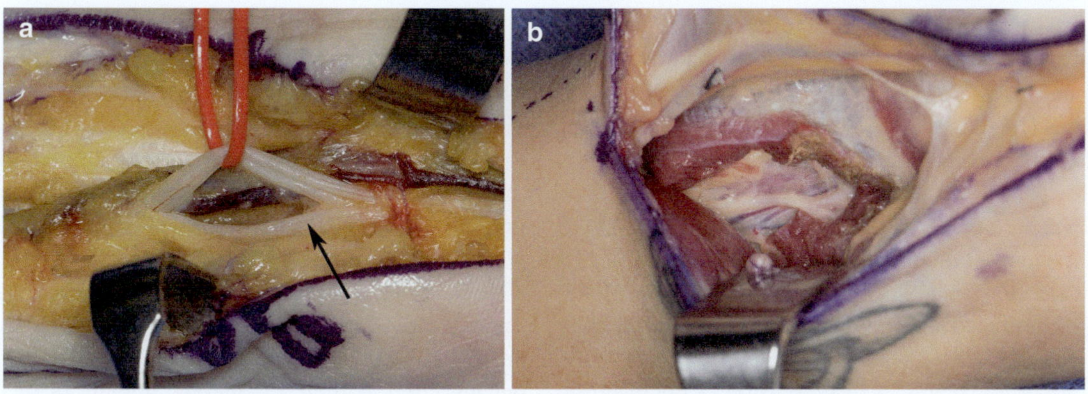

Fig. 18.3 Technique for AIN transfer. Isolation of ulnar motor branch in forearm should be performed distal to dorsal sensory branch take off. (**a**) Intraoperative case showing red vessel loop around more radial sensory component while arrow points to motor branch. If there is any question of orientation, dissection can be performed retrograde after release of Guyon's canal. (**b**, **c**) A spate case showing isolation and dissection of AIN through the cut portion of the pronator quadratus muscle. The nerve should be dissected terminally to obtain longus possible graft length. (**d**) An End to side neuroraphy is performed with aid of operating room microscope. Figure (**e**) shows AIN transfer (small arrow) and deep course of motor branch as it enters Guyon's canal

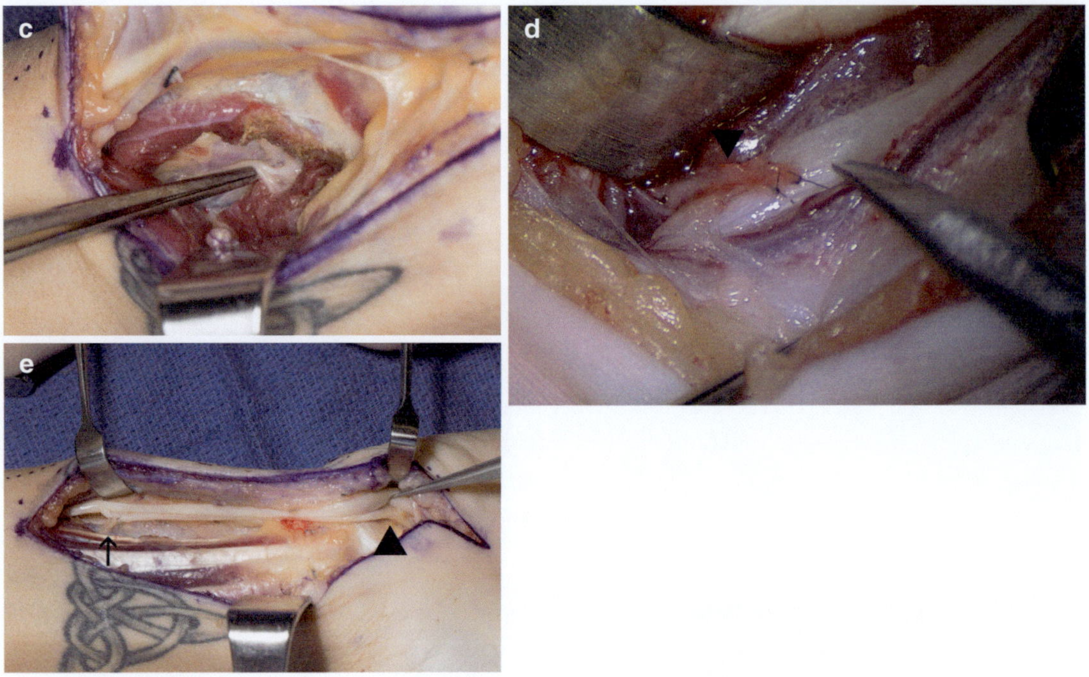

Fig. 18.3 (continued)

ensure there is no recovery or function prior to transfer. A formal internal neurolysis is not typically necessary or recommended. The point of the coaptation is typically just distal to the DCBUN branch point.

The finger flexor muscle bellies are retracted radially to expose the pronator quadratus (PQ) and the AIN motor branch and anterior interosseous artery as they enter the proximal aspect of the pronator (Fig. 18.3). The AIN is dissected distally by using bipolar cautery to release the muscle as it lies on top of the AIN. The AIN is dissected until it begins branching, ensuring to maximize the diameter of the nerve for coaptation. The AIN is then divided at this point and dissected proximally until it is able to transpose ulnarly to the ulnar motor nerve area. A distal portion of the insertion of the flexor digitorum profundus can be released to improve the reach of the AIN. The area of coaptation is identified and an epineurial and perineurial window is made on the ulnar aspect of the ulnar motor branch. This will avoid the need for internal neurolysis and potential coaptation into the sensory branch of the ulnar nerve. The AIN is sutured end to side to the deep ulnar motor branch using 9-0 nylon sutures and is then bathed in fibrin glue (Fig. 18.3). Fibrin glue should be placed along the margins of the PQ dissection to prevent bleeding. The tension on the coaptation should be checked with range of motion of the wrist and elbow.

Sensory Reconstruction

The target nerves for reconstruction of the low ulnar nerve palsy sensory deficits are the branch to the 4th webspace [6], the ulnar digital nerve to the little finger [17] or the ulnar sensory nerve proper [6]. The common donor are the 3rd webspace nerve from the median nerve [6, 18, 19], the radial digital nerve of the middle or ring finger [20], the lateral antebrachial cutaneous nerve (LABC) [17, 18, 21], the DCBUN (in low palsies), the palmar cutaneous branch of the median or ulnar nerve [17] and end to side into the median nerve [6]. In addition, Mackinnon has recently reported a side to side bridging nerve graft, similar to that described Sherif and Amr, to restore sensation in the ulnar digits [5] (Fig. 18.1).

A commonly described transfer combination to restore full ulnar sensation is as follows: (1) median nerve branch to the 3rd webspace end-to-end to the ulnar sensory branch (2) DCBUN end-to-side to the median nerve (3) distal stump of the 3rd webspace donor nerve placed end-to-side back to the median nerve to minimize the donor deficit [6, 19, 22, 23]. This is typically performed in conjunction with an AIN transfer to the deep motor branch and can be performed at the wrist level to avoid painful scars in the palm or injury to the palmar arches. The third webspace branch can be readily identified and neurolysed from the median nerve to provide length for transfer, ensuring to preserve interfascicular branches [22] (Fig. 18.4). Another option to restore sensation to the volar aspect of the ulnar nerve would be to cut the ulnar sensory nerve and take the distal stump end-to-side to the 3rd webspace median nerve fascicle, which would be the most ulnar aspect of the median nerve. Few studies report on the outcomes of these transfers. It is felt that they provide protective sensation and may take up to 2 years to reach maximal benefit [19].

The use of the radial digital nerve of the middle or ring finger to the ulnar digital nerve was studied by Brunelli, who achieved S2+ (tactile sensation with associated allodynia) in two patients and S1 (protective sensation) in a third patient. Bertelli described the transfer of the palmar cutaneous branch of the median nerve to the ulnar digital nerve of the little finger in patients with lower brachial plexus injuries to restore sensation [17]. Two patients had an additional transfer from the ulnar digital nerve of the index. They achieved recovery of two-point discrimination <10 mm in three of eight patients (S3+), five had >S3 recovery (perceived contact from a 33.1-g/mm^2 monofilament) [17]. Oberlin described the LABC transfer to the DCBUN with an interpositional graft to restore protective sensation in patients with a lower brachial plexus injury [24]. Felder et al. have introduced the idea of the bridging nerve graft for recovery of sensation, which they term a "cross-

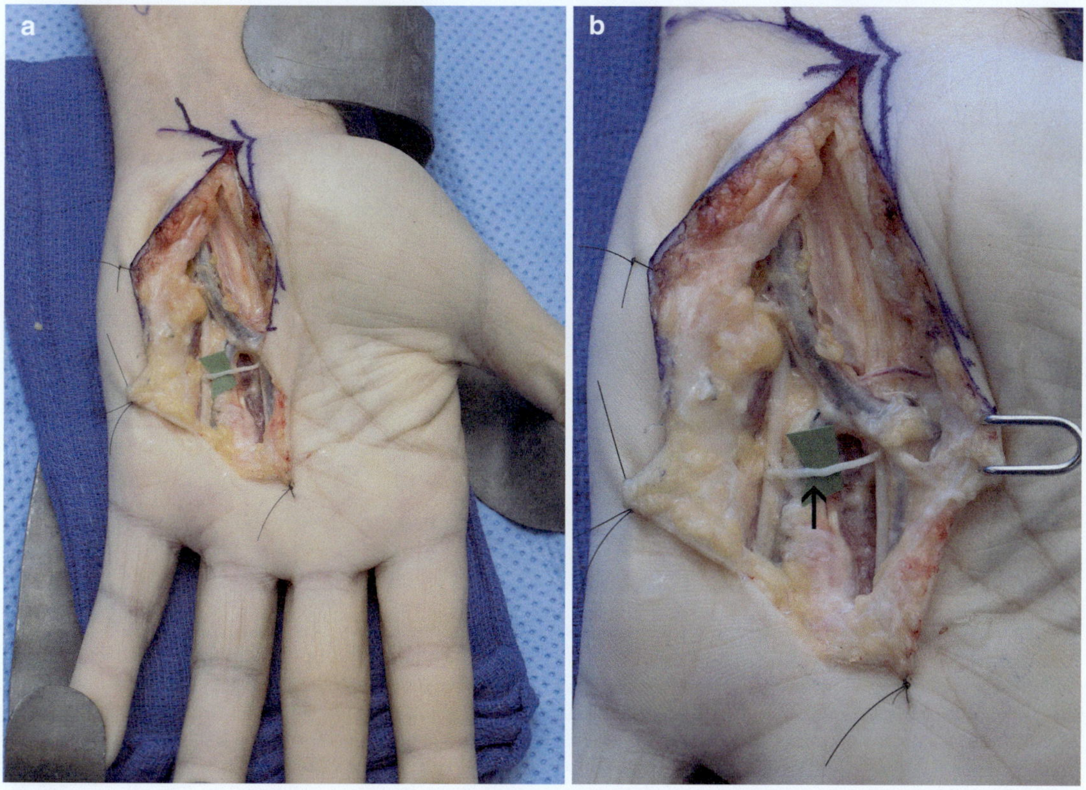

Fig. 18.4 Figure (**a**) shows a case of distal transfer of median nerve branch to 3rd web space to common digital nerve of ring and small finger for improvement in sensory recovery. (**b**) Arrow points to nerve branch of 3rd web space following coaptation to common digital nerve to ulnar ring and small finger

cross graft" [5]. In their series, 48 patients had one or more bridging nerve grafts, consisting of both allograft and autograft, placed between the ulnar and median sensory components in the palm. In this study 20 of these patients had severe cubital tunnel syndrome, 60% of which were revision cases. Of the 24 patients with complete data, 21 (87%) recovered protective sensation within 1 year [5]. Due to the limited donor site morbidity of this procedure, this is our transfer of choice in patients with severe ulnar nerve compression and severe sensory loss (Figs. 18.1 and 18.5).

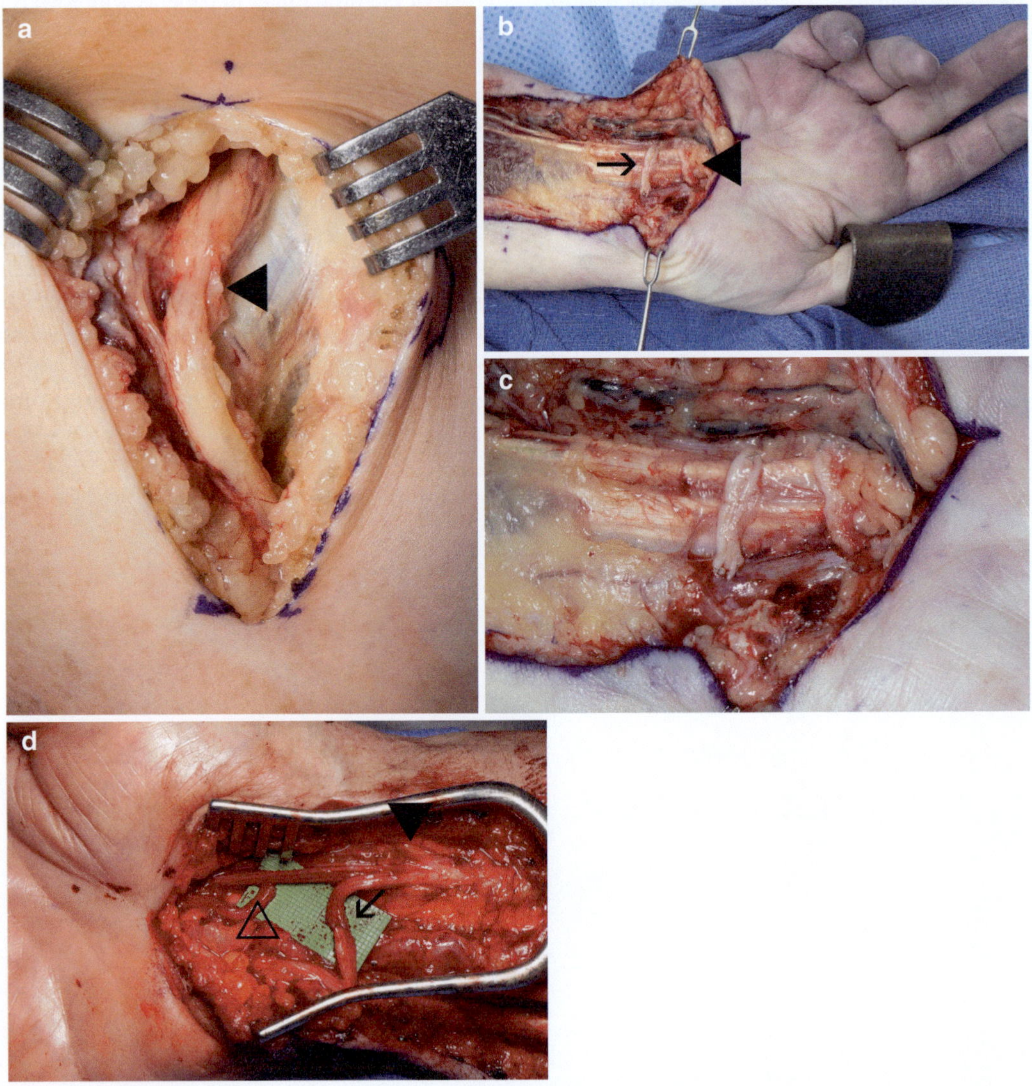

Fig. 18.5 Examples of cross-cross grafts for restoration of ulnar nerve function. Image (**a**) shows a case of severe ulnar nerve compression occurring at the elbow in a 58 year old man with >12 mm pre-operative 2 point sensation in small and ring finger. (**a**) Arrow points to visible compression of nerve following nerve release at cubital tunnel. (**b**, **c**) Show image of cross-cross graft with arrow pointing to proximal allograft running from median sensory of 3rd web to the ulnar aspect of the ulnar sensory nerve and the distal graft (arrowhead) running to radial component of ulnar sensory nerve. (**d**) Severe damage to the ulnar nerve may necessitate the use of an ETE nerve transfer of the 3rd web space branch of the median nerve to the sensory branch to the small and ring finger. Image (**d**) shows such a transfer. The sensory component of the median nerve has been isolated with a green micro background from larger median nerve (Solid arrow head). 3rd web space branch is sewn end to end into the sensory component of ulnar nerve (black arrow), while the distal sensory stump of the median nerve sensory branch with be sewn ETS into the main sensory branch of the median nerve (Clear arrowhead)

High Ulnar Neuropathy

In high ulnar nerve injuries, in addition to the deficits of a low injury, there is a loss of FCU and FDP function. There is loss of sensation of the dorsal hand and digits from the DCBUN. This sensation can be lost in a low ulnar nerve palsy, as well, if the injury is proximal to the takeoff of the DCBUN. The claw deformity is less severe as there is reduced pull from the ulnar FDP muscle belly [13].

Motor Reconstruction

The same options are present as for a low ulnar nerve palsy, and the SETS AIN to deep motor branch transfer is still considered the gold standard. Additional reconstruction of the FCU or FDP branches of the ulnar nerve are not typically attempted, as the FCR tendon can adequately power wrist flexion, and a side-to-side tenorrhaphy of the ring and little finger FDP tendons to the long finger FDP tendon (excluding the index to preserve independent function) produces adequate function.

Sallam et al. performed an AIN to ulnar motor branch in conjunction with sensory transfers from the 3rd webspace branch of the median nerve to the ulnar sensory branch with an end-to-side transfer of the DCBUN and the donor nerve stump to the median nerve in patients with high ulnar nerve injuries [23]. This group was compared to a group where nerve grafting of the nerve injury was performed without transfers. They had 83% M3 or greater recovery of intrinsic function in the nerve transfer group versus 57% in those with only nerve grafts. There was no difference in sensory recovery, with 58% and 54% of patients achieving S3 or greater sensation in the transfer and graft group, respectively [23]. In terms of sensory donor morbidity, two patients were aware of the loss of sensation and all patients regained at least protective sensation (S1).

Sensory Reconstruction

The same options would be available for a high ulnar nerve lesion, as described previously. A high ulnar nerve injury would definitively affect the DCBUN, which may or may not be affected in a low palsy. The reconstruction of the DCBUN is not considered a critical sensory area, but can be important as the ulnar side of the hand acts as a support while the radial side performs manipulation [17].

Median Nerve Compression

Low Median Neuropathy

A low median neuropathy produces a loss of motor function distal to the branch point of the AIN; thus, the motor function of the pronator teres, FCR, FDS, palmaris longus (PL) are preserved. The palmar cutaneous branch is also spared. Weakness of loss of thumb thenar function results in limited thumb opposition, palmar abduction and pronation. Some function of the flexor pollicus brevis may remain due to ulnar nerve innervation, but pinch strength has been shown to be limited to 60% and 70% of the contralateral side [25]. The sensory loss in these injuries is extremely disabling due to the use of the radial digits for fine manipulation. Sensory loss to the thumb can result in a 20% global functional loss to the entire hand [26]. There are few reports in the literature commenting on SETS transfers in cases of severe median neuropathies, however in the section below we present the nerve transfers which can be used to resort both motor and sensory function.

Motor Reconstruction

The recipient nerve for reconstruction of intrinsic hand function after a low median nerve injury is the recurrent motor branch of the median nerve. The typical donor nerves are the AIN [6], FDS, FCR, PL, abductor digiti minimi (ADM) branch of the ulnar nerve [25], or the 3rd lumbrical branch from the ulnar nerve [27].

The AIN and recurrent motor branch have comparable axon counts of 900 and 1050, respectively, and given that it is predominately a motor branch at this level, it is a good choice as a donor nerve. However, it is necessary to perform an interpositional graft. It is approached through an extended carpal tunnel release with neurolysis of the recurrent motor branch as proximal as possible, after which the resulting gap is grafting with an interpositional graft. Wang and Zhu transferred the AIN to the recurrent motor branch in 14 patients with a low median nerve palsy at an average of 5 years and 8 months, with 3 patients obtaining M5, 6 with M4, 3 with M3 and 2 with M2 [28]. The transfer from ulnar nerve branches of the ADM or 3rd lumbrical can allow direct coaptation due to their proximity and are beneficial in high median nerve injuries when the AIN is not a usable donor and nerve recovery may be prolonged with nerve repair or grafting (Fig. 18.6).

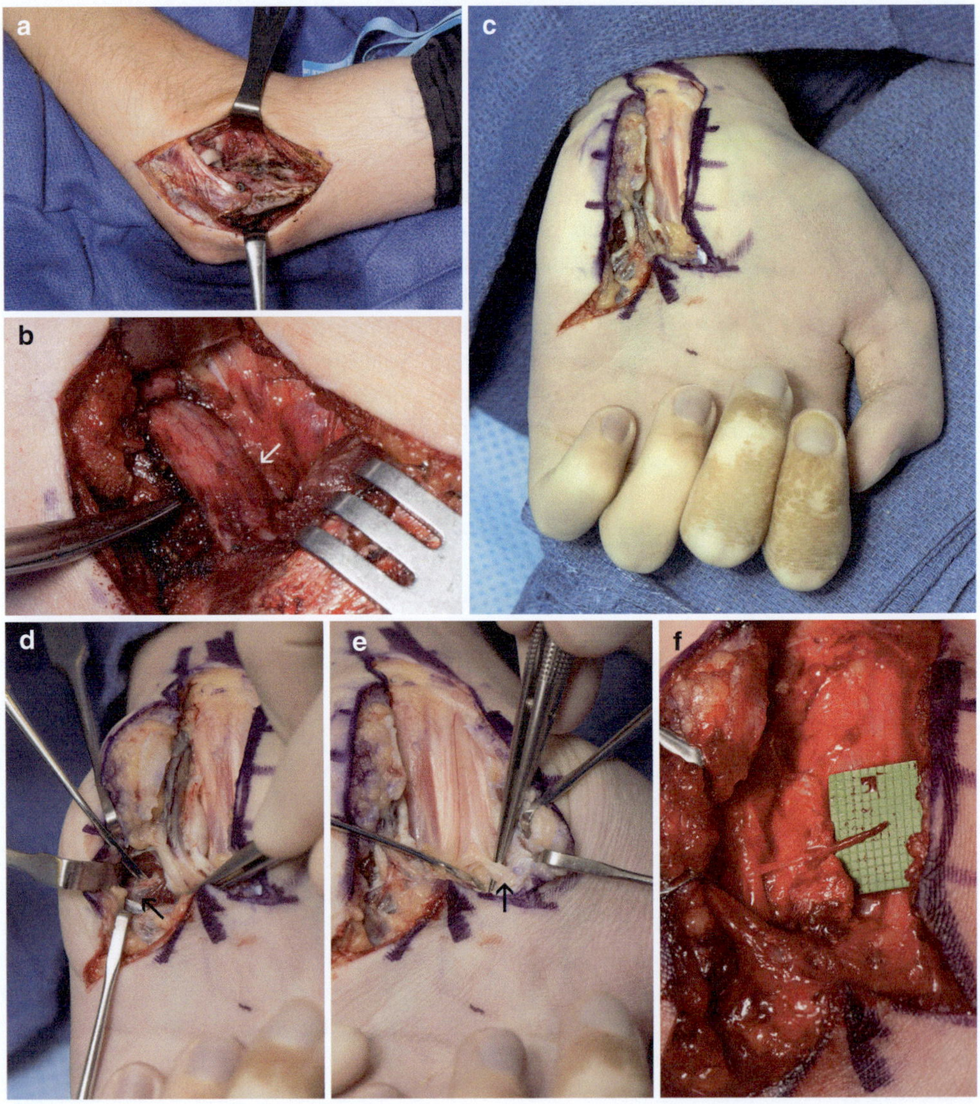

Fig. 18.6 A case of an ADM SETS transfer to median nerve motor branch in 15 year old who suffered supracondylar fracture with no thenar function at 4 months and evidence of decreased CMAPs to that muscle. (**a**) The median nerve was explored at the elbow. (**b**) Exploration of nerve and intraoperative nerve stimulation revealed intact nerve with evidence of partial axonal injury (arrow points to area of severe nerve contusion). (**c**) ADM motor branch transfer was performed to help preserve thenar function. (**d**) ADM was isolated and motor branch dissected back to the deep motor branch of the ulnar nerve. Arrow points to ADM motor branch. The median nerve motor branch was identified after carpal tunnel release (**e**) (arrow points to motor branch). And SETS transfer was then performed as close to thenar muscle as possible (**f**)

This transfer will be discussed further as a SETS transfer in the high median nerve injury section.

Sensory Reconstruction

To restore critical median nerve sensation, the radial digital nerve of the index and ulnar digital nerve of the thumb should be restored [6]. Common donor nerves are the 4th webspace branches of the ulnar nerve (ulnar digital nerve of the ring and radial digital nerve of the little finger) [6, 26], the DCBUN [22], and the superficial branch of the radial nerve [26, 29–31], which are less critical sensory areas. The 4th webspace branch is identified in the palm around the metacarpal head and transferred end-to-end to the 1st webspace branches of the median nerve, while the distal stump of the 4th webspace branch of the ulnar nerve is transferred end-to-side back to intact sensory branches to attempt to preserve donor site sensation [6]. A similar technique can be performed with the DCBUN by tracing it as distal as possible, transferring it to the thumb and radial aspect of the index sensory branches, and transferring the distal stump end to side to intact ulnar nerve fascicles [22]. To restore sensation to the second and third webspace, these can be transferred end-to-side to the ulnar digital nerve of the little finger. Brunelli performed a transfer of the DCBUN to the 1st webspace in two patients with a brachial plexus injury, however, both did not regain any sensation (S0) [20]. When he used the 4th webspace nerve to the 1st webspace in two patients, they regained tactile sensation (S2) [20].

The use of the radial nerve was first reported by Harris in 1921 to restore median nerve sensation in with a low median nerve injury with recovery beginning around 3 months postoperative [31]. Brunelli performed 12 cases of transfer from the radial sensory branches of the 1st webspace to the thumb and index finger at the 1st webspace and 2 similar transfers in the wrist in patients with a brachial plexus injury [20]. He had 6 patients with S2+, 6 with S2, 1 with S1 (protective sensation) and 1 patient with S0 (no sensation). Additionally, he had three patients where he transferred digital nerves from the ring and little to the thumb and index, in which they achieved S2 function [20]. Ozkan et al. performed various digital nerve transfers for both median and ulnar nerve injuries. They were able to achieve two-point discrimination of less than 10 mm in 15 of their 25 patients [26]. Of these patients, 7 had a median nerve injury of which all recovered >S3 sensation after a transfer to either an index or thumb digital nerve from the digital nerves of the ring or long finger [26].

High Median Neuropathy

In addition to the motor deficits of a low median neuropathy of the thenar musculature, a high median neuropathy also affects pronator teres, FCR, FDS, PL and AIN (FDP, pronator quadratus and flexor pollicis longus) function. The AIN and the branches to pronator teres now become a priority to provide proper hand function as tendon transfers to restore thumb opposition are well described and successful, while there are few successful tendon transfers to restore pronation [32]. The sensory deficit of a high median neuropathy includes the palmar cutaneous branch of the median nerve. It can be more difficult to regain sensation in a high median nerve injury versus a low injury. In a low injury, the sensation can be restored more predictably through direct suturing or repair with nerve grafting. With a high injury, there is a longer distance to reinnervate the target area and thus less chance of recovering protective sensation or motor function [29]. It can also be more difficult to line up the proper fascicular pattern to reinnervate distal targets when the injury is more proximal.

Motor Reconstruction

In addition to reinnervating the recurrent motor branch, the AIN and pronator teres branch are additional targets in a high median nerve injury and are no longer available donors. The common transfers are as follows: (1) ECRB, brachioradialis, supinator or FCU transferred to the pronator teres branch (2) Supinator, ECRB or brachialis branch of the musculocutaneous nerve to the AIN [22]. The use of ECRB for pronator teres is a synergistic transfer typically performed end-to-end and is preferred by some authors [6]. Hsiao et al. described a case of a high median nerve injury after a humeral fracture where a supinator to AIN and ECRB to pronator teres was performed [32]. The patient progressed from M0 AIN and pronator function to M4+ pronator teres and flexor pollicis longus and M4-FDP function at 18 months [32].

If the injury is not a complete high median neuropathy, then FCR, FDS or PL branches can be used to reconstruct the AIN, if available. As stated previously reconstruction of high median nerve injuries can be performed using a bridging nerve graft sutured end to side into both the median and ulnar nerve [16]. This allows axon sprouting between the nerves and recovery of the damaged recipient nerve function through the donor nerve both clinically and on EMG studies has been demonstrated.

Shultz and Aiache described the transfer of the ulnar nerve fascicle to the 3rd lumbrical to the recurrent motor branch in a patient with a high median nerve laceration [6]. The ulnar nerve branch was detached just proximal to the myoneural junction and the recurrent motor was neurolysed to allow tension free coaptation as close to the thenar musculature as possible. The patient recovered thumb abduction at 11 weeks postoperatively and regained pinch motion between his thumb, index and small fingers. EMG studies showed conduction from the ulnar nerve into the abductor pollicis brevis [6]. Bertelli et al. performed a cadaveric study and case series describing the transfer of the ADM branch of the ulnar nerve, which is the first branch of the deep motor branch of the ulnar nerve, to the recurrent motor branch of the median nerve. This was performed in five patients with a high median nerve injury, three of which had a concomitant ECRB to AIN transfer. All patients recovered M4 thumb and index finger flexion and an average grasp and pinch strength of 77% and 75% of the contralateral hand, respectively. The ABP strength improved from an average of M1.8 to M4 [25]. Our experience with this transfer has also been favorable (Fig. 18.6).

Sensory Reconstruction

As with low median nerve palsies, the target for reconstruction is the 1st webspace branches of the median nerve. Typically, the additional deficit of the palmar branch of the median nerve is not a priority for reconstruction as ulcers and injuries occur usually at the fingertips and not on the palm [29]. It has been reported that protective sensation to the palm and proximal aspects of the thumb and long finger are typically preserved by the palmar branches of the radial nerve after a median nerve injury and reconstruction should be focused on the tips of the thumb and index [20]. The options exist as per a low median nerve palsy, using the radial sensory nerve, the 4th webspace, DCBUN or LABC. Bertelli and Ghizoni performed transfer of the dorsal branches of the radial sensory nerve to the proper digital nerves of the index and thumb at the digital level in eight patients with a high median nerve injury [29]. Within 3–4 months, all thumbs recovered protective sensation and at 6 months, the index fingers recovered protective sensation in seven of eight patients (ability to feel a 2.0 g Semmes-Weinstein monofilament). At 12 months, three of eight patients had normal sensation in the thumb (ability to feel a 0.05 g filament) with no donor site deficit [29].

Summary

The indications for nerve transfers in cases of severe nerve compression are evolving. The use of SETS transfers may offer the benefit of more rapid motor recovery and improved sensory recovery long term. While not all patients with compressive neuropathies are candidates, we would recommend considering SETS transfers for patients with ulnar nerve compression at the elbow with evidence of decreased CMAP to the hand intrinsic muscles. Crossing bridge grafts may also be a means of improving sensation with little donor site morbidity. The use of nerve transfers in median nerve compression requires additional study; however, transfers can be considered in cases of high median nerve compression where critical sensation and thenar function are significantly affected (Fig. 18.7).

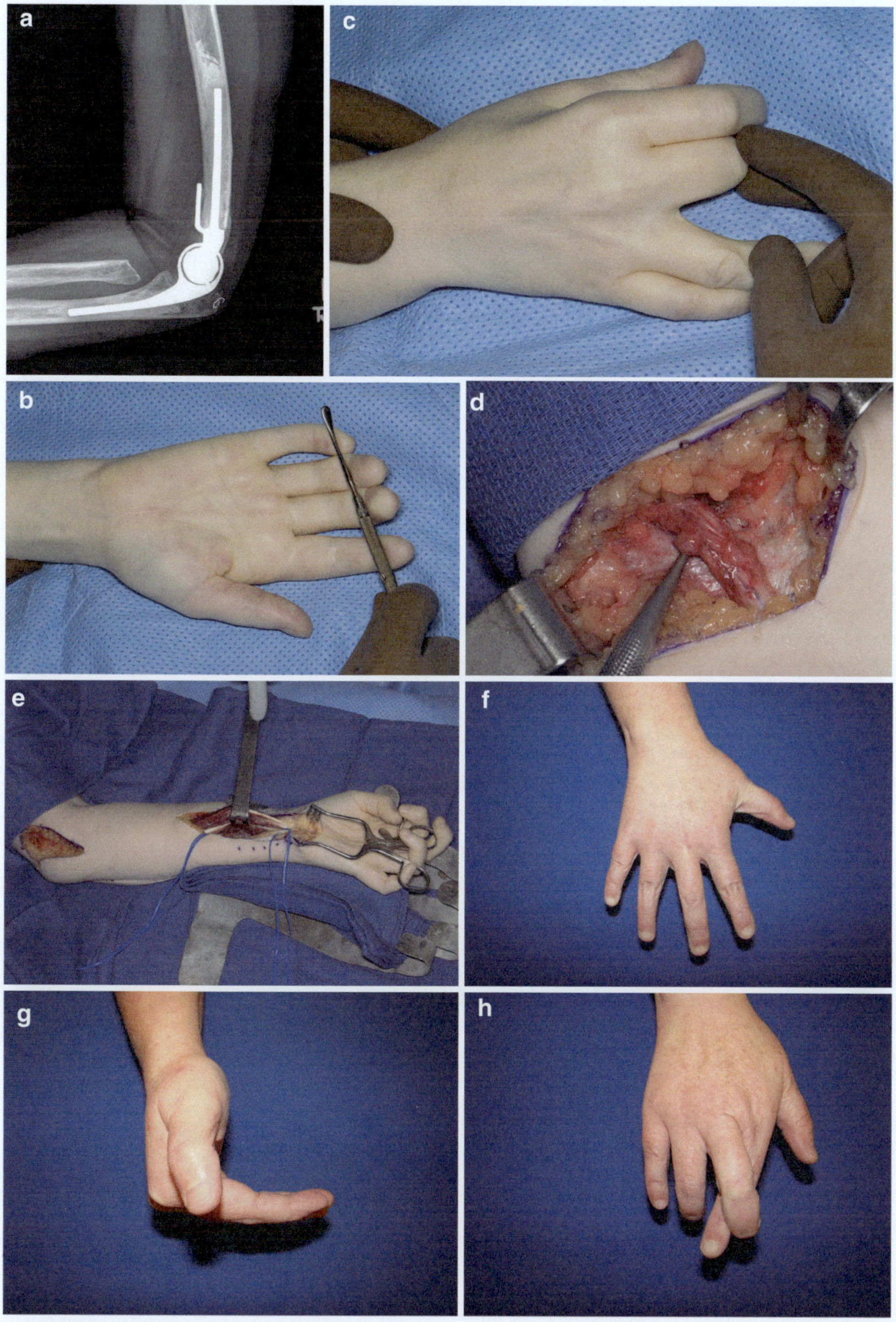

Fig. 18.7 (**a**) A case of a 63 year old woman with history of rheumatoid arthritis and previous total elbow replacement with recurrent ulnar nerve compression following release done elsewhere. (**b**, **c**) Pre-operatively the hand had evidence of intrinsic atrophy and decreased CMAPs within the ulnar intrinsic muscles to the hand. (**d**) At time of cubital tunnel release the patient was found to have significant scaring and fibrosis around the nerve. (**e**) AIN SETS transfer was performed in conjunction with a proximal neurolysis. Good intrinsic function was obtained at 5 months following the surgery and continued to improve for 12 months (**f**–**h**)

References

1. Tung TH, Barbour JR, Gontre G, Daliwal G, Mackinnon SE. Transfer of the extensor digiti minimi and extensor carpi ulnaris branches of the posterior interosseous nerve to restore intrinsic hand function: case report and anatomic study. J Hand Surg Am. 2013;38(1):98–103.
2. Farber SJ, Glaus SW, Moore AM, Hunter DA, Mackinnon SE, Johnson PJ. Supercharge nerve transfer to enhance motor recovery: a laboratory study. J Hand Surg Am. 2013;38(3):466–77.
3. Isaacs J, Patel G, Mallu S, et al. Effect of reverse end-to-side (supercharging) neurotization in long processed acellular nerve allograft in a rat model. J Hand Surg Am. 2019;44(5):419.e1–419.e10.
4. Baltzer H, Woo A, Oh C, Moran SL. Comparison of ulnar intrinsic function following supercharge end-to-side anterior interosseous-to-ulnar motor nerve transfer: a matched cohort study of proximal ulnar nerve injury patients. Plast Reconstr Surg. 2016;138(6):1264–72.
5. Felder JM, Power H, Hill E, Hasak J, Mackinnon SE. Cross-cross sensory nerve grafts to enhance sensory recovery in complex ulnar neuropathy [abstract]. Paper presented at: American Society of Peripheral Nerve Annual Meeting, Phoenix, Arizona; 12–14 Jan 2018.
6. Brown JM, Mackinnon SE. Nerve transfers in the forearm and hand. Hand Clin. 2008;24(4):319–40, v.
7. Moran SL, Steinmann SP, Shin AY. Adult brachial plexus injuries: mechanism, patterns of injury, and physical diagnosis. Hand Clin. 2005;21(1):13–24.
8. Gordon T, Tyreman N, Raji MA. The basis for diminished functional recovery after delayed peripheral nerve repair. J Neurosci. 2011;31(14):5325–34.
9. Sammer DM, Chung KC. Tendon transfers: part I. Principles of transfer and transfers for radial nerve palsy. Plast Reconstr Surg. 2009;123(5):169e–77e.
10. Schreiber JJ, Byun DJ, Khair MM, Rosenblatt L, Lee SK, Wolfe SW. Optimal axon counts for brachial plexus nerve transfers to restore elbow flexion. Plast Reconstr Surg. 2015;135(1):135e–41e.
11. Power HA, Sharma K, El-Haj M, Moore AM, Patterson MM, Mackinnon SE. Compound muscle action potential amplitude predicts the severity of cubital tunnel syndrome. J Bone Joint Surg Am. 2019;101(8):730–8.
12. Davidge KM, Yee A, Moore AM, Mackinnon SE. The supercharge end-to-side anterior interosseous-to-ulnar motor nerve transfer for restoring intrinsic function: clinical experience. Plast Reconstr Surg. 2015;136(3):344e–52e.
13. Woo A, Bakri K, Moran SL. Management of ulnar nerve injuries. J Hand Surg Am. 2015;40(1):173–81.
14. Barbour J, Yee A, Kahn LC, Mackinnon SE. Supercharged end-to-side anterior interosseous to ulnar motor nerve transfer for intrinsic musculature reinnervation. J Hand Surg Am. 2012;37(10):2150–9.
15. Novak CB, Mackinnon SE. Distal anterior interosseous nerve transfer to the deep motor branch of the ulnar nerve for reconstruction of high ulnar nerve injuries. J Reconstr Microsurg. 2002;18(6):459–64.
16. Magdi Sherif M, Amr AH. Intrinsic hand muscle reinnervation by median-ulnar end-to-side bridge nerve graft: case report. J Hand Surg Am. 2010;35(3):446–50.
17. Bertelli JA. Distal sensory nerve transfers in lower-type injuries of the brachial plexus. J Hand Surg Am. 2012;37(6):1194–9.
18. Ray WZ, Chang J, Hawasli A, Wilson TJ, Yang L. Motor nerve transfers: a comprehensive review. Neurosurgery. 2016;78(1):1–26.
19. Brown JM, Yee A, Mackinnon SE. Distal median to ulnar nerve transfers to restore ulnar motor and sensory function within the hand: technical nuances. Neurosurgery. 2009;65(5):966–77; discussion 977-968
20. Brunelli GA. Sensory nerves transfers. J Hand Surg Br. 2004;29(6):557–62.
21. Ruchelsman DE, Price AE, Valencia H, Ramos LE, Grossman JA. Sensory restoration by lateral antebrachial cutaneous to ulnar nerve transfer in children with global brachial plexus injuries. Hand (N Y). 2010;5(4):370–3.
22. Moore AM, Franco M, Tung TH. Motor and sensory nerve transfers in the forearm and hand. Plast Reconstr Surg. 2014;134(4):721–30.
23. Sallam AA, El-Deeb MS, Imam MA. Nerve transfer versus nerve graft for reconstruction of high ulnar nerve injuries. J Hand Surg Am. 2017;42(4):265–73.
24. Oberlin C, Teboul F, Severin S, Beaulieu JY. Transfer of the lateral cutaneous nerve of the forearm to the dorsal branch of the ulnar nerve, for providing sensation on the ulnar aspect of the hand. Plast Reconstr Surg. 2003;112(5):1498–500.
25. Bertelli JA, Soldado F, Rodrigues-Baeza A, Ghizoni MF. Transfer of the motor branch of the abductor digiti quinti for thenar muscle reinnervation in high median nerve injuries. J Hand Surg Am. 2018;43(1):8–15.
26. Ozkan T, Ozer K, Gulgonen A. Restoration of sensibility in irreparable ulnar and median nerve lesions with use of sensory nerve transfer: long-term follow-up of 20 cases. J Hand Surg Am. 2001;26(1):44–51.
27. Schultz RJ, Aiache A. An operation to restore opposition of the thumb by nerve transfer. Arch Surg. 1972;105(5):777–9.
28. Wang Y, Zhu S. Transfer of a branch of the anterior interosseus nerve to the motor branch of the median nerve and ulnar nerve. Chin Med J. 1997;110(3):216–9.
29. Bertelli JA, Ghizoni MF. Very distal sensory nerve transfers in high median nerve lesions. J Hand Surg Am. 2011;36(3):387–93.
30. Turnbull F. Restoration of digital sensation after transference of nerves. J Neurosurg. 1963;20:238–40.
31. Harris RI. The treatment of irreparable nerve injuries. Can Med Assoc J. 1921;11(11):833–41.
32. Hsiao EC, Fox IK, Tung TH, Mackinnon SE. Motor nerve transfers to restore extrinsic median nerve function: case report. Hand (N Y). 2009;4(1):92–7.

19 Ulnar Tunnel Syndrome (Guyon Canal)

Elizabeth P. Wahl and Marc J. Richard

Introduction

Jean Casimir Felix Guyon, a French urologist practicing in the mid-nineteenth century, first described the distal ulnar tunnel at the wrist in 1861 in the *Bulletin de la Societe de Anatomique de Paris* [1, 2]. In this bulletin, he described the projection of 'petits lobules' that appeared when he compressed the volar-ulnar aspect of his wrist. He pursued this further with anatomic dissections and discovered and described an intra-aponeurotic space now known as the distal ulnar tunnel. He further described the course of the ulnar artery and nerve in this space [1]. More than a century later in 1969, Shea and McClain described three types of compression syndromes of the wrist and hand depending on where in the wrist and hand the nerve was being compressed [3]. Later, Gross and Gelberman divided the distal ulnar tunnel into three zones based on the local anatomy of the ulnar nerve as it coursed through the tunnel [4]. The three-zone system is the most commonly used classification system today as it allows the treating physician to localize the site of the compression based on symptoms.

E. P. Wahl · M. J. Richard (✉)
Duke University Medical Center, Department of Orthopaedic Surgery, Durham, NC, USA
e-mail: elizabeth.wahl@duke.edu; marc.richard@duke.edu

Compressive neuropathy of the ulnar nerve (UN) at the wrist, ulnar tunnel syndrome (UTS), is less common than compression of the UN at the elbow, cubital tunnel syndrome (CuTS). These two syndromes often have similar and sometimes overlapping symptoms. However, there are key differences that can help differentiate the two diagnoses. Distinguishing between these two syndromes, as well as other sensory and motor neuropathies affecting the wrist and hand, requires a thorough understanding of the anatomy of the ulnar nerve.

Anatomy

The UN originates from the eighth cervical (C8) and first thoracic (T1) nerve roots. C8 and T1 merge to become the inferior trunk of the brachial plexus. The inferior trunk then branches into an anterior and posterior division. Fibers from the anterior division become the medial cord and the UN is the terminal branch of the medial cord [5]. Rarely, the UN receives some contributions from the lateral cord and middle trunk. After the axilla, the nerve travels in the anterior compartment of the arm, lying posteromedial to the brachial artery. In the brachium, the UN does not give off any branches. Approximately 8–10 cm proximal to the medial epicondyle, the UN pierces the intramuscular septum, traveling through the Arcade of Struthers, to course posterior to the septum along the medial head of the triceps.

D. G. Sotereanos, L. K. Papatheodorou (eds.), *Compressive Neuropathies of the Upper Extremity*, https://doi.org/10.1007/978-3-030-37289-7_19

The UN then enters the cubital tunnel posterior to the medial epicondyle and medial to the olecranon. The nerve travels between the ulnar and humeral head of the flexor carpi ulnaris (FCU) muscle as it enters the forearm. It then travels between the muscle bellies of the FCU and the flexor digitorum profundis (FDP) and at the junction of the middle and distal third of the forearm, the nerve passes ulnar to the ulnar artery. In the forearm, the nerve provides motor branches to the FCU and the ulnar half of the FDP and two sensory branches. The palmar cutaneous branch, sometimes known as the 'nerve of Henle', originates 16 cm proximal to the ulnar styloid [6], and the dorsal cutaneous branch of the ulnar nerve, branching approximately 3–5 cm proximal to the distal ulna [5].

The forearm is also the site of a potential Martin-Gruber anastomosis; an anomalous connection between the median and UN. This connection occurs anywhere from 2 to 10 cm distal to the medial epicondyle in the forearm and it is estimated to be found in 17% of the population [7]. This finding may account for preserved intrinsic function despite proximal UN pathology.

As the UN approaches the wrist it becomes more superficial and it travels into the wrist via the narrow distal ulnar tunnel, or Guyon's canal, accompanied by the ulnar artery (UA). At this level, the ulnar nerve is located dorsal and ulnar to the ulnar artery (Fig. 19.1). The distal ulnar tunnel is a fibro-osseous tunnel that is 1–2 cm proximal and deep to the distal wrist crease and is 4–4.5 cm in length. It begins at the proximal edge of the volar carpal ligament (VCL) and ends at the fibrous arch of the origin of the hypothenar muscles [4]. The tunnel does not have distinct borders through the entirety of the canal as the UN and UA take a tortuous path.

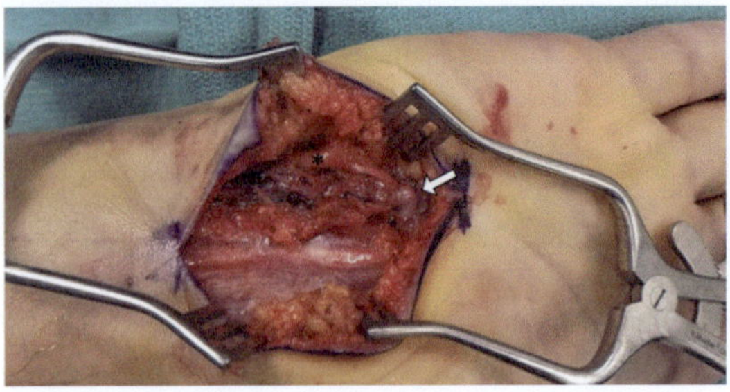

Fig. 19.1 Intraoperative photograph demonstrating the ulnar nerve (asterisk) traveling ulnar and dorsal to the ulnar artery (arrow) as it enters the wrist

The proximal and ulnar border is the pisiform and the radial and distal border is the hook of the hamate. The entrance of the tunnel is triangular, with a radial apex. From proximal to distal, the roof is the VCL, followed by the palmaris brevis and finally the fatty/fibrous tissue of the hypothenar eminence. The floor is made from the tendons of the FDP, the transverse carpal ligament (TCL), the pisohamate and pisometacarpal ligaments and the opponens digiti minimi (ODM) muscle. The radial boundary is defined by the extrinsic flexor tendons, the TCL and the hook of the hamate while the ulnar boundary is made of the tendon of the FCU, the pisiform and the abductor digiti minimi (ADM) [4]. Within the tunnel are the UN, UA as well as the venae comitantes and connective fatty tissue [8].

The UN lies slightly dorsal and ulnar to the UA within the canal. The UN bifurcates into the superficial sensory branch and deep motor branch [5]. The superficial sensory branch travels distally as a pure sensory nerve with the exception of motor branches that supply the palmaris brevis. It provides sensation to the palmar hypothenar eminence, the small finger and the ulnar aspect of the ring finger. The deep motor branch arises from the ulnar aspect of the UN. It travels distally and radially to the hook of the hamate. This motor nerve provides innervation to the hypothenar muscles (flexor digiti minimi [FDM], ADM, ODM), the ulnar two lumbricals, the interosseous muscles, the adductor pollicis and half of the flexor pollicis brevis [9]. The Riche-Cannieu anastomosis is a communication between the recurrent motor branch of the median nerve (MN) and the deep motor branch of the UN in the palm. This connection has been reported in up to 77% of patients and can lead to confusing clinical and electrodiagnostic findings [10]. For example, the MN may innervate the third and sometimes fourth lumbrical or the UN may innervate the thenar muscles.

The distal ulnar tunnel was divided into three zones by Gross and Gelberman for the purposes of making compression lesions of the UN easier

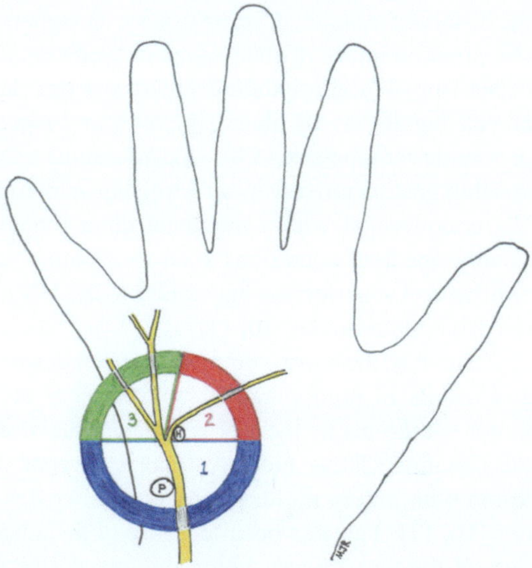

Fig. 19.2 Schematic drawing of the course of the ulnar nerve (yellow) through the three zones of Guyon's canal. Blue is zone 1, red is zone 2, and green is zone 3. Red is zone 2 and green is zone 3. P, pisiform; H, hook of the hamate

to diagnose and treat [4]. Each zone is identified by a specific part of the UN as well as the anatomic structures surrounding it (Fig. 19.2). Zone 1 is the area proximal to the bifurcation of the UN, zone 2 is the area surrounding the deep motor branch of the UN and zone 3 is the area surrounding the superficial branch of the UN [4].

Zone 1 is slightly more than 3 cm in length. It begins at the proximal aspect of the ulnar tunnel and extends to the bifurcation of the nerve. The UN and UA pass under the VCL with the tendons of the FDP forming the floor of zone 1. The VCL originates ulnarly from the tendon of the FCU and inserts radially to the TCL. The most distal fibers of the VCL curve radially and dorsally to merge with the fibers of the TCL, thereby wrapping the UN and UA and forming the radial wall of zone 1. As the UN and UA course distally in zone 1, the TCL travels ulnarly to insert on the base of the pisiform and becomes the floor of the tunnel. Similarly, the palmaris brevis becomes the roof of zone 1 distal to the VCL. The palmaris brevis is approximately 2.5 cm in length, making it the roof at the distal extent of zone 1 along with the pisohamate and pisometacarpal ligaments as the floor.

Zone 2 starts at the bifurcation of the UN and encompasses the deep branch of the UN to the fibrous arch of the hypothenar muscles [2]. The roof of zone 2 proximally is the palmaris brevis and distally is the fibrous arch of the hypothenar muscles. The UN follows a dorsal and radial course around the hamate as it dives deep to the fibrous arch. The UN passes under the fibrous arch and between the ADM and the FDM, innervating both of these muscles before it pierces and innervates the ODM as it curves radially and dorsally around the hook of the hamate. The UA enters zone 2 radially and volarly to the UN. The artery follows the UN in this zone as it passes under the fibrous arch [4]. After the motor fibers have exited zone 2, the fibers course parallel to the deep palmar arch radially, innervating the third and fourth lumbrical, the adductor pollicis, flexor pollicis brevis and the interossei [10].

Zone 3 begins slightly distal to the bifurcation of the UN and contains the superficial branch of the UN. The proximal boundaries of zone 3 consist of the palmaris brevis volarly (roof), the ADM ulnarly, the pisometacarpal ligament and the triquetro-hamate joint capsule dorsally (floor) and the border of zone 2 radially [4]. In contrast to the motor fibers in zone 2, the sensory fibers of zone 3 take a volar-ulnar course after the bifurcation. As the nerve courses distally, two motor branches pierce and innervate the palmaris brevis within the first 10 mm of zone 3. The remainder of the nerve is purely sensory and becomes the proper digital nerve to the ulnar side of the small finger and the common digital nerve to the web space of the ring and small fingers. The superficial branch of the UN exits zone 3, and consequentially the ulnar tunnel, by passing volar to the fibrous arch of the hypothenar muscles. The UA lies volar and radial to the UN. At the distal extent of the zone, the UN lies between the hypothenar fascia dorsally and the UA with an associated fibrofatty layer volarly.

Pathoetiology

The true incidence and prevalence of UTS are not truly known. The presenting signs and symptoms can help the clinician to localize where the nerve is being compressed. In their 1969 work, Shea and McClain reported that the most common cause of UN compression of the wrist in all zones was ganglion cysts (39%) followed closely by occupational neuritis (32%) [3]. More recent studies report that ganglia remain the most common cause of identifiable compression, however idiopathic compression with no identifiable cause is the most common etiology of compression [11, 12]. Other less common causes include tumors of the hand, anomalous muscles, hypothenar hammer syndrome, cyclist's palsy, fractures, carpal tunnel syndrome, iatrogenic neuropraxias during wrist arthroscopy, opponensplasty or tendon transfers, burns and medical conditions such as rheumatoid or osteoarthritis [3, 8, 11, 12].

A thorough occupational, recreational and medical history may also suggest etiologies of nerve compression. Repeated trauma from vibratory occupational tasks (jackhammering), hammer wielding or recreational activities like racquet or club sports can result in fractures of the hook of the hamate or thrombosis of the UA (Fig. 19.3) [8, 10]. Hypothenar hammer syndrome is injury to the UA due to entrapment between the hamate (hammer) and a fixed object (anvil) with repetitive contact. A direct hit from the external force results in "hammering" of the UA against the hook of the hamate. The injury to the UA may lead to enlargement with thrombosis of the UA at this level with subsequent occlusion and ischemia leading to nerve symptoms [11, 13]. Recreations such as cycling, baseball or carpentry may result in chronic injuries of the ulnar side of the wrist leading to UN compression in the distal ulnar tunnel. Cyclist's palsy, an isolated compression injury of zone 2 seen in cyclists, can occur from chronic external pressure from the bicycle handles to the ulnar palm after prolonged continuous compression [14, 15]. Adhesions may develop postoperatively as an iatrogenic cause of UN compression within the distal ulnar tunnel. Finally, medical conditions such as rheumatoid arthritis and scleroderma may injury to the UN in the distal ulnar tunnel [10, 11].

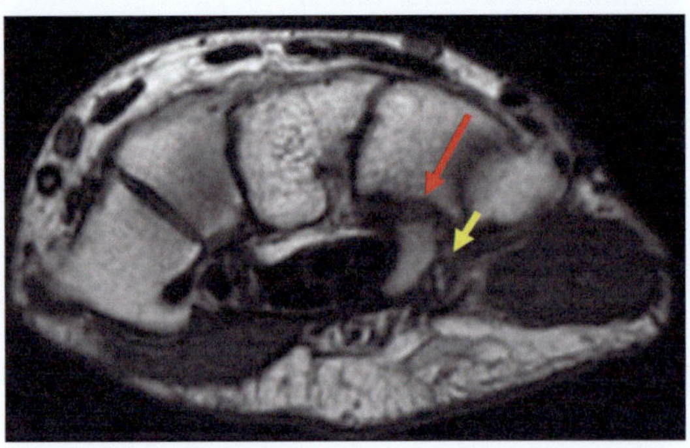

Fig. 19.3 Axial cut of a T1-weighted MRI of a left wrist. Long arrow pointing to a hook of the hamate fracture and short arrow pointing to the ulnar nerve

Zone 1 is the most commonly affected zone and results in predominantly both sensory and motor symptoms as the UN is a mixed nerve at this location. There are rare reports of zone 1 lesion with purely motor or purely sensory deficits [16, 17]. This can occur because of the anatomy of the nerve fibers within the mixed UN at this location. The motor fibers lie dorsally while the sensory fibers lie volarly. Thus, a small lesion arising dorsally may only affect the motor fibers, while a small, superficial volar lesion may affect isolated sensory fibers [4, 11]. The source of compression in zone 1 can be from the VCL volarly and TCL dorsally in the proximal aspect. Additionally, ganglia are commonly a cause of compression. The ganglia usually arise dorsally from the carpal bones, causing tethering of the nerve proximally and distally [4].

Zone 2 compression is also commonly caused by ganglion cysts. In zone 2, the majority of UTS occurs by compression of the UN against the fibrous arch of the hypothenar muscles. Unique causes of UN compression in zone 2 include hook of the hamate fractures and a thickened pisohamate ligament. The most common cause of compression in zone 3 is UA thrombosis and aneurysm [4].

In cases of unusual clinical findings, the treating clinician should consider concurrent pathologies. Importantly, MN neuropathy and UN neuropathy are not mutually exclusive. A study of 53 cases of UTS that underwent electrodiagnostic testing demonstrated 22 cases of concomitant mild to moderate MN lesions at the wrist. Of these 22 cases, 13 had symptoms of MN compression at the wrist [18]. Similarly, studies have shown that the converse is also true. Specifically, patients with electrodiagnostic evidence of CTS also had evidence of compression of the ulnar nerve at the wrist [19, 20]. In fact, one study reported that CTS and UTS co-occurrence was significantly more common than its absence [21]. Therefore, when the history and exam findings are not straight forward, the clinician should consider simultaneous compressive neuropathies as well as Martin-Gruber or Riche-Cannieu connections.

Clinical Findings

In suspected cases of UTS, the entire upper extremity should also be evaluated for all other potential causes of UN compression, including foraminal stenosis of C8 and T1, thoracic outlet syndrome and CuTS. Furthermore, the contralateral upper extremity should also be evaluated to assess muscle atrophy and symmetry. Ideally, the history and physical examination should rule out proximal sites of UN compression [22].

Ulnar neuropathy may be demonstrated by clawing of the ring and small finger with the hand in a resting position, hyperextension of the metacarpophalangeal (MCP) joints as well as wasting of the first dorsal interosseous muscle [22]. These findings are only present with significant compression of the motor fibers. Visible masses of the volar or dorsal wrist may suggest the presence of space-occupying lesions though the majority of ganglia causing UTS are not identifiable by physical examination. Palpation may reveal tenderness over the hook of the hamate. Additionally, palpation may reveal a bruit or thrill, suggesting an underlying vascular aneurysm. An Allen test should be performed to evaluate the patency of the ulnar artery.

The Tinel and Phalen tests of the UN at the elbow and wrist and of the MN at the wrist respectively are commonly performed, however their sensitivity and specificity are unclear [10, 11, 22]. Grundberg reported 92% of 31 cases with zone 1 compression had a positive Phalen test and 44% had a positive Tinel sign [23]. However, the Tinel and Phalen test can be helpful in identifying concurrent CTS and/or CuTS.

The Semmes-Weinstein monofilament test and the 2-point static discrimination test may both provide useful information about the severity of the disease. Typically, compressive neuropathies are best evaluated by using a threshold test that measures a single nerve fiber innervating a receptor. Threshold tests, such as Semmes-Weinstein monofilament test and vibration tests are more sensitive in measuring a gradual, progressive change in nerve function as more fibers are lost. Innervation density tests such as static and moving 2-point discrimination measure multiple overlapping receptive fields and are best used for evaluating functional nerve regeneration. Pathology in zone 1 will demonstrate sensory deficits over the volar-ulnar hand, hypothenar eminence, the small finger and the ulnar half of the ring finger [3, 8]. Importantly, sensation to the dorsal ulnar hand will be intact as this area is innervated by the dorsal cutaneous branch of the ulnar nerve, which originates approximately 3–5 cm proximal to the ulnar styloid.

Testing of the intrinsic and extrinsic motor function in the MN and UN distribution can provide useful information about the location of the compression. Testing should include comparison of grip and pinch strength in each hand as well as testing of the affected muscles. Interossei, lumbricals, hypothenar and thenar muscles as well as extrinsic flexors should be tested. Special tests that are provocative for ulnar nerve dysfunction can be helpful to determine pathology. For example, electrodiagnostic studies can take advantage of the dorsal cutaneous branch of the UN as it does not travel through the distal ulnar tunnel and will be normal in UTS, however may be abnormal in CuTS.

The Froment sign (Fig. 19.4), substitution of thumb interphalangeal and index finger distal interphalangeal joint flexion to maintain pinch while attempting key pinch, suggests dysfunction of the adductor pollicis. The flexor pollicis longus and flexor digitorum profundus to the index finger are innervated by the anterior interosseous nerve and compensate for the loss of ulnar nerve innervated muscles responsible for key pinch. The Wartenberg sign, abduction of the small finger due to unopposed pull of the abductor action of the radial nerve innervated extensor digiti quinti, may be present. This is due to loss of func-

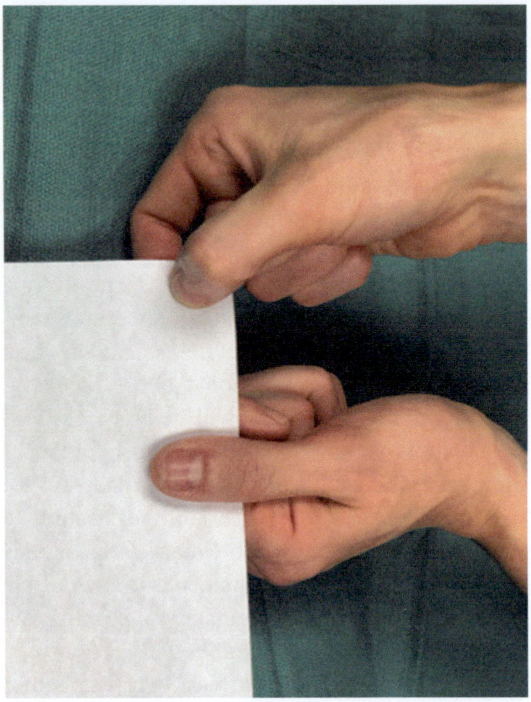

Fig. 19.4 Clinical photograph of the Froment sign. The left hand demonstrates normal function of the adductor pollicis (innervated by the ulnar nerve) while the right hand demonstrates compensation by the flexor pollicis longus and flexor digitorum profundus (innervated by AIN) when attempting key pinch

tion of the palmar interosseous to the small finger, an ulnar nerve innervated muscle. Finally, the palmaris brevis sign, sparing of the palmaris brevis muscle with concurrent weakness of the hypothenar muscles, suggest an isolated lesion to zone 2 as the motor innervation to palmaris brevis comes from the superficial sensory branch of the UN in zone 3 [8, 11, 22].

Diagnostics

Further studies for the evaluation of UTS include electrodiagnostic studies, radiographs and advanced imaging, including MRI and CT scans.

Electrodiagnostic studies are useful to help differentiate UTS from other compressive neuropathies of the upper extremity that can manifest similarly to UTS. Nerve conduction studies (NCS) and electromyography (EMG) can discern between CuTS, CTS, thoracic outlet syndrome, cervical radiculopathy or even peripheral neuropathy [24]. Specifically, needle EMG may show denervation of the hypothenar muscles with sparing of the FCU in cases of UTS [25]. Zone 1 lesions are characterized by diminished sensory responses and prolonged latency to the first dorsal interosseous and ADM muscles with preserved conduction velocity across the elbow [10, 11]. Zone 2 injures will also show normal conduction across the elbow and may show preserved latency of the hypothenar muscles, if the lesion is distal, with diminished latency of the first dorsal interosseous muscle [11, 26]. Zone 3 lesions will demonstrate diminished evoked sensory responses in the superficial sensory branch of the UN [25].

Radiographic evaluation should include standard PA and lateral radiographs of the wrist to assess for fractures of the distal radius and ulna and carpal bones as well as the carpal tunnel view to assess for a hook of the hamate fracture. Similarly, a CT scan of the wrist and hand can further identify hook of the hamate fractures as well as fractures of other carpal bones or of the ring and small finger proximal metacarpals. CT scans can also define ectopic calcifications of the distal ulnar tunnel. MRI can be a powerful tool in diagnosing space-occupying lesions like ganglion cysts or hand tumors. Furthermore, MRI can better define the branching pattern of the UN and UA within the distal ulnar tunnel as well as the presence of anomalous muscles [27, 28].

Doppler examination or arteriography may be of use in identifying and further characterizing vascular pathology in the ulnar artery [10, 22]. Finally, ultrasonography is a noninvasive method that can be used for evaluation of vascular, soft-tissue and nerve structures without the cost and invasiveness of more advanced imaging modalities [19, 29–31].

Treatment

Initial treatment of UTS should consist of a trial of nonsurgical management for cases caused by repetitive activities [8, 10, 11, 22]. Modalities such as protective splinting, nonsteroidal anti-inflammatory medication and activity modification are the mainstay of treatment. Cyclists may find improvement in symptoms by changing the handle bars, wearing protective gloves and ensuring the bicycle seat is positioned such that excessive weight is not placed on the hands [8, 14, 15]. Alternatively, cyclists may find relief by avoiding cycling for a period of time. Likewise, people affected by playing racquet or club sports or other repetitive activities may also trial a period of activity modification to see if symptoms improve [8, 30]. Aspiration of ganglion cysts has been described and can be successful, however aspiration with or without image-guidance does place the UA and UN at risk and should only be performed in the hands of an experienced ultrasonographer [31].

Surgical treatment should be pursued if symptoms persist despite a 2–4 month trial of nonsurgical treatment [10, 32, 33]. Additionally, surgery should be considered if initial findings demonstrate intrinsic muscle atrophy, denervation or weakness [8, 10, 11]. Surgical treatment should seek to address the causative pathology, e.g. removal of space-occupying lesions, as well as decompress the entire ulnar tunnel with exposure of the UN from its proximal to distal boundaries [11].

In general, surgical treatment can be performed under general, regional or local anesthesia. Some authors advise avoidance of local anesthesia as infiltration of the surgical area can obscure anatomic landmarks [22]. The bony landmarks of the pisiform and hook of the hamate are palpated, and the incision is carried obliquely between these two structures. The typical incision will be approximately 4–5 cm in length, starting 6 mm ulnar to the thenar crease and extend 1–2 cm proximal and 2–3 cm distal from the volar wrist crease (Fig. 19.5) [9, 11]. An S- or Z- shaped incision is used to cross the volar wrist crease to avoid contracture [10, 11]. The FCU is identified and retracted ulnarly to expose the UA and UN. Distally, there may be an ulnar palmar cutaneous branch crossing the incision that is present in about 15% of patients [9, 22]. This should be identified and protected. Then, incising the distal antebrachial fascia over the proximal wrist, the VCL and the palmaris brevis will decompress and expose the UN proximal to the bifurcation.

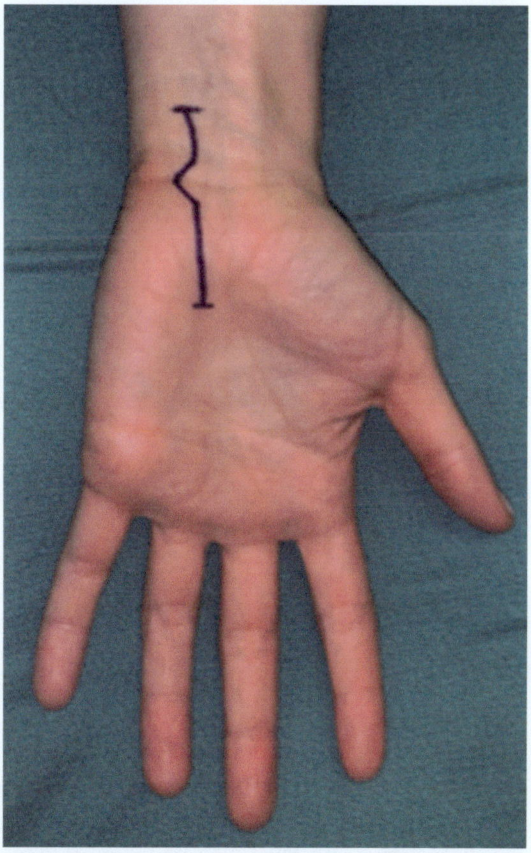

Fig. 19.5 Skin marking of the incision release of the distal ulnar tunnel

The UA and UN are gently retracted ulnarly, exposing the hook of the hamate and the fibrous arch of the hypothenar muscles is identified originating from the hook of the hamate [22]. The hypothenar fascia is identified by noting the oblique pattern of the fascia along the surface of the hypothenar muscles [9]. To decompress the deep motor branch in zone 2, the tendinous hypothenar muscle origin is carefully released near the hook of the hamate. This ensures protection of the superficial sensory branch that courses ulnar and volar to the hypothenar muscles. All fascial attachments around the hook of the hamate should be released, with care taken to avoid injury to the thin-walled vessels that run with the deep motor branch [9, 11, 22]. Finally, the UA

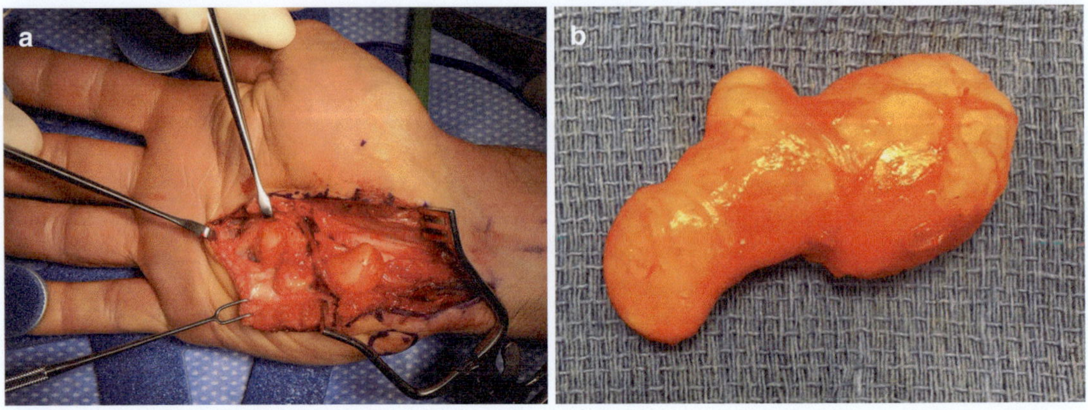

Fig. 19.6 (**a**) Intra-operative photograph of a large lipoma that compresses the ulnar nerve at the Guyon canal. (**b**) The lipoma gross specimen. (Photo courtesy of Dr. Dean Sotereanos)

should be inspected along its course to evaluate for aneurysms or thromboses. Any ganglion cyst or tumor that compresses the UN should be excised (Fig. 19.6).

Surgical decompression of the distal ulnar tunnel does place the UN and UA at risk for iatrogenic injury. Preservation of the vascular supply to the UN is important as well as preservation of the crossing sensory branch of the UN during the dissection. Care must also be taken to avoid injury to the structures in the carpal tunnel as the distal ulnar tunnel and the carpal tunnel are in very close proximity to each other. Currently, there are no large, long-term studies on the outcomes of treatment of UTS, however small retrospective series have reported good to excellent results with decompression of the distal ulnar tunnel [10, 12, 22].

Summary

Diagnosis and treatment of UTS requires a complete understanding of the anatomy and function of the ulnar nerve from its origin in the neck to its distal branches in the hand. UTS is less common than CTS and CuTS and is commonly caused by space-occupying lesions, acute or repetitive trauma or underlying medical conditions. A thorough history and examination can elucidate the underlying cause of the presenting symptoms in most cases and further diagnostic studies can be helpful when the diagnosis remains unclear. Nonsurgical management should be the mainstay of initial treatment unless there are initial signs of motor involvement. When treating UTS surgically, a thorough understanding of the complex anatomy and potential sites of compression is required for safe and successful management.

References

1. Guyon F. Note on the anatomical condition affecting the underside of the wrist not previously reported. 1861. J Hand Surg Br. 2006;31(2):147–8.
2. Maroukis BL, Ogawa T, Rehim SA, Chung KC. Guyon canal: the evolution of clinical anatomy. J Hand Surg Am. 2015;40(3):560–5.
3. Shea JD, McClain EJ. Ulnar-nerve compression syndromes at and below the wrist. J Bone Joint Surg Am. 1969;51(6):1095–103.
4. Gross MS, Gelberman RH. The anatomy of the distal ulnar tunnel. Clin Orthop Relat Res. 1985;196:238–47.
5. Polatsch DB, Melone CP Jr, Beldner S, Incorvaia A. Ulnar nerve anatomy. Hand Clin. 2007;23(3):283–9, v.
6. McCabe SJ, Kleinert JM. The nerve of Henle. J Hand Surg Am. 1990;15(5):784–8.
7. Leibovic SJ, Hastings H 2nd. Martin-Gruber revisited. J Hand Surg Am. 1992;17(1):47–53.
8. Chen SH, Tsai TM. Ulnar tunnel syndrome. J Hand Surg Am. 2014;39(3):571–9.
9. Mackinnon SE, Novak CB. Compressive neuropathies. In: Wolfe SW, Hotchkiss RN, Pederson WC, Kozin SH, Cohen MS, editors. Green's operative hand surgery. 7th ed. Philadelphia: Elsevier; 2017. p. 921–58.

10. Earp BE, Floyd WE, Louie D, Koris M, Protomastro P. Ulnar nerve entrapment at the wrist. J Am Acad Orthop Surg. 2014;22(11):699–706.
11. Waugh RP, Pellegrini VD Jr. Ulnar tunnel syndrome. Hand Clin. 2007;23(3):301–10, v.
12. Murata K, Shih JT, Tsai TM. Causes of ulnar tunnel syndrome: a retrospective study of 31 subjects. J Hand Surg Am. 2003;28(4):647–51.
13. Yuen JC, Wright E, Johnson LA, Culp WC. Hypothenar hammer syndrome: an update with algorithms for diagnosis and treatment. Ann Plast Surg. 2011;67(4):429–38.
14. Capitani D, Beer S. Handlebar palsy--a compression syndrome of the deep terminal (motor) branch of the ulnar nerve in biking. J Neurol. 2002;249(10):1441–5.
15. Patterson JM, Jaggars MM, Boyer MI. Ulnar and median nerve palsy in long-distance cyclists. A prospective study. Am J Sports Med. 2003;31(4):585–9.
16. Dupont C, Cloutier GE, Prevost Y, Dion MA. Ulnar-tunnel syndrome at the wrist. A report of four cases ulnar-nerve compression at the wrist. J Bone Joint Surg Am. 1965;47:757–61.
17. Boyes JH. Repair of the motor branch of the ulnar nerve in the palm. J Bone Joint Surg Am. 1955;37-A(5):920–4.
18. Seror P. Electrophysiological pattern of 53 cases of ulnar nerve lesion at the wrist. Neurophysiol Clin. 2013;43(2):95–103.
19. Ginanneschi F, Filippou G, Reale F, Scarselli C, Galeazzi M, Rossi A. Ultrasonographic and functional changes of the ulnar nerve at Guyon's canal after carpal tunnel release. Clin Neurophysiol. 2010;121(2):208–13.
20. Ginanneschi F, Milani P, Mondelli M, Dominici F, Biasella A, Rossi A. Ulnar sensory nerve impairment at the wrist in carpal tunnel syndrome. Muscle Nerve. 2008;37(2):183–9.
21. Kiylioglu N, Akyildiz UO, Ozkul A, Akyol A. Carpal tunnel syndrome and ulnar neuropathy at the wrist: comorbid disease or not? J Clin Neurophysiol. 2011;28(5):520–3.
22. Bachoura A, Jacoby SM. Ulnar tunnel syndrome. Orthop Clin North Am. 2012;43(4):467–74.
23. Grundberg AB. Ulnar tunnel syndrome. J Hand Surg Br. 1984;9(1):72–4.
24. Werner RA. Electrodiagnostic evaluation of carpal tunnel syndrome and ulnar neuropathies. PM R. 2013;5(5 Suppl):S14–21.
25. Campion D. Electrodiagnostic testing in hand surgery. J Hand Surg Am. 1996;21(6):947–56.
26. Cavallo M, Poppi M, Martinelli P, Gaist G. Distal ulnar neuropathy from carpal ganglia: a clinical and electrophysiological study. Neurosurgery. 1988;22(5):902–5.
27. Andreisek G, Crook DW, Burg D, Marincek B, Weishaupt D. Peripheral neuropathies of the median, radial, and ulnar nerves: MR imaging features. Radiographics. 2006;26(5):1267–87.
28. Andreisek G, Burg D, Studer A, Weishaupt D. Upper extremity peripheral neuropathies: role and impact of MR imaging on patient management. Eur Radiol. 2008;18(9):1953–61.
29. Harvie P, Patel N, Ostlere SJ. Prevalence and epidemiological variation of anomalous muscles at guyon's canal. J Hand Surg Br. 2004;29(1):26–9.
30. Ginanneschi F, Filippou G, Milani P, Biasella A, Rossi A. Ulnar nerve compression neuropathy at Guyon's canal caused by crutch walking: case report with ultrasonographic nerve imaging. Arch Phys Med Rehabil. 2009;90(3):522–4.
31. Nakamichi K, Tachibana S. Ganglion-associated ulnar tunnel syndrome treated by ultrasonographically assisted aspiration and splinting. J Hand Surg Br. 2003;28(2):177–8.
32. Kim DH, Han K, Tiel RL, Murovic JA, Kline DG. Surgical outcomes of 654 ulnar nerve lesions. J Neurosurg. 2003;98(5):993–1004.
33. Almeida V, de Carvalho M. Lesion of the deep palmar branch of the ulnar nerve: causes and clinical outcome. Neurophysiol Clin. 2010;40(3):159–64.

Radial Tunnel Syndrome - Posterior Interosseous Nerve Compression Syndrome

20

Ioannis K. Sarris and Ilias D. Alafropatis

Introduction

Compression of the radial nerve through the anatomic space called radial tunnel is believed to be the cause of two separately described clinical conditions.

Radial tunnel syndrome is a syndrome characterized by forearm and wrist pain with no motor weakness manifestations. The fact that the posterior interosseous nerve is believed to be a motor-only nerve has been the cause of controversy whether the RTS even exists as a pathological entity [1, 2]. However, surgeons who have historically supported the diagnosis have reported relief of the symptoms with radial nerve decompression [3, 4].

The posterior interosseous nerve compression syndrome (PINCS) on the other hand is a compressive neuropathy caused either by normal anatomical structures or pathological structures (lipomas, ganglia, fibrous adhesions, rheumatoid synovium) in the radial tunnel [4–8]. The PINCS is characterized by progressive weakness of fingers and thumb metacarpophalangeal joints extension. Atrophy of extensor muscle bellies may be present if the condition is left untreated. Pain is absent or might be mild in the vast majority of the cases and sensory deficits are never encountered.

I. K. Sarris (✉) · I. D. Alafropatis
3rd Orthopaedic Department, Papageorgiou General Hospital, Aristotle University of Thessaloniki Medical School, Thessaloniki, Greece

Anatomy

The Radial Nerve

The radial nerve originates from the posterior cord of the brachial plexus and carries fibers of C6, C7, and C8 nerve roots. Following a spiral course in the upper arm it innervates most of the triceps brachii muscle and the anconeus. It then pierces the lateral intermuscular septum approximately 10 cm proximal to the lateral epicondyle and innervates the brachialis, brachioradialis, extensor carpi radialis longus (ECRL) and in 90% of the cases the extensor carpi radialis brevis (ECRB). The nerve then crosses the elbow anterior to the lateral epicondyle and divides into the superficial branch of the radial nerve and the posterior interosseous nerve. The bifurcation lies 6–10 cm distal to the lateral intermuscular septum and 3–4.5 cm proximal to the leading edge of the supinator [9].

The PIN, which is primarily motor, passes then under the dorsal surface of the radial neck, courses under the arcade of Fröhse and enters the forearm between the two heads of the supinator muscle. Exiting the supinator muscle the PIN is divided into its terminal medial and lateral branches which innervate the extensor carpi ulnaris (ECU), extensor digitorum communis (EDC), extensor digitorum quinti (EDQ), abductor pollicis longus (APL), extensor pollicis

D. G. Sotereanos, L. K. Papatheodorou (eds.), *Compressive Neuropathies of the Upper Extremity*,
https://doi.org/10.1007/978-3-030-37289-7_20

longus (EPL), extensor pollicis brevis (EPB) and extensor indicis proprius (EIP) in that order [10].

The terminal branches of the PIN also carry unmyelinated (group IV) fibers from the wrist capsule and small myelinated (group IIA) fibers from muscles along its distribution.

The Radial Tunnel

The radial tunnel is a musculo-aponeurotic tunnel that extends from the lateral epicondyle of the humerus proximally, to the distal edge of the supinator muscle distally (Fig. 20.1). Proximally, the radial nerve passes between the brachioradialis and the extensor carpi radialis longus posteriorly and between the brachialis and the biceps brachii muscles anteriorly. The floor of the tunnel is formed by the anterior aspect of the radiocapitellar joint capsule and the deep portion of the supinator muscle. The superficial head of the supinator muscle, aponeurotic fibers stretching from the lateral epicondyle and the extensor carpi radialis brevis insertion constitute the roof of the tunnel [11, 12].

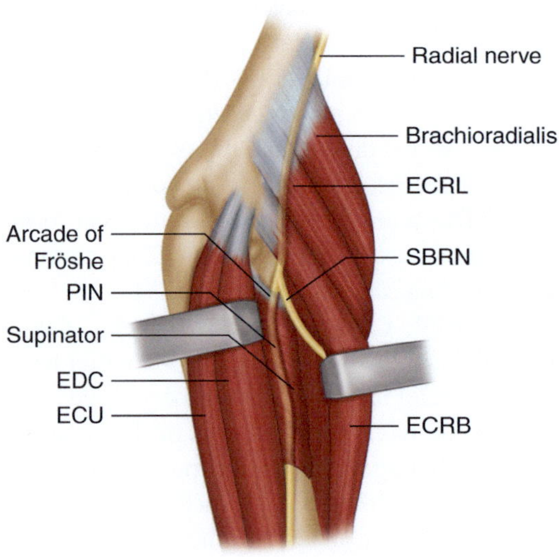

Fig. 20.1 Schematic representation of the radial nerve and the PIN as it courses through the radial tunnel. ECRL = extensor carpi radialis longus, ECRB = extensor carpi radialis brevis, SBRN = superficial branch of radial nerve, PIN = posterior interosseous nerve, EDC = extensor digitorum communis, EDU = extensor carpi ulnaris

Etiology

Both RTS and PINCS are thought to be clinical manifestations of compression of the PIN in the radial tunnel. The incidence of PIN compression is estimated at 0.03% per year whereas the carpal tunnel syndrome, which represents the most common compression neuropathy, has an estimated 0.1–0.35% annual incidence rate [1, 13, 14].

Increased pressure on the nerve may reduce venous blood flow, cause ischemia or even block axonal transport [15, 16]. The PIN may be mechanically constricted due to normal anatomical structures as it crosses the radial tunnel. Five possible sites of compression of the PIN have been identified through its course in that area: fibrous bands between the brachialis and brachioradialis anterior to the radiocapitellar joint, recurrent radial vessels at the radial neck level also known as the "leash of Henry", the supero-medial edge of the ECRB, the proximal edge of the superficial portion of the supinator also reffered to as "arcade of Fröhse" and the distal edge of the supinator muscle. The arcade of Fröhse is mentioned as the most frequent site of PIN entrapment [17–21].

Other space-occupying pathological structures such as lipomas, adhesions, ganglia or cysts and inflammatory synovium caused by rheumatoid arthritis have also been reported as mechanically compressing the PIN [4–6, 22].

Traditionally, repetitive alternating forearm pronation and supination has been considered as a causative factor of PIN neuropathy [23–27]. Intra-operative measurements of pressures exerted on the PIN by the proximal edge of the supinator during passive forearm pronation and tetanic nerve stimulation have been found to be comparable with pressures responsible of nerve fibers' functional compromise. Passive forearm pronation stretches the supinator whereas tetanic nerve stimulation produces active contraction of muscles innervated by the PIN. Excessive, prolonged and repetitive use of those muscles is thought to have an obstructive effect in nerve conduction [28]. Manual laborers who use tools with full elbow extension or use forces with frequent pronosupination and elbow extension between 0° and 45° are also reported to have increased chance of developing RTS [29–30].

Controversy

Given the fact that the PIN is thought of as an absolute motor nerve, muscle weakness or dropped fingers should be typical symptoms of PIN compression neuropathy [31]. In 1972, Roles and Maudsley were the first to report an association between forearm pain and PIN neuropathy in a series of cases with persistent "tennis elbow" [3]. They proposed the term "Radial Tunnel Syndrome" which was adapted by subsequent studies to describe pain in the proximal radial aspect of the forearm over the course of the PIN, with no motor deficit which is believed to be due to PIN compression. Lack of motor manifestations, radiologic findings, electrodiagnostic criteria and standardized clinical tests in addition to unpredictable outcomes after surgery are the main arguments against identifying PIN neuropathy as the cause of RTS [2, 32]. Localized tenderness over the course of the PIN and subjective clinical tests are on the other hand the hallmark of RTS diagnosis [16, 33].

To support the idea of mechanical constriction of the PIN as the cause of RTS, understanding the PIN function as of not being purely motor has been proposed. The PIN carries unmyelinated Group IV and small myelinated Group IIA afferent fibers from muscles along its distribution. Group IV fibers are associated with nociception and pain and Group IIA fibers are associated with temperature sensation. Moderate pressure on that kind of fibers may produce the pain and discomfort associated with the RTS without affecting the large myelinated fibers of the PIN which transfer motor stimuli. Another interesting fact in favor of that theory is that unmyelinated and small myelinated fibers cannot be evaluated by nerve-conduction studies, giving a possible explanation to the lack of specific electrodiagnostic findings in patients with RTS [34].

Physical Examination

Radial Tunnel Syndrome

Pain in the proximal anterior radial aspect of the forearm, which in some cases may radiate to the dorsum of wrist and fingers, is the sole clinical finding in RTS. Radial tunnel proximity to the lateral epicondyle, concomitant lateral epicondylitis and the fact that the syndrome was firstly reported as a persistent tennis elbow syndrome may be confusing when assessing patients who present with RTS symptomatology. Exact localization of the pain is of paramount importance in order to differentiate from other elbow pathology. Typically, pain and tenderness in palpation over the PIN, approximately 5 cm distal to the lateral epicondyle, is diagnostic of RTS [16, 33].

The "Rule-of-Nine test" is a test proposed to improve RTS related pain localization. A large square box is drawn over the anterior aspect of the proximal forearm with its sides determined by the width of the elbow crease with the forearm in full extension and supination. The square is then divided in 3 columns and 3 rows which creates 9 equal smaller squares. Tenderness involving the 2 proximal squares of the lateral column is indicative of PIN irritation [35] (Fig. 20.2).

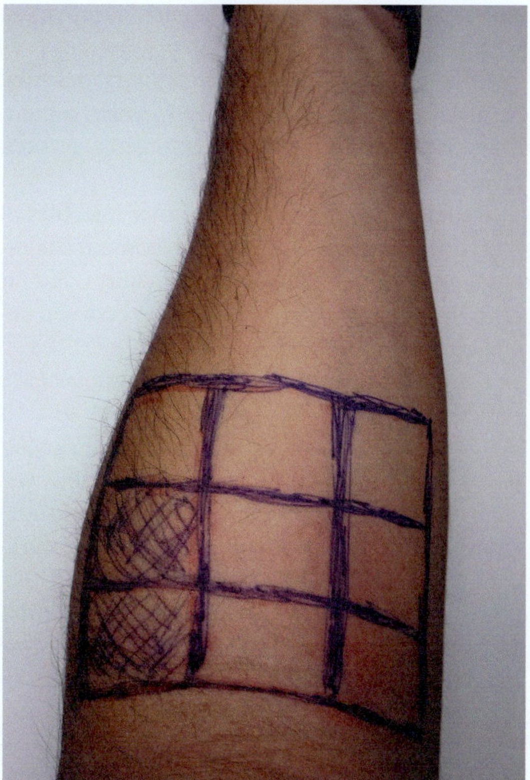

Fig. 20.2 The "Rule-of-Nine" test. Tenderness with palpation over the proximal 2 squares of the lateral column (highlighted in the photograph) is proposed as diagnostic of radial tunnel syndrome

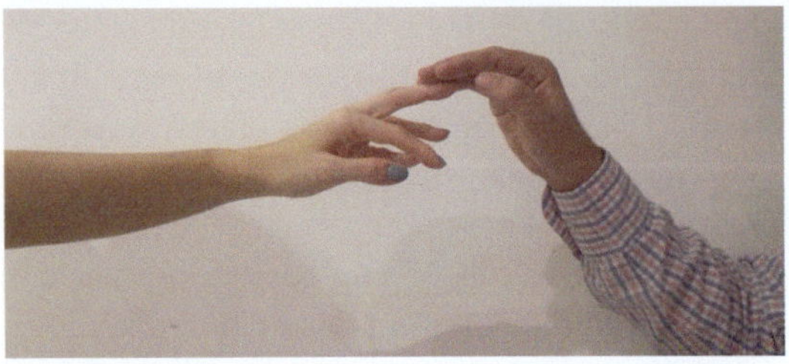

Fig. 20.3 Active extension of the middle finger with the forearm in pronation, against resistance. Pain provoked with that maneuver is characteristic in patients suffering from the radial tunnel syndrome

Other clinical tests may also be utilized, with Lister in 1979 being the first to describe a provocative test for diagnosing RTS. The test consists of active extension of the middle finger against resistance with the forearm in pronation (Fig. 20.3). That way the ECRB, which contributes to the formation of the radial tunnel and has its insertion on the base of the third metacarpal, becomes tensed. If pain is provoked with that maneuver the test is characterized as positive for RTS [36]. Other authors describe pain exacerbation with resisted forearm supination or resisted wrist hyperextension as confirming of the diagnosis [33, 37].

Relief of pain or discomfort after injection of local anesthetic into the area of maximum tenderness is another diagnostic modality and is described as useful in differentiating between lateral epicondylitis and RTS [38, 39].

Clinical tests utilized for RTS diagnosis have not been assessed in depth or verified so it is highly unlikely to specify or falsify the diagnosis based on a single clinical test [1, 2]. However, since RTS is an almost exclusively clinically diagnosed pathologic condition, physical examination should be careful and thorough. Other elbow pathology must be excluded and clinical indication of the diagnosis must be high before treatment decision-making.

Posterior Interosseous Nerve Compression Syndrome

Patients with PINCS present with dropped fingers and thumb without a history of previous trauma. Wrist extension is preserved with radial deviation because the ECRL and in most cases the ECRB innervation is not affected by constriction of the PIN. Weakness of the APL, EPB, EPL and EIP is indicative of compression on the lateral branch of the PIN, whereas weakness of the ECU, EDQ and EDC points at involvement of the medial branch of the PIN [10]. If PINCS is left untreated, atrophy of the forearm extensor muscles becomes obvious within a matter of weeks.

Sensory deficits are typically absent, although some patients may report mild pain or discomfort radiating in the forearm or wrist. Wrist extension ability and lack of paraesthesia are useful at excluding compression or lesions of the radial nerve proximally to the radial tunnel. If severe pain precedes or coexists with PIN palsy and sensory disturbance in other areas of the arm is present neuralgic amyotrophy/Parsonage – Turner syndrome may be the cause of paralysis. In those cases an history of viral infection, toxic exposure, vaccination, systemic diseases or major surgery may be recalled and physical examination should aim to reveal multiple nerve involvement [40].

Imaging Studies

Plain radiographs that are routinely ordered in cases of forearm pain are of no diagnostic use in cases of suspected RTS. Magnetic resonance imaging (MRI) techniques have been utilized and described as diagnostic of RTS with controversial findings. Ferdinand et al reported that in 52% of patients with RTS who underwent MRI examination, denervation edema or muscle atrophy within the supinator or the extensor muscles innervated by the PIN were present. An additional 28% of the patients also had findings such as thickening of the proximal edge of the ECRB, abnormal radial recurrent vessels or swelling of the epineurium [41]. Those findings however are disputed by other authors and their validity remains controversial, supporting the idea that RTS has no specific imaging characteristics [9].

In cases of true PIN palsy, MRI is highly sensitive in identifying secondary alterations of denervated muscles. A specially designed MRI protocol with the use of microscopy coil has been reported as to have directly depicted nerve swelling associated with PINCS in addition to those secondary changes owing to nerve dysfunction [42]. MRI is in addition a gold-standard method of revealing space occupying lesions within the radial tunnel. The vast majority of tumors or tumor-like lesions causing compression neuropathy have been found to be of extraneural origin [43]. Intramuscular or parosteal lipomas are reported as being the most common extrinsic factor causing PIN compression [6, 44–51] (Fig. 20.4). Ganglia rising from the anterior capsule, chondromatosis, vasculitis, septic arthritis and rheumatoid pannus have also been identified with MRI as nerve irritating factors [5, 8, 52–63]. In a recent study however, defined masses compressing the PIN were found in only 27% of patients suffering from isolated PIN palsy [64].

Another imaging modality which may be of use is modern high resolution ultrasonography. In a small case series of patients suffering from PINCS examined with ultrasonography, swelling of the PIN just proximal to the arcade of Fröhse implying constriction at that level was found in 40% of the cases. Swelling distal to the radial tunnel was found in 10% and soft tissue masses were observed in 40% of the patients. The examiners were also able to identify denervation atrophy of the supinator and the extensors in 20% of the patients and the mean anteroposterior diameter of pathologic nerves was significantly larger than that of the contralateral side [65]. Such findings underline the potential benefit of the use of ultrasonography in PIN entrapment pathology, since ultrasonography has also the advantage of allowing dynamic examination in different forearm positions.

Electrodiagnostic Testing

Electromyography and nerve-conduction velocity studies are typically believed to be of no use for the diagnosis of RTS. In an attempt to identify possible electrodiagnostic alterations in RTS and combine them with a proposed pathophysiological explanation of the syndrome, studies were designed with the nerve being examined in different positions of the forearm or dynamically with active forearm maneuvers. When Rosen et al compared motor latency at rest and with active supination no difference was recorded in the results [66]. In another study including 25 patients with RTS diagnosis, PIN motor latency

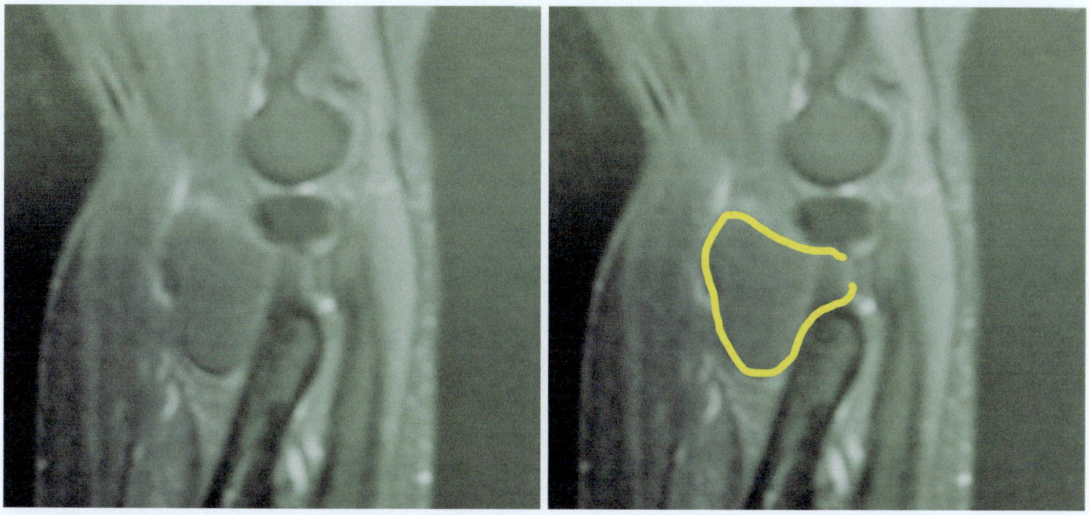

Fig. 20.4 MRI of the right elbow of a patient who presented with dropped index finger and thumb. Weakness of the rest of the digits was present but wrist extension was spared. A soft tissue mass (later identified as a parosteal lipoma) is depicted in contact with the radial neck

was recorded in three different forearm positions: neutral, passive supination and passive pronation. Differential motor latencies of the patients were greater than that of controls. The investigators proposed that a differential motor latency of 0.3 ms or more is a sensitive diagnostic criterion in patients with RTS [67]. Furthermore, the difference in motor latency between the nerve to the BR and the nerve to ECU has been utilized as a diagnostic method of RTS [68].

Electromyographic evidence of PIN innervated muscles denervation in patients with RTS diagnosis is almost always absent and sensory conduction studies are constantly normal. However, neurophysiological testing must be part of the overall evaluating process, since it can provide useful information or help in ruling out other pathological conditions (e.g. cervical radiculopathy, neuralgic amyotrophy).

In cases of PINCS electrodiagnostic testing is used not only as an objective confirmation method of the otherwise obvious clinical presentation, but also as a prognostic tool, providing information about re-innervation potential [8]. Nerve conduction investigation is always performed bilaterally for comparison reasons. Typical findings in motor conduction studies are delayed conduction velocity, prolonged distal latency and reduced amplitude. Sensory conduction studies are always normal, as in the RTS. Electromyographic evaluation may reveal positive sharp waves and fibrillations which are characteristic of abnormal spontaneous activity, decreased recruitment intervals and discrete recruitment pattern in muscles innervated by the PIN [69, 70]. Neurophysiological findings in PIN entrapment must be carefully evaluated, since abnormalities not related to the PIN distribution have been found in up to 36% of patients diagnosed with "isolated" PIN palsy, when reviewed carefully retrospectively [64].

Treatment

Pain relief and rehabilitation to the previous activity level are the therapeutic goals for patients with RTS [71]. Conservative treatment is the first line of treatment. Every patient with RTS symptomatology should follow a course of nonoperative treatment with a duration of up to 6 months [39, 72]. Wrist immobilization in the form of casting, non steroid anti-inflammatory medication and activity modification are the most commonly used methods of conservative treatment. Activity modification consists of avoidance of the pain provoking activity, which typically is repetitive pronosupination or manual labor with extended elbow and flexed wrist. Such modifications may require ergonomic retraining [71]. Physical therapy is advised and muscle stretching, nerve gliding excercises, cryotherapy, thermotherapy and ultrasound massaging all have been used with variable results. Successful treatment of clinical diagnosed RTS has also been reported after following a dry needling program with complete pain resolution maintained for 6 months of follow-up [73]. However, the efficacy of such therapeutic methods is generally in doubt and there is no consensus or guidance on which method may provide better results. Generally, symptom relief is expected in only about 30% of the patients with RTS following conservative treatment [74, 75]. Cortico-steroid injections have also been used in treatment of RTS. According to Sarhadi et al, a single injection of 2 ml 1% lidocaine and 40 mg of triamcinolone in 1 ml of carrier has been shown to provide pain resolution in 72% of the patients within a 6-week period and a 2 year symptom-free period in 62% of the patients. Injection is performed at the site of maximal tenderness [39]. Most recently in a published prospective study the utility of a single corticosteroid injection in the proximal forearm in 35 patients suffering from RTS was assessed. 0.25 ml of lidocaine 1% and 0.75 ml of Celestone 6 mg/ml was administered in the area of maximal tenderness, typically within the mobile wad of the extensors. No specific attempt was made to block the PIN. Tenderness to palpation and pain in the proximal forearm with resisted forearm supination or middle finger extension subsided immediately after injection in all patients. During the first year of follow up only 23% of the patients proceeded on to surgical decompression of the PIN, rendering corticosteroid injection a therapeutic measure with potential long-term benefits in the treatment of RTS [76].

Since conservative treatment is of doubtful effectiveness in RTS and if pain does not improve after following non-operative measures for a period of 3–6 months, operative treatment with surgical PIN decompression is offered. Surgical treatment is recommended with caution and after thoroughly explaining to the patient that outcomes may not always be excellent [77–79].

In cases of PINCS, it is obvious that if a causative factor can be identified, immediate surgical decompression is recommended. More specifically, if a structural malformation or space occupying lesion is present within the radial tunnel, prompt removal is highly indicated, because further obstruction of nerve stimuli will lead to irreversible damage to the nerve and thus complete and irreversible muscle paralysis. However, there are cases that such decision is difficult to be made, mainly for two reasons. The first is that PINCS may be misdiagnosed or confused with other PIN palsy causes, such as neuralgic amyotrophy and spontaneous hourglass constriction of the PIN (SHGC). Thresholds for surgical exploration differ between true entrapment neuropathy and neuralgic amyotrophy. Entrapment neuropathy generally has a low threshold for surgical intervention whereas in neuralgic amyotrophy a longer period of non-operative treatment and observation is accepted owing to the conditions' high possibility of spontaneous recovery. The second is that in many cases and even if clinical and neurophysiological findings are characteristic of PINCS, no structural cause can be identified. A short period of anticipation for spontaneous recovery is accepted in those cases. Physical therapy and very close observation is recommended and even complete resolution of PIN compression symptoms using soft tissue manipulation therapy has been reported [80]. No consensus has been reached as to the duration of that observational period. Studies suggest that prolonged conservative treatment of PINCS negatively affects results after surgical decompression. Those studies imply that if the syndrome remains untreated for a period of over 4.7 months, the possibility for full recovery drops to 74% compared to a 94% possibility of full recovery if surgical decompression is performed in less than 2.2 months after the onset of symptoms [81, 82]. Neglected cases for over 12–18 months have no potential of muscle re-innervation since muscle fibrosis occurs and the only way to restore hand function is by tendon transfers.

A reasonable period of spontaneous recovery should not exceed 6 weeks and should be combined with strict activity modifications, arm splinting, physical therapy and close patient observation. If no signs of recovery are present after that period, surgical decompression is the only way to increase full recovery possibility [7, 72, 83].

Surgical Approaches

Although the two syndromes present with completely different clinical manifestations and the RTS is not recognized as a true entrapment neuropathy by many upper extremity surgeons, surgical decompression of the PIN is utilized for treatment of both RTS and PINCS. The PIN can be surgically explored and released via various approaches.

Anterior Approach [84]

General or regional anaesthesia is provided and the arm is positioned in a supinated position on a hand table. Tourniquet is applied after exsanguination of the arm. The approach starts with a curvilinear incision over the elbow crease. The proximal part of the incision starts 3–5 cm proximal to the elbow crease along to the lateral border of the biceps brachii. It is curved and extended transversely over the elbow crease for 2–3 cm and then curved again to a distal direction for another 4–5 cm along the medial border of the brachioradialis. Cephalic vein which lies in the subcutaneous fat may be ligated or preserved depending on exposure demands. The lateral antebrachial cutaneous nerve (LACN) is typically identified lateral to the biceps tendon and protected. Failure to recognize and protect the LACN may cause its intraoperative laceration which then may be the cause of neurinoma formation and disturbing sensory complaints. The fascia is divided along the brachioradialis and the muscle is then retracted laterally. The brachialis in the proximal wound and the biceps and pronator teres in the distal wound are retracted medially. The radial nerve is then identified proximally between the brachialis and the brachioradialis. The BR branch may be visible at that level. Following the nerve distally branches to the ECRL and ECRB may be encountered with variable origins. In 97% of the cases the radial nerve bifurcates just proximal to the radiocapitellar joint level in its two terminal branches. The SBRN travels along the medial border of the BR and the PIN continues on the deeper layers distally. Recurrent branches of the radial artery and muscular vessel branches are meticulously ligated and divided. Fibrous adhesions between the brachialis and brachioradialis and the fibrous leading edge of the ECRB are then divided since they represent potential sites of compression. Next the proximal insertion of the supinator which in most cases is tendinous is released under direct vision and with respect to the branch of the PIN which innervates the supinator itself, a branch arising from the PIN just proximal to the arcade of Fröhse. The PIN is traced distally in the supinator and fibrous bands of the muscle are released along its entire length. In order to visualize the full length of the supinator, the mobile wad of the extensors must be elevated and retracted. Space occupying lesions such as ganglia or lipomas are separated from surrounding tissues and excised if present. The subcutaneous fat and skin is then sutured after tourniquet release and careful haemostasis.

Posterior Approach [85]

After preparation and positioning with the arm in pronation, the approach starts a with longitudinal skin incision of approximately 5–8 cm. The incision starts distal to the lateral humeral epicondyle at the radial neck region and extends distally and dorsally following an imaginary line connecting the lateral epicondyle with the distal radioulnar joint. The lateral cutaneous nerves of the arm are protected. Dissection follows the interval of the extensors mobile wad and the EDC, most specifically the plane between ECRB and EDC. The supinator muscle is revealed underneath by developing that plane at the proximal edge of the EDC. In contrary to the EDC muscle fibers that run parallel to the forearm, supinator muscle fibers have an oblique course, a fact that can be helpful in orientation. If additional exposure is needed the EDC insertion may be detached off the lateral epicondyle. The PIN can be identified at the distal edge of the supinator and followed proximally. Under direct vision, the superficial head of the supinator, the leash of Henry, the fibrous edge of the ECRB and the arcade of Frohse are released. The possible advantage of such an approach is the ability to address pathology around the lateral epicondyle such as persistent tennis elbow [86]. Haemostasis and wound closure follows.

Lateral Approaches

Between BR and ECRL

With this approach the interval between BR and ECRL is developed. The incision is made over the mobile wad and the posterior antebrachial cutaneous nerve is identified and protected. The fascia is incised longitudinally over the level of that interval. The two muscles are separated with blunt dissection and the radial tunnel becomes directly visible underneath.

Transbrachioradialis [36] (Fig. 20.5)

Incision starts 3 cm lateral of the biceps brachii tedon and just proximal to the radial head level and is extended for 6–8 cm. The fascia over BR is incised over the muscle, in parallel with its fibers. The muscle's belly is then bluntly split and a part of the muscle belly is retracted medially with the remainder retracted laterally. By splitting the BR parallel to its course, the PIN will become visible at the proximal edge of the supinator which lies

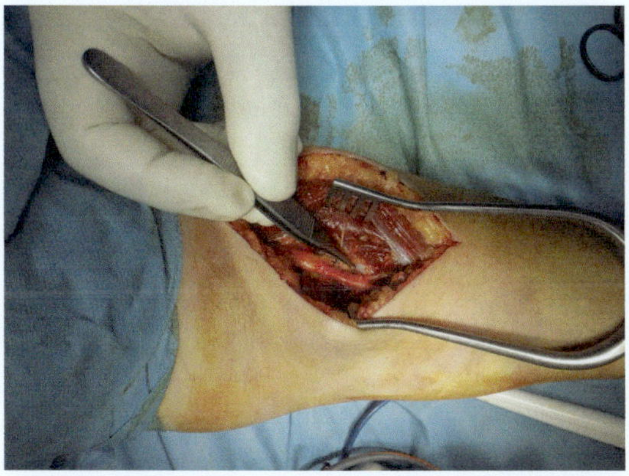

Fig. 20.5 Transbrachioradiallis approach. A forceps is used to point at the tendinous proximal edge of the supinator

underneath, surrounded by fat tissue. By moving the blunt retractors proximally and distally the leading edge of ECRB and radial recurrent vessels and the distal part of the supinator can be identified respectively. The PIN is then released and mobilized under direct vision. This approach provides the possible benefit of being less traumatic since only blunt dissection of the BR is performed and only blunt retractors are used. It has also been shown that through that approach all possible sites of PIN compression can be identified and released [87].

Endoscopic Assisted Methods

Endoscopic or endoscopic assisted methods of nerve decompression are gaining in popularity with possible advantages in terms of earlier rehabilitation, lower morbidity and improved cosmesis. Endoscopic carpal tunnel release and endoscopic assisted cubital tunnel release are utilized in an ongrowing number of cases [88, 89]. The past few years endoscopic assisted methods of PIN decompression have been developed.

Leclēre et al in 2013 described a procedure where a 2–3 cm incision is made 5 cm proximal to the elbow in line with the imaginary line connecting the deltoid insertion to the lateral epicondyle. Dissection to the fascia follows and the fascia is incised. The radial nerve is inspected through the endoscope and the lateral intermuscular septum is also opened. The radial nerve is neurolysed with the elbow in extension position up to 5 cm distal to the elbow joint. A second incision is then made at the point, where the endoscope light is visible through the skin, on the lateral surface of the forearm utilizing the interval between the BR and ECRL. The PIN which was previously identified through the first approach is exposed. The endoscope is then introduced through the second approach and the neurolysis is completed by releasing any pathological structure [90].

Ertem et al most recently described a different endoscopic assisted method of PIN decompression. The operation starts with a 2–3 cm incision 6–8 cm distal to the lateral epicondyle as part of the posterior approach incision. The interval between EDC and ECRB is dissected and the PIN is exposed as it emerges of the distal supinator. The endoscope then is inserted and the superficial supinator belly and other structures that compress the PIN are then dissected proximally. If necessary the radial nerve may be released even more proximally. That operation makes use of a single incision to decompress the radial nerve [91].

Outcomes

The generally low incidence of the PINCS makes the study of effectiveness of different treatment choices problematic. In cases of mechanical PIN constriction with motor deficit, good outcomes have been reported even with delayed surgical decompression and pre-operative neurological testing showing poor re-innervation potential. Complete or partial resolution is usually gradual and may demand 2 or even 4 years after the onset of symptoms [69, 92, 93]. Rates of 74–95% of excellent results have been reported with timing of surgery being of paramount importance, since better results are obtained with earlier intervention [81, 82]. In a systematic review by Huisstede et al., no randomized controlled trials were found about the effectiveness of other treatment choices. Of the studies included, the conclusion drown is that surgical decompression of the PIN is effective for patients with PINCS. None of high-quality studies report on the effectiveness of conservative treatment of PINCS. Even in studies that mention conservative treatment of PINCS, no further information about the kind of such treatment is given. Higher quality studies and further research must be conducted in order to assess the effectiveness of non-operative treatment [94].

PIN decompression indications for PIN palsy also extend beyond true compression neuropathy, like in cases of neuralgic amyotrophy. It is believed by some surgeons that surgical treatment with interfascicular neurolysis may promote nerve recovery, if Parsonage – Turner patients do not show signs of recovery within the first month of the onset of symptoms [92]. Surgical decompression with interfascicular neurolysis is also thought of providing good to excellent results in the majority of patients with SHGC with an age younger than 50 years, a pre-operative wait of less than 7 months and only mild to moderate constrictions [8, 92].

As in PINCS, there are no published randomized controlled trials or controlled clinical trials studying the effectiveness of different treatment modalities for patients with RTS. The effectiveness of conservative treatment is questionable and no methodology or program has been proposed as the cornerstone of non-operative treatment. The analysis of studies of the best quality by Huisstede et al in 2008, found that 67–92% of patients with RTS treated with surgical decompression reported good to excellent results. There are, however, controversial results in the literature concerning surgical treatment in RTS. Earlier studies had encouraging outcomes reporting success rates of 81–95% after radial tunnel surgical release [28, 33, 36].

Reports that followed, on the other hand, showed a low percentage of about 40% of patient satisfaction after surgical treatment of RTS, regardless of sex, hand dominance, employment, duration of symptoms, surgeon or operative findings [95, 96]. Outcomes of endoscopic assisted methods of PIN decompression for the treatment of RTS are promising but in a small number of patients. Leclēre et al report pain relief in three out of four patients and Ertem et al report good and excellent results in eight out of ten patients [90, 91].

Concomitant pathology may be of critical importance when operatively treating RTS patients. If RTS is the sole pathological condition in the patient's upper extremity, a success rate of 86% may be anticipated. That rate drops to 57% if another entrapment neuropathy co-exists and even in 40% if the patient also suffers from lateral epicondylitis [75].

Outcomes also vary depending on whether the patients operated on were receiving workers' compensation benefits. In a study published in 1997, there was no difference in outcome between workers' compensation patients and non-workers' compensation patients, but the study was criticized as of having a low number of patients [38]. Sotereanos and colleagues reported an extremely disappointing success rate of 32% in workers' compensation patients or patients in litigation. In the same study, overall results were excellent or good in 64% of the patients [97]. Comparing patients receiving workers' compensation with others not, Lee et al also demonstrated a lower success rate in the former category. Only 58% of patients receiving workers' compensation had optimal results, with 73% of patients with no compensation claims having excellent outcome in a series of 33 patients [75].

The aforementioned controversies in outcomes, define patient selection as of major importance when deciding surgical treatment for RTS. Published data supports that patients who suffer from concomitant upper extremity conditions such as lateral epicondylitis or other neuropathies and patients that are likely to receive workers' compensation benefits, may probably have less successful outcomes. That fact should be kept in mind when offering surgical decompression to RTS patients, since the syndrome is exclusively clinically diagnosed and the only indication for surgery is failure of conservative treatment.

Conclusion

RTS and PINCS both share surgical decompression as the definite treatment, although they present with completely different symptomatology. The unknown connection between the two syndromes' pathophysiology – if any connection exists – may lie in the void of our complete understanding of how the PIN functions. It is possible that intermediate repetitive and intermittent compressive forces on the PIN provoke pain and discomfort by irritating proprioceptive and pain transmitting nerve fibers only, whereas higher prolonged pressure on the nerve blocks motor stimuli as in the PINCS. The inability to test every nerve conduction parameter via electrodiagnostics may be responsible for lack of objective findings in the RTS.

In terms of deciding the right treatment for both syndromes, controversies still exist. High quality controlled randomized trials or clinical controlled trials are needed in order to clarify the effectiveness of conservative treatment and which non-operative remedy is the most suitable for each condition. The low reported incidence of PIN entrapment renders planning and conduction of such studies even more problematic.

Prompt surgical decompression holds a key role in the treatment of PINCS which is thought of as a true compressive neuropathy. For RTS, even skeptics agree that surgical treatment should be offered to patients with persistent non-resolving symptoms [1]. However, due to the fact that RTS is diagnosed exclusively clinically, surgeons should proceed to surgical exploration cautiously. Concomitant pathology in the upper extremity, misdiagnosed conditions and workers' compensation claims may have a negative impact on outcomes of an otherwise justifiable operation.

References

1. Van den Ende K, Steinmann SP. Radial tunnel syndrome. J Hand Surg Am. 2010;35:1004–6.
2. Rosenbaum R. Disputed radial tunnel syndrome. Muscle Nerve. 1999;22(7):960–7.
3. Roles NC, Maudsley R. Radial tunnel syndrome: resistant tennis elbow as a nerve entrapment. J Bone Joint Surg Br. 1972;54:499–508.
4. Sharrard WJ. Posterior interosseous neuritis. J Bone Joint Surg Br. 1966;48:777–80.
5. Bowen TL, Stone KH. Posterior interosseous nerve paralysis caused by a ganglion at the elbow. J Bone Joint Surg Br. 1966;48(4):774–6.
6. Fitzgerald A, Anderson W, Hooper G. Posterior interosseous nerve palsy due to parosteal lipoma. J Hand Surg Br. 2002;27(6):535–7.
7. Wu P, Yang J, Yu C. Surgical treatment of spontaneous posterior interosseous nerve palsy with hourglass-like constriction. J Hand Surg Eur Vol. 2014;40(6):646–7.
8. Hashizume H, Inoue H, Nagashima K, Hamaya K. Posterior interosseous nerve paralysis related to focal radial nerve constriction secondary to vasculitis. J Hand Surg Br. 1993;18(6):757–60.
9. Thomas SJ, Yakin DE, Parry BR, Lubahn JD. The anatomical relationship between the posterior interosseous nerve and the supinator muscle. J Hand Surg Am. 2000;25(5):936–41.
10. Elgafy H, Ebraheim NA, Rezcallah AT, Yeasting RA. Posterior interosseous nerve terminal branches. Clin Orthop Relat Res. 2000;376:242–51.
11. Portilla Molina AE, Bour C, Oberlin C, et al. The posterior interosseous nerve and the radial tunnel syndrome: an anatomical study. Int Orthop. 1998;22:102–6.
12. Riffaud L, Morandi X, Godey B, Brassier G, Guegan Y, Darnault P, et al. Anatomic bases for the compression and neurolysis of the deep branch of the radial nerve in the radial tunnel. Surg Radiol Anat. 1999;21:229–33.
13. Dang AC, Rodner CM. Unusual compression neuropathies of the forearm, part I: radial nerve. J Hand Surg Am. 2009;34(10):1906–14.
14. Barnum M, Mastey RD, Weiss AP, Akelman E. Radial tunnel syndrome. Hand Clin. 1996;12(4):679–89.
15. Rydevik B, Lundborg G, Bagge U. Effects of graded compression on intraneural blood blow: an in vivo study on rabbit tibial nerve. J Hand Surg. 1981;6:3–12.
16. Bentley FH, Schlapp W. The effects of pressure on conduction in peripheral nerve. J Physiol. 1943;102:72–82.
17. Derkash RS, Niebauer JJ. Entrapment of the posterior interosseous nerve by a fibrous band in the dorsal edge of the supinator muscle and erosion of a groove in the proximal radius. J Hand Surg Am. 1981;6(5):524–6.
18. Capener N. The vulnerability of the posterior interosseous nerve of the forearm. J Bone Joint Surg Br. 1966;48(4):770–3.
19. Clavert P, Lutz JC, Adam P, et al. Frohse's arcade is not the exclusive compression site of the radial nerve in its tunnel. Orthop Traumatol Surg Res. 2009;95:114–8.
20. Prasartritha T, Liupolvanish P, Rojanakit A. A study of the posterior interosseous nerve (PIN) and the radial tunnel in 30 Thai cadavers. J Hand Surg. 1993;18(Am):107–12.
21. Fuss F, Wurzl G. Radial nerve entrapment at the elbow: surgical anatomy. J Hand Surg. 1991;16(Am):742–7.
22. Moon N, Marmor L. Parosteal lipoma of the proximal part of the radius. A clinical entity with frequent radial-nerve injury. J Bone Joint Surg Am. 1964;46:608–14.
23. Hobhouse N, Heald C. A case of posterior interosseous paralysis. BMJ. 1936;1:841.
24. Silverstein A. Progressive paralysis of the dorsal interosseous nerve. Arch Neurol Psychiatr. 1937;38:885.
25. Weinberger L. Non-traumatic paralysis of the dorsal interosseous nerve. Surg Gynecol Obstet. 1939;69:358.
26. Kruse F. Paralysis of the dorsal interosseous nerve not due to direct trauma: a case showing spontaneous recovery. Neurology. 1958;8:307.

27. Sonna LA, Scott BR. Posterior interosseous nerve palsy in a machine gunner. Mil Med. 1995;160:364–6.
28. Werner CO, Haeffner F, Rosén I. Direct recording of local pressure in the radial tunnel during passive stretch and active contraction of the supinator muscle. Arch Orthop Trauma Surg. 1980;96(4):299–301.
29. Van Rijn RM, Huisstede BM, Koes BW, et al. Associations between work-related factors and specific disorders at the elbow: a systematic literature review. Rheumatology. 2009;48:528–36.
30. Roquelaure Y, Raimbeau G, Saint-Cast Y, et al. Occupational risk factors for radial tunnel syndrome in factory workers. Chir Main. 2003;22:293–8.
31. Suematsu N, Hirayama T. Posterior interosseous nerve palsy. J Hand Surg. 1998;23B:104–6.
32. Verhaar J, Spaans F. Radial tunnel syndrome. An investigation of compression neuropathy as a possible cause. J Bone Joint Surg Am. 1991;73:539–44.
33. Hagert CG, Lundborg G, Hansen T. Entrapment of the posterior interosseous nerve causing forearm pain. Scand J Plast Reconstr Surg. 1977;11:205–12.
34. Lin YT, Berger RA, Berger EJ, et al. Nerve endings ofthe wrist joint: a preliminary report of the dorsal radiocarpal ligament. J Orthop Res. 2006;24:1225–30.
35. Loh YC, Lam WL, Stanley JK, et al. A new clinical test for radial tunnel syndrome – the Rule-of-Nine test: a cadaveric study. J Orthop Surg. 2004;12:83–6.
36. Lister GD, Belsole RB, Kienert HE. The radial tunnel syndrome. J Hand Surg. 1979;4:52–9.
37. Bolster MA, Bakker XR. Radial tunnel syndrome: emphasis on the superficial branch of the radial nerve. J Hand Surg Eur. 2009;34(3):343–7.
38. Jebson PJ, Engber WD. Radial tunnel syndrome: long-term results of surgical decompression. J Hand Surg Am. 1997;22:889–96.
39. Sarhadi NS, Korday SN, Bainbridge LC. Radial tunnel syndrome: diagnosis and management. J Hand Surg Br. 1998;23:617–9.
40. Smith CC, Bevelaqua AC. Challenging pain syndromes: parsonage-turner syndrome. Phys Med Rehabil Clin N Am. 2014;25(2):265–77.
41. Ferdinand BD, Rosenberg ZS, Schweitzer ME, Stuchin SA, Jazrawi LM, Lenzo SR, et al. MR Imaging features of radial tunnel syndrome: initial experience. Radiology. 2006;240(1):161–8.
42. Furuta T, Okamoto Y, Tohno E, Minami M, Nishiura Y, Ohtomo K. Magnetic resonance microscopy imaging of posterior interosseous nerve palsy. Jpn J Radiol. 2009;27(1):41–4.
43. Martínez-Villén G, Badiola J, Alvarez-Alegret R. Mayayo ENerve compression syndromes of the hand and forearm associated with tumours of non-neural origin and tumour-like lesions. J Plast Reconstr Aesthet Surg. 2014;67(6):828–36.
44. Blakemore ME. Posterior interosseous nerve paralysis caused by a lipoma. J R Coll Surg Edinb. 1979;24:113–6.
45. Eralp L, Ozger H, Ozkan K. Posterior interosseous nerve palsy due to lipoma. Acta Orthop Traumatol Turc. 2006;40:252–4.
46. Ganapathy K, Winston T, Seshadri V. Posterior interosseous nerve palsy due to intermuscular lipoma. Surg Neurol. 2006;65:495–6.
47. Mosser JJ, Deflassieux M, Aupecle P, Piganiol G. Compression of the posterior branch of the radial nerve by a benign tumour of the elbow region: report of three cases. J Chir (Paris). 1978;115:515–21.
48. Nishida J, Shimamura T, Ehara S, Shiraishi H, Sato T, Abe M. Posterior interosseous nerve palsy caused by parosteal lipoma of proximal radius. Skelet Radiol. 1998;27:375–9.
49. Pidgeon KJ, Abadee P, Kanakamedala R, Uchizono M. Posterior interosseous nerve syndrome caused by an intermuscular lipoma. Arch Phys Med Rehabil. 1985;66:468–71.
50. Richmond DA. Lipoma causing a posterior interosseous nerve lesion. J Bone Joint Surg. 1953;35B:83.
51. Wu KT, Jordan FR, Eckert C. Lipoma, a cause of paralysis of deep radial (posterior interosseous) nerve: report of a case and review of the literature. Surgery. 1974;75:790–5.
52. Hashizume H, Nishida K, Nanba Y, Inoue H, Konishiike T. Intraneural ganglion of the posterior interosseous nerve with lateral elbow pain. J Hand Surg. 1995;20B:649–51.
53. Mass DP, Tortosa R, Newmeyer WL, Kilgore ES Jr. Compression of posterior interosseous nerve by a ganglion: case report. J Hand Surg. 1982;7:92–4.
54. McCollam SM, Corley FG, Green DP. Posterior interosseous nerve palsy caused by ganglions of the proximal radioulnar joint. J Hand Surg. 1988;13A:725–8.
55. Steiger R, Vogelin E. Compression of the radial nerve caused by an occult ganglion: three case reports. J Hand Surg. 1998;23B:420–1.
56. Tonkin MA. Posterior interosseous nerve axonotmesis from compression by a ganglion. J Hand Surg. 1990;15B:491–3.
57. Tsurushima H, Matsumura A, Meguro K, Nakata Y, Fujita T. Posterior interosseous nerve paralysis caused by ganglion: a case report. No Shinkei Geka. 1991;19:443–5.
58. Yamazaki H, Kato H, Hata Y, Murakami N, Saitoh S. The two locations of ganglions causing radial nerve palsy. J Hand Surg. 2007;32B:341–5.
59. Marmor L, Lawrence JF, Dubois EL. Posterior interosseous nerve palsy due to rheumatoid arthritis. J Bone Joint Surg. 1967;49A:381–3.
60. Kato H, Iwasaki N, Minami A, Kamishima T. Acute posterior interosseous nerve palsy caused by septic arthritis of the elbow: a case report. J Hand Surg. 2003;28A:44–7.
61. Field JH. Posterior interosseous nerve palsy secondary to synovial chondromatosis of the elbow joint. J Hand Surg. 1981;6:336–8.
62. Jones JR, Evans DM, Kaushik A. Synovial chondromatosis presenting with peripheral nerve compression: a report of two cases. J Hand Surg. 1987;12B:25–7.
63. Yanagisawa H, Okada K, Sashi R. Posterior interosseous nerve palsy caused by synovial chondromatosis of the elbow joint. Clin Radiol. 2001;56:510–4.

64. Maldonado AA, Amrami KK, Mauermann ML, Spinner RJ. Nontraumatic "isolated" posterior interosseous nerve palsy: reinterpretation of electrodiagnostic studies and MRIs. J Plast Reconstr Aesthet Surg. 2017;70(2):159–1.
65. Kim Y, Ha D, Lee SM. Ultrasonographic findings of posterior interosseous nerve syndrome. Ultrasonography. 2017;36(4):363–9.
66. Rosén I, Werner CO. Neurophysiological investigation of posterior interosseous nerve entrapment causing lateral elbow pain. Electroencephalogr Clin Neurophysiol. 1980;50(1–2):125–33.
67. Kupfer DM, Bronson J, Lee GW. Differential latency testing: a more sensitive test for radial tunnel syndrome. J Hand Surg Am. 1998;23:859–64.
68. Seror P. Posterior interosseous nerve conduction. A new method of evaluation. Am J Phys Med Rehabil. 1996;75:35–9.
69. Bevelaqua AC, Hayter CL, Feinberg JH, Rodeo SA. Posterior interosseous neuropathy: electrodiagnostic evaluation. HSS J. 2012;8(2):184–9.
70. Werner CO. Radial nerve paralysis and tumor. Clin Orthop Relat Res. 1991;268:223–5.
71. Cleary CK. Management of radial tunnel syndrome: a therapist's clinical perspective. J Hand Ther. 2006;19(2):186–91.
72. Eaton CJ, Lister GD. Radial nerve compression. Hand Clin. 1992;8:345–57.
73. Anandkumar S. Effect of dry needling on radial tunnel syndrome: a case report. Physiother Theory Pract. 2019;35(4):373–82.
74. Moss SH, Switzer HE. Radial tunnel syndrome: a spectrum of clinical presentations. J Hand Surg Am. 1983;8(4):414–20.
75. Lee JT, Azari K, Jones NF. Long term results of radial tunnel release: the effect of co-existing tennis elbow, multiple compression syndromes and workers' compensation. J Plast Reconstr Aesthet Surg. 2008;61(9):1095–9.
76. Marchese J, Coyle K, Cote M, Wolf JM. Prospective evaluation of a single corticosteroid injection in radial tunnel syndrome. Hand (N Y). 2019;14(6):741–5. https://doi.org/10.1177/1558944718787282.
77. Sarris IK, Papadimitriou NG, Sotereanos DG. Radial tunnel syndrome. Tech Hand Up Extrem Surg. 2002;6:209–12.
78. Stanley J. Radial tunnel syndrome: a surgeon's perspective. J Hand Ther. 2006;19:180–4.
79. Kalb K, Gruber P, Landsleitner B. Compression syndrome of the radial nerve in the area of the supinator grove. Experiences with 110 patients. Handchir Mikrochir Plast Chir. 1999;31:303–10.
80. Saratsiotis J, Myriokefalitakis E. Diagnosis and treatment of posterior interosseous nerve syndrome using soft tissuemanipulation therapy: a case study. J Bodyw Mov Ther. 2010;14(4):397–402.
81. Hashizume H, Nishida K, Nanba Y, Shigeyama Y, Inoue H, Morito Y. Non-traumatic paralysis of the posterior interosseous nerve. J Bone Joint Surg. 1996;78B:771–6.
82. Vrieling C, Robinson P, Geertzen J. Posterior interosseous nerve syndrome: literature review and report of 14 cases. Eur J Plast Surg. 1998;21:196–202.
83. Huisstede BMH, van Opstal T, de Ronde MT, Verhaar JA, Koes BW. Interventions for treating radial tunnel syndrome: a systematic review of observational studies. J Hand Surg. 2008;33A:72–8.
84. Henry AK. Extensile exposure. 3rd ed. Edinburgh: Churchill Livingstone; 1957. p. 100e106.
85. Campbell WC, Canale ST, Beaty JH. Campbell's operative orthopaedics, vol. 1. 11th ed. Philadelphia: Mosby Elsevier; 2008. p. 111e112.
86. Froimson AI. Tenosynovitis and tennis elbow. In: Green DP, editor. Operative hand surgery. New York: Churchill Livingstone; 1993. p. 1989–2006.
87. Ummel JR, Coury JG, Lum ZC, Trzeciak MA. Transbrachioradialis approach to the radial tunnel: an anatomic study of 5 potential compression sites. Hand (N Y). 2019;14(3):329–32. https://doi.org/10.1177/1558944717750916.
88. Sayegh ET, Strauch RJ. Open versus endoscopic carpal tunnel release: a meta-analysis of randomized controlled trials. Clin Orthop Relat Res. 2015;473(3):1120–32.
89. Hoffmann R, Siemionow M. The endoscopic managementof cubital tunnel syndrome. J Hand Surg Br. 2006;31:23–9.
90. Leclère FM, Bignion D, Franz T, Mathys L, Vögelin E. Endoscopically assisted nerve decompression of rare nerve compression syndromes at the upper extremity. Arch Orthop Trauma Surg. 2013;133(4):575–82.
91. Ertem K, Aslantürk O, Ergen E, Karakaplan M, Canbay A, Ferrero MAM. Endoscopic assisted retrograde release of posterior interosseous nerve: preliminary results of new technique. J Plast Reconstr Aesthet Surg. 2018;71(12):1816–34. https://doi.org/10.1016/j.bjps.2018.08.005.
92. Ochi K, Horiuchi Y, Tazaki K, et al. Surgical treatment of spontaneous posterior interosseous nerve palsy. J Bone Joint Surg Br. 2011;93(2):217–22.
93. Takao O, Akira N, Hideyuki M, Masaaki T, Hiroaki O, Kumiko O. Simultaneous anterior and posterior interosseous nerve paralysis with several hourglass-like fascicular constrictions in both nerves. J Hand Surg Am. 2001;26(6):1088–92.
94. Huisstede BM, Miedema HS, van Opstal T, de Ronde MT, Kuiper JI, Verhaar JA, Koes BW. Interventions for treating the posterior interosseus nerve syndrome: a systematic review of observational studies. J Peripher Nerv Syst. 2006;11(2):101–10.
95. Atroshi I, Johnsson R, Ornstein E. Radial tunnel release. Unpredictable outcome in 37 consecutive cases with a 1–5 year follow-up. Acta Orthop Scand. 1995;66:255–7.
96. De Smet L, Van Raebroeckx T, Van Ransbeeck H. Radial tunnel release and tennis elbow: disappointing results? Acta Orthop Belg. 1999;65:510–3.
97. Sotereanos DG, Varitimidis SE, Giannakopoulos PN, et al. Results of surgical treatment for radial tunnel syndrome. J Hand Surg Am. 1999;24:566–70.

Pronator Teres Syndrome: Anterior Interosseous Nerve Compressive Neuropathy

21

Konstantinos Anagnostakos,
Nikolaos P. Zagoreos, and Nickolaos A. Darlis

Introduction

Pronator teres Syndrome (PS) is characterized by vague volar forearm pain associated with median nerve paresthesias. Originally described by Seyffarth in 1951 [1], classic PS refers to compression of the median nerve as it passes between the two heads of the Pronator Teres (PT) muscle or at the proximal arch of the Flexor Digitorum Superficialis (FDS) muscle. Despite its name, this syndrome is, in general, a proximal median nerve dysfunction that may also result from compression of the nerve under the ligament of Struthers, the bicipital aponeurosis (lacertus fibrosus), or under an accessory head of the Flexor Pollicis Longus (FPL) muscle (i.e., the Gantzer muscle). Entrapment at any of these anatomic sites may produce the constellation of symptoms that characterize PS. The PS diagnosis is rare; hence, its incidence and prevalence has not been firmly established. It is thought to be more common in women, in fifth decade and has also been associated with well-developed forearm muscles.

Palsy of the anterior interosseous nerve (AIN) was first described by Tinel in 1918 under the title "Dissociated paralysis of the median nerve" and is characterized exclusively by motor deficits only with no cutaneous sensory changes. AIN neuropathy's epidemiology is equally uncertain.

Anatomy

The median nerve receives contributions from C5, C6, C7, C8 and T1 nerve roots and is formed as the medial and lateral cords of the brachial plexus converge, emerging on the anterolateral side of the brachial artery. Then, it crosses over the brachial artery from lateral to medial and continues on the medial side of the arm between the biceps brachii and brachialis muscles. Typically, the nerve has no muscle branches above the elbow; however, there may be a variable branch innervating the PT muscle.

The median nerve then may pass deep to the ligament of Struthers, if present, and enters into the antecubital region. The ligament of Struthers is present in 1–2% of the population and is an anatomic variant that extends from a small, supracondylar process on the humeral shaft to the medial epicondyle of the humerus [1–4].

As the median nerve traverses the elbow, it travels under the bicipital aponeurosis (lacertus fibrosus) into the antecubital fossa, remaining medial to the biceps tendon and brachial artery

K. Anagnostakos
Bioclinic Athens, Athens, Greece

N. P. Zagoreos · N. A. Darlis (✉)
Metropolitan Hospital, Athens, Greece

D. G. Sotereanos, L. K. Papatheodorou (eds.), *Compressive Neuropathies of the Upper Extremity*,
https://doi.org/10.1007/978-3-030-37289-7_21

Table 21.1 Potential sites of median nerve entrapment at the elbow and proximal forearm

Osseous supracondylar process
Ligament of Struthers
Bicipital aponeurosis (lacertus fibrosus)
Between the ulnar and humeral heads of pronator teres
Flexor Digitorum Superficialis aponeurotic arch

and volar to the brachialis muscle muscle and its tendon insertion. The nerve then passes between the two heads of the PT muscle, deep to the proximal fibrous arch of the FDS muscle, and continues distally through the forearm between the FDS and flexor digitorum profundus (FDP) muscles. Distal to the elbow, the median nerve provides motor branches for the innervation of the PT, FDS, palmaris longus, and flexor carpi radialis (FCR) muscles. Further distal in the forearm, the nerve provides two main branches (the AIN and the palmar cutaneous branch of the median nerve (PCBMN)) before entering in the carpal tunnel at the wrist [5].

Pathoanatomy

Potential sites of entrapment in PS (and possibly in AIN Palsy) are summarized in Table 21.1 and Fig. 21.1. Other possible compressing structures include an accessory head of FPL muscle (i.e., the Gantzer's muscle), an accessory muscle from FDS to FDP muscles and aberrant forearm muscles (Flexor Carpi Radialis Brevis, Palmaris Profundus) [6–8].

Clinical Manifestations

PS patients typically present with proximal forearm pain at rest or during activities. In the distal forearm and hand, they demonstrate the same symptoms with carpal tunnel syndrome (CTS) patients, as both syndromes are the result of median nerve dysfunction. Both syndromes are characterized by numbness and paresthesias in the palmar side of the radial three and one half digits and pain in the distal forearm and volar wrist [6, 9, 10]. However, PS patients may report decreased sensation in the PCBMN distribution over the thenar eminence, symptom not reported in the CTS patients.

On the other hand, AIN syndrome patients present with vague forearm pain and spontaneous weakness or complete absence of FPL function. Functions of the FDP of the index and middle fingers are also generally affected, although function of the FDP of the middle finger may be preserved due to cross innervation by the ulnar nerve. A typical patient with complete AIN palsy should have no motor function to all muscles innervated by AIN. Patients with incompletes palsies or with Martin-Gruber anastomosis [11] (nerve branch connecting the median and ulnar nerves in the forearm, present in 10–15% of the population) may present with intrinsic weakness alone. Since the AIN does not provide any cutaneous innervation, sensory deficits do not present with an isolated AIN palsy. However, altered sensation may be seen if other nerves are involved in the setting of Parsonage – Turner syndrome [12]. Presence of prodromal viral infection symptoms and acute onset of pain are thought to strengthen attribution of AIN syndrome to neuritis (as in Parsonage – Turner syndrome).

Diagnosis

Pronator Syndrome

Three main diagnostic tests are performed during the physical examination to evaluate for PS [6, 13–15] (Fig. 21.1). The first is the pronator compression test, performed by applying pressure proximal and lateral to the proximal edge of the PT muscle belly on the volar forearm. A positive test is the most common sign of PS reproducing pain or paresthesias within 30 seconds of compression. The second is the resisted pronation and supination test, which can reproduce median nerve compression symptoms by the PT or the lacertus fibrosus. The third test is the resisted flexion of the proximal interphalangeal joint of the middle finger, which may cause pain and paresthesias in patients with PS because the median nerve is compressed by the aponeurotic arch of the FDS mus-

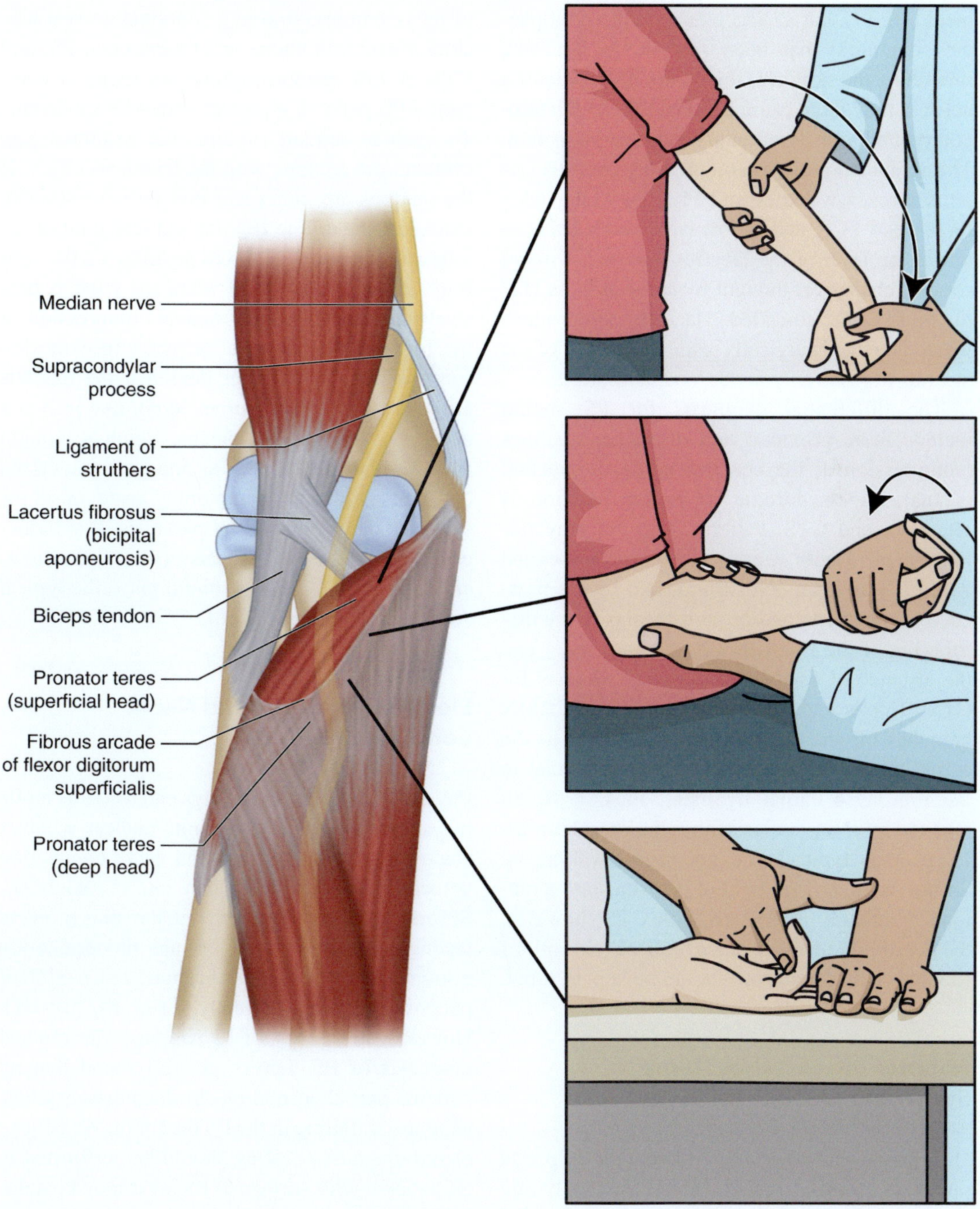

Fig. 21.1 Illustration of potential sites of entrapment and physical exam tests for pronator teres syndrome

cle; however, this finding may also be positive in CTS patients. In addition to the above tests, symptoms elicited by resisted flexion of the forearm in full supination are thought to indicate compression of the median nerve at the more proximal level of the lacertus fibrosus. Finally, a positive Tinel sign over the proximal volar forearm has also been reported to be indicative of PS.

The "scratch-collapse" test has also been described for localization of the site of the entrapment [16, 17], but its acceptance in the orthopaedic community has been modest. In this test, scratching the skin over the compression site of a nerve is thought to cause a spinal reflex with temporary inhibition of voluntary muscle contraction. The combination of pain on pressure over the lacertus fibrosus, weakness of FPL, FDP of the index finger, and FCR and a positive scratch collapse test at the level of the lacertus fibrosus, without sensory changes is thought by some authors [17] to signify the so-called "lacertus syndrome", which is treated surgically with the release of the lacertus fibrosus only under local anesthesia.

The differential diagnosis for PS should include more proximal and distal neuropathies (compression at the cervical spine or brachial plexus), AIN syndrome (if motor function is affected), and CTS. Patients with PS may initially present with similar symptoms associated with CTS and can be distinguished by the presence of numbness and/or paresthesias in the distribution of the PCBMN (thenar eminence) and the absence of findings of provocative tests for CTS (Tinel's and Phalen's tests). The PCBMN branches off the median nerve proximal to the carpal tunnel and enters the wrist superficial to the transverse carpal ligament; thus, it is not affected by compression within the carpal tunnel. PS patients typically do not report waking up during the night with pain or paresthesias, symptoms frequently associated with CTS; however, the possibility of coexistence of these two entities (double crush syndrome) should be kept in mind.

Anterior Interosseous Nerve Syndrome

On clinical examination weakness of grip and pinch are observed, specifically of the the thumb, index and middle finger with their flexion being weak or absent. Patients typically are unable to make the "OK" sign with the thumb and index finger [6, 18, 19]. Pronator quadratus weakness is also expected and can be appreciated by weak resisted pronation when the elbow is fully flexed.

Differential diagnosis of AIN syndrome includes trauma, tendon rupture, proximal sites of nerve compression (e.g., cervical nerves, brachial plexus), thoracic outlet syndrome, PS, and CTS. A FPL tendon rupture can mimic a complete FPL palsy in a patient with AIN syndrome. To exclude tendon rupture, the examiner can evaluate the tendons with the tenodesis effect. If the tendons are intact and the wrist is passively extended, the thumb IP joint and DIP joint of the index finger assume a flexed position; on the contrary, these joints extend when the wrist is passively flexed. Moreover, manual compression of the forearm flexors with the wrist in extension can produce slight finger flexion if the tendons are intact. Parsonage-Turner Syndrome [12] is a neuritis of the brachial plexus, which is thought to be similar to AIN neuritis and is characterized by viral prodrome symptoms, acute onset of shoulder pain followed by paralysis of shoulder girdle muscles and AIN palsy (sometimes bilateral). It is a self limiting condition (as the typical AIN palsy is thought to be).

Electromyography and Nerve Conduction Studies

Physical examination findings can be quite subtle in patients with PS. It remains unclear whether electromyography (EMG) and nerve conduction velocity (NCV) studies can aid in diagnosis. Several studies have reported that results of nerve testing in patients with PS are predominantly normal, with abnormalities reported in 7–31% of patients treated surgically [13, 14, 18–21]. However, in a study of 13 patients with clinical diagnosis of PS, Lee et al. [22] found that all patients had abnormal electrodiagnostic studies, an unusual finding in the PS literature. We believe electrodiagnostic testing should be performed in all patients with suspected PS, as it may be helpful in ruling out other sites of compression, especially in patients with distal sensory symptoms.

Electrodiagnostic studies serve an important role in the workup for AIN syndrome; these studies can support the diagnosis [19, 23, 24]. The affected muscles may exhibit fibrillations, sharp waves, abnormal latency, and abnormal compound motor action potentials on EMG/NCV testing. Nerve testing may also help ruling out other lesions as a cause of symptoms. For example, in a patient with rheumatoid arthritis, it may be difficult to assess an intact tenodesis effect secondary to limited wrist motion. In this case, EMG can be helpful to distinguish AIN syndrome from an attritional flexor tendon rupture.

Imaging Studies

Radiographic series of the elbow should be obtained initially to assess the presence of bony pathology; the appearance of a supracondylar process can indicate the presence of a ligament of Struthers. Ultrasound examination can help rule out space occupying lesions in the vicinity of the nerve and MRI should be reserved for patients with palpable or ultrasound detected soft tissue masses. MRI may show edema in the AIN innervated muscles, which can be attributed to either compression of the AIN or to brachial neuritis. However, unless a mass or tendon rupture is revealed, MRI can rarely guide surgical treatment.

It should be emphasized that PS is a controversial diagnosis among many orthopaedic surgeons. Patients who present with aching proximal forearm pain, occasional paresthesias, and symptoms that are not reliably reproduced by clinical examination represent a puzzling clinical situation that may not necessarily merit a more specific label or diagnosis. Therefore, diagnosis of nonspecific arm pain is preferable to diagnosis of tendinitis or PS, if consistent evidence is lacking. On the other hand, AIN syndrome has more evident diagnosis with clear motor symptoms that can be also demonstrated by EMG/NCV studies.

Treatment

Nonsurgical Management

Evidence regarding treatment outcomes in patients with PS is limited. The few small studies that follow nonsurgical cases report that 29–100% of patients improve with nonsurgical treatment [13, 18]; however, no randomized controlled studies have been performed. Additionally, no studies have compared the duration or effectiveness of the different nonsurgical modalities for management of PS. Since high-level clinical outcome data are lacking, we recommend an initial conservative approach to management that includes rest, forearm flexor muscle stretching exercises, activity modification, and anti-inflammatory medication. The duration of conservative treatment can be as long as 6 months depending on clinical findings in repeated clinical examinations [16]. A significantly shorter waiting time is reserved only for patients with evidence of PS, when an adequate transverse carpal ligament release fails to improve symptoms attributed initially to carpal tunnel or in patients with a space occupying lesion in the vicinity of the nerve at the forearm.

Since the natural history of AIN syndrome has not yet been fully determined, controversy exists regarding its management. No randomized controlled trials have compared non-surgical and surgical management methods, and only limited data exist regarding the duration of nonsurgical management. Hence, it is difficult to make evidence-based recommendations on the timing of surgical intervention. It is generally accepted to be more prolonged (in the 9–12 month timeframe), unless it is associated with blunt trauma or a space occupying mass. Proposed conservative approach involves observation, rest, anti-inflammatory medication, maintaining supple joints and splinting [19, 20, 23, 24].

Surgical Management

Like its diagnosis, surgical management of PS is controversial. No controlled trials and few outcome studies have evaluated the effectiveness of surgical treatment. In fact, small case series and technique papers comprise most of the literature.

Although consensus on the optimal surgical technique for surgical management of PS is lacking, most authors have traditionally recommended complete decompression of the median nerve throughout its course in the proximal forearm (Fig. 21.2). The same approach applies for AIN syndrome release.

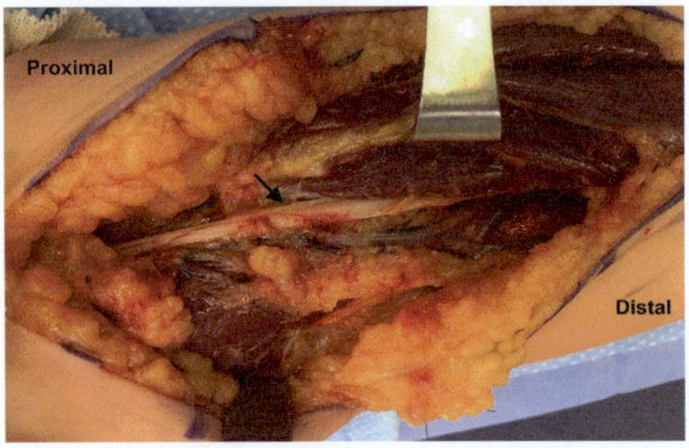

Fig. 21.2 Intra-operative photograph of decompression of the median nerve (black arrow). (Photo courtesy of Dr. Dean Sotereanos)

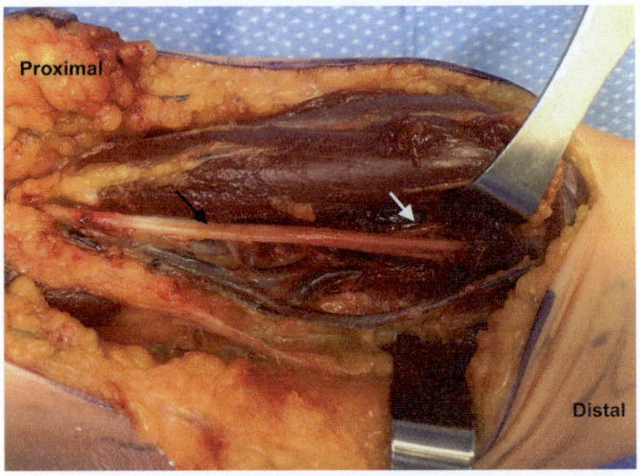

Fig. 21.3 Intra-operative photograph of decompression of the median nerve (black arrow) and AIN (white arrow). (Photo courtesy of Dr. Dean Sotereanos)

Various skin incision have been described, including oblique, transverse [25] and lazy S-shaped incisions. We prefer a lazy S-shaped incision running medial to the biceps tendon and just distal to the elbow crease. The dissection is carried out through the subcutaneous tissue, preserving superficial sensory nerves and ligating crossing veins. The lacertus fibrosus, proximally, and the radial artery, distally, are identified. The lacertus is released and the median nerve is identified lying medial to the lacertus fibrosus proximally and medial and deep to the radial artery more distally.

Following this point, the dissection and release are carried along the median nerve. Proximally, the nerve is released under direct vision and finger dissection verifies an unobstructed course. If there is an osseous supracondylar process visible on x-ray, proximal extension of the incision will permit release of the median nerve under direct vision. Distal dissection continues on the median nerve. Crossing vessels are ligated with hemoclips and the superficial and deep heads of PT muscle are released with tenotomy of any compressing tendinous bands. The radial artery, superficial radial nerve and motor branches of the median nerve should be protected. It should be noted that the motor branches of the median nerve (including the motor branch to the pronator teres) emerge from the median nerve medially whereas the AIN emerges on the lateral side of the median nerve (Fig. 21.3). The final structure that should be released distally is the superficial arch of FDS muscle. Any space occupying lesions are removed and the tourniquet is deflated followed by meticulous hemostasis. A drain should be used if there is doubt about hemostasis or in cases of a concurrent bleeding disorder. Following surgery, we encourage early active range of motion with full return to activity by 6–8 weeks.

Recently there have been described alternative techniques including an endoscopic-assisted release [22], an open technique in which only the lacertus fibrosus is being released [17], and a minimally invasive approach [26], in which only the deep fascia of the superficial head of the PT muscle is released.

Outcomes of surgical decompression are variable with approximately 70–80% of patients experiencing relief or significant amelioration of symptoms. The majority, though, of the published studies are retrospective, lacking control groups, having no clear inclusion and/or exclusion criteria, and having limited use of validated outcome measures.

References

1. Seyffarth H. Primary myoses in the M. pronator teres as cause of lesion of the N. medianus (the pronator syndrome). Acta Psychiatr Neurol Scand Suppl. 1951;74:251–4.
2. Smith RV, Fisher RG. Struthers ligament: a source of median nerve compression above the elbow. Case report. J Neurosurg. 1973;38(6):778–9.

3. Barnard LB, McCoy SM. The supra condyloid process of the humerus. J Bone Joint Surg Am. 1946;28(4):845–50.
4. Suranyi L. Struthers ligament: median nerve compression. J Neurol Neurosurg Psychiatry. 1983;46(11):1047–9.
5. Bezerra AJ, Carvalho VC, Nucci A. An anatomical study of the palmar cutaneous branch of the median nerve. Surg Radiol Anat. 1986;8(3):183–8.
6. Johnson RK, Spinner M, Shrewsbury MM. Median nerve entrapment syndrome in the proximal forearm. J Hand Surg Am. 1979;4(1):48–51.
7. Seitz WH Jr, Matsuoka H, McAdoo J, Sherman G, Stickney DP. Acute compression of the median nerve at the elbow by the lacertus fibrosus. J Shoulder Elb Surg. 2007;16(1):91–4.
8. Al-Qattan MM. Gantzer's muscle: an anatomical study of the accessory head of the flexor pollicis longus muscle. J Hand Surg Br. 1996;21(2):269–70.
9. Fuss FK, Wurzl GH. Median nerve entrapment: pronator teres syndrome. Surgical anatomy and correlation with symptom patterns. Surg Radiol Anat. 1990;12(4):267–71.
10. Tulwa N, Limb D, Brown RF. Median nerve compression within the humeral head of pronator teres. J Hand Surg Br. 1994;19(6):709–10.
11. Rodriguez-Niedenführ M, Vazquez T, Parkin I, Logan B, Sañudo JR. Martin-Gruber: anastomosis revisited. Clin Anat. 2002;15(2):129–34.
12. Parsonage MJ, Turner JW. Neuralgic amyotrophy: the shoulder-girdle syndrome. Lancet. 1978;1(6513):973–8.
13. Hartz CR, Linscheid RL, Gramse RR, Daube JR. The pronator teres syndrome: compressive neuropathy of the median nerve. J Bone Joint Surg Am. 1981;63(6):885–90.
14. Olehnik WK, Manske PR, Szerzinski J. Median nerve compression in the proximal forearm. J Hand Surg Am. 1994;19(1):121–6.
15. Gainor BJ. The pronator compression test revisited: a forgotten physical sign. Orthop Rev. 1990;19(10):888–92.
16. Mackinnon SE, Novak CB. Compression neuropathies. In: Green DP, Wolfe SW, editors. Green's operative hand surgery. Philadelphia: Elsevier/Churchill Livingston; 2011. p. 977–1014.
17. Hagert E. Clinical diagnosis and wide-awake surgical treatment of proximal median nerve entrapment at the elbow: a prospective study. Hand (N Y). 2013;8(1):41–6.
18. Morris HH, Peters BH. Pronator syndrome: clinical and electrophysiological features in seven cases. J Neurol Neurosurg Psychiatry. 1976;39(5):461–4.
19. Rodner C, Tinsley B, O'Malley M. Pronator syndrome and anterior interosseous nerve syndrome. J Am Acad Orthop Surg. 2013;21:268.
20. Koo JT, Szabo RM. Compression neuropathies of the median nerve. J Am Soc Surg Hand. 2004;4:156–75.
21. Presciutti S, Rodner CM. Pronator syndrome. J Hand Surg Am. 2011;36(5):907–9.
22. Lee AK, Khorsandi M, Nurbhai N, Dang J, Fitzmaurice M, Herron KA. Endoscopically assisted decompression for pronator syndrome. J Hand Surg Am. 2012;37(6):1173–9.
23. Nagano A. Spontaneous anterior interosseous nerve syndrome. J Bone Joint Surg Br. 2003;85(3):313–8.
24. Schantz K, Riegels-Nielsen P. The anterior interosseous nerve syndrome. J Hand Surg Br. 1992;17(5):510–2.
25. Tsai TM, Syed SA. A transverse skin incision approach for decompression of pronator teres syndrome. J Hand Surg Br. 1994;19(1):40–2.
26. Zancolli ER III, Zancolli EP IV, Perrotto CJ. New mini-invasive decompression for pronator teres syndrome. J Hand Surg Am. 2012;37(8):1706–10.

22 Lateral Antebrachial Nerve Entrapment

Filippos S. Giannoulis, Nikolaos G. Papoulidis, and Anastasia V. Krexi

Lateral Antebranchial Cutaneous Neuropathy

Lateral antebrachial cutaneous nerve (LABCN) is the sensory branch of musculocutaneous nerve supplying the lateral aspect of forearm. Entrapment neuropathy of LABCN is a syndrome that is well defined, yet relatively uncommon. It was first described by Narasanagi in 1972 and later by Hale as "handbag paresthesia" [1]. Due to the rarity of this entity, it is infrequently recognized but it leads to debilitating symptoms for the patients. The most characteristic of them is paresthesia along the volar radial aspect of the distal forearm [2–5]. Most of the published articles in the literature are case reports [2, 6–9]. Only 2 large series of 11 (15 patients when it was republished by the same authors) and 23 patients respectively, have been published so far [4, 10].

Anatomy

The LABCN originates from the musculocutaneous nerve. It passes behind or parallel to the cephalic vein, within the subcutaneous fat, emerges from beneath the lateral margin of the biceps about 2–5 cm proximal to the elbow flexion crease, where it pierces the branchial fascia and becomes subcutaneous (Figs. 22.1, 22.2, 22.3, and 22.4). After that it separates into two terminal divisions (volar and dorsal). The volar

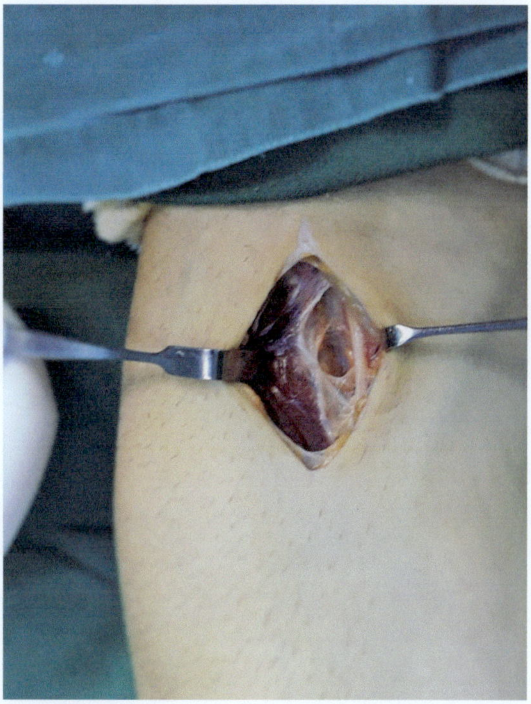

Fig. 22.1 Recognition of the lateral antebrachial cutaneous nerve at approximately 2.5 cm distance from the elbow crease

F. S. Giannoulis (✉) · N. G. Papoulidis · A. V. Krexi
Hand, Upper Extremity and Microsurgery Department, KAT Hospital, Athens, Greece

D. G. Sotereanos, L. K. Papatheodorou (eds.), *Compressive Neuropathies of the Upper Extremity*,
https://doi.org/10.1007/978-3-030-37289-7_22

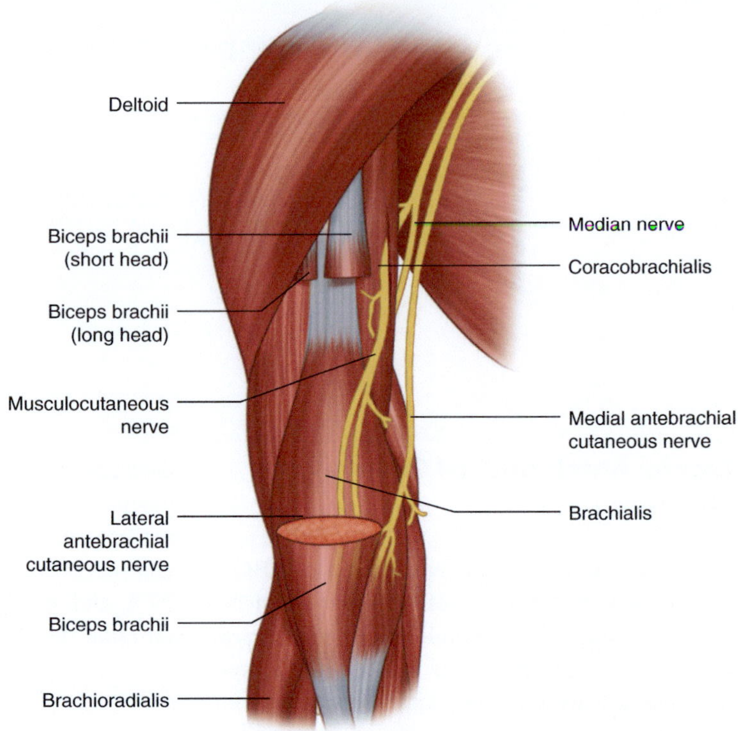

Fig. 22.2 Anatomical landmarks of the lateral antebrachial cutaneous nerve

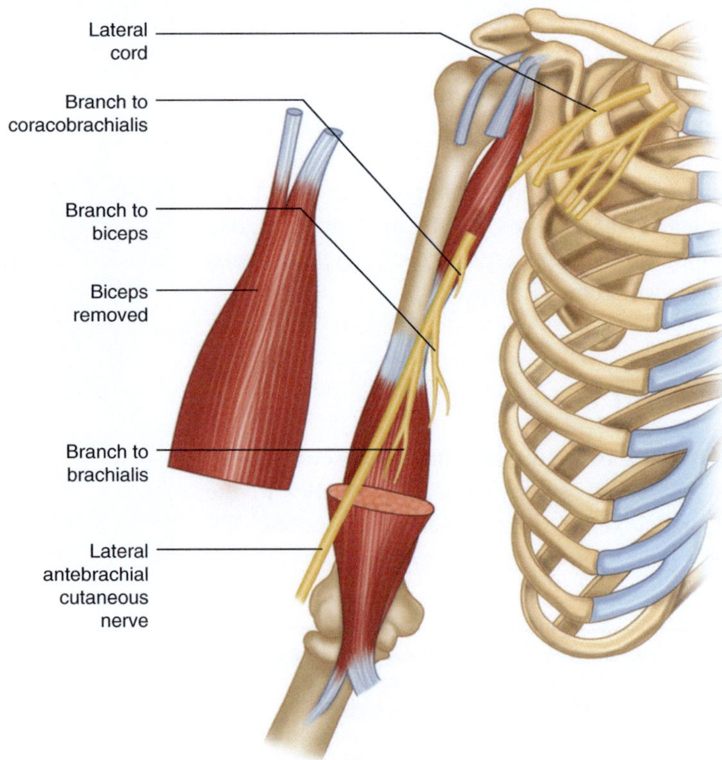

Fig. 22.3 Course of musculocutaneus and lateral antebrachial cutaneous nerve

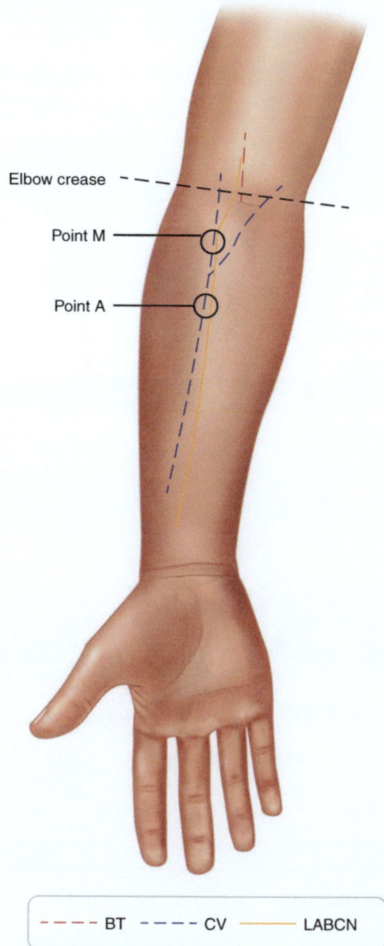

Fig. 22.4 Schematic relationship of the lateral antebrachial cutaneous nerve and the cephalic vein

branch runs distally along radial border of forearm, supplying lateral volar forearm skin sensation. It ends in communicating branches to superficial branch of the radial nerve (dorsal radial thumb innervation) and to palmar cutaneous branch of median nerve (volar thumb innervation). On the other hand, the dorsal branch runs distally along dorsal radial forearm, supplying dorsal-lateral cutaneous innervations and it ends in communicating branches to superficial radial nerve and dorsal antebrachial cutaneous branch of radial nerve. The LABCN is a pure sensory nerve, without any motor function or participation to any reflexes [4, 5, 11, 12]. Various studies have reported several variations in the anatomic course of the nerve. Rosen et al., in a study of 33 upper extremities in 22 adult cadavers, found that the LABCN pierced the brachial fascia an average of 3.2 cm proximal to the lateral epicondyle and was located an average of 4.5 cm medial to the lateral epicondyle, as it crosses the interepicondylar line. Bourne et al., dissected 20 specimens and found that the LABCN emerged from the lateral aspect of the biceps tendon and pierced the deep fascia at the level of the interepicondylar line. They confirmed their findings by injecting 10 volunteers with 1.5 mL of 1% lidocaine at the defined point along the interepicondylar line. Wongkerdsook et al., dissected 96 upper extremities from 26 males and 22 females and found that the LABCN consistently emerged from the lateral margin of biceps branchii tendon. It then pierced the deep fascia distal to the interepicondylar line in 84.4%. At that level, the LABCN in all cases was medial to the lateral epicondyle. Belzile and Cloutier, reported a case of an anatomic variation of the nerve, piercing the deep fascia distal to the usual site. Mackinnon and Dellon, reported on the overlap pattern of the sensory distribution of the LABCN and the superficial branch of the radial nerve (70%). Mok et al., also demonstrated an actual intraneural connection between the radial nerve and the LABCN in 33% of cadavers [2, 13–17].

Clinical Presentation

Primary features of lateral antebrachial cutaneous neuropathy include lateral forearm paresthesia, without any motor deficit and pain over the lateral aspect of the ipsilateral lower arm and elbow (Fig. 22.5). Despite the fact that the LABCN is strictly a sensory nerve, most patients complaint of pain rather than dysaesthesia or paresthesia. Patients report worsening pain along with paresthesia, when arm is in pronation or extension. This is probably because at this position the pressure on the nerve at the elbow site is increased. The patient's symptoms can be acute or chronic at the time of examination. However, most often the onset of symptoms is gradual and

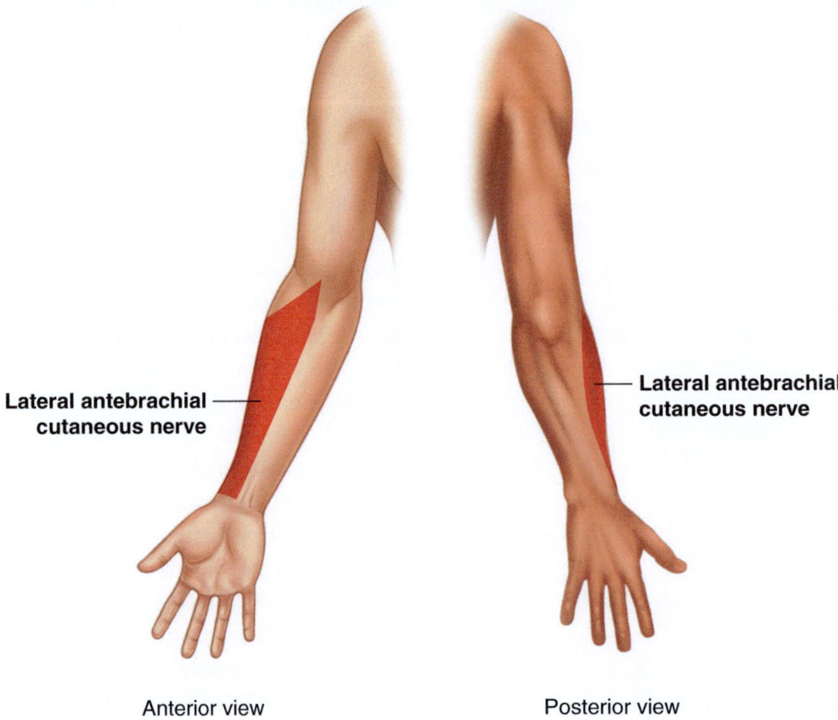

Fig. 22.5 Distribution of pain in lower arm in lateral antebrachial cutaneous nerve entrapment

only progressive aggravation causes the patients to seek medical advice. Clinical examination reveals localized painful tenderness or hyperesthesia to palpation at the anterolateral aspect of the elbow about 3–5 cm proximal to the elbow flexion crease, along the lateral margin of the biceps muscle. Symptoms can also be reproduced by bringing the forearm into full pronation and extension. There are no pathological findings from the cervical spine, neither weakness of the biceps muscle. There is full painless range of motion in elbow and wrist, unless the forearm is fully pronated and extended. Grip and pinch strength vary to 80–100% of the contralateral side. Tinel's sign may be positive, if there is a gentle tapping at the location of the LABCN at the level of elbow. In this case, the patient complaints about paresthesia along the volar radial aspect of the forearm and even an electric feeling, like shock radiating to the ipsilateral shoulder [2–5, 18, 19].

Epidemiology

According to the literature, the lateral antebrachial cutaneous neuropathy is more common in males than in females. Its occurrence is commonly unilaterally, with a peak age range of 25–40 years, although it occurs in all age groups. The prevalence of lateral antebrachial cutaneous neuropathy is higher in dominant hand and also in manual workers. There seems to be a correlation with low BMI but it is not proved. There is no racial prevalence [2–5, 20].

Socioeconomic Effects

Despite the fact that there are no official statistics of the average number of days away from work due to lateral antebrachial cutaneous neuropathy, it seems to be a burden on the National Health Service of any country to provide care for lateral antebrachial cutaneous neuropathy patients, in the form of clinicians' time, diagnosis, and conservative management and treatment options. Almost 74% of patients were workers' compensation cases and the mean time spent in order for them to return to work is 5 months according to literature [2, 4].

Risk Factors

There are certain risk factors that have been associated with this condition. The most significant of these, are prolonged or repetitive postures in extremes of pronation and elbow extension. Activities that can incite this kind of neuropathy include vigorous backstroke swimming, a forceful overhead tennis stroke with the forearm pronated, a backhand stroke in racquetball with the elbow extended, slam-dunking a basketball and hanging on the rim, windsurfing with the arm flexed. Also there have been reports of onset of symptoms due to carrying heavy handbags, trays or rolled carpets with the forearm flexed. Previous injuries or fractures at the site of elbow can play major role. Furthermore, injury by antecubital phlebotomy, wrong positioning while under general anesthesia and venipuncture are iatrogenic risk factors that are related to lateral antebrachial cutaneous neuropathy. More rare risk factors are traumatic rupture of long head of biceps, inappropriate use of tourniquet, restraining strap or improperly placed blood pressure cuff that can cause compression of the LABCN [3, 4, 8, 19, 21, 22].

Pathophysiology

The LABCN does not have a well defined distribution to the elbow or the lateral epicondyle. Nevertheless compression of the nerve at the lateral edge of the biceps produces pain and localized tenderness at the site of entrapment. The cause of this phenomenon is not well known. However this can be aggravated by the movements of abduction and external rotation, in the site where the LABCN enters the coracobrachialis muscle. Another way is by the movements of pronation and supination with the elbow extended at the site where it emerges from the lateral side of the biceps tendon, before piercing the deep fascia. With the extension of the elbow, the lateral margin of the biceps aponeurosis exerts a compression force on the LABCN and it is caught between the biceps tendon and the branchialis fascia. Even with all anatomic variations that were described above, the most commonly reported area of entrapment is the second one. Both motor and sensory disorders are observed in cases of compression at the level of coracobrachialis, whereas purely sensory symptoms are noted after entrapment of the terminal branch [1, 4, 22].

Diagnosis

Diagnosis of LABCN entrapment depends on a good history and physical examination with good knowledge of the anatomic landmarks of the location of the nerve. Electrodiagnostic studies, using the special technique recommended by Spindler and Felsenthal [23], document either a prolonged distal latency or decrease in amplitude of the evoked response of the lateral cutaneous nerve of the forearm in the symptomatic arm. Diagnostic injection of local anesthetic, according to the technique described by Olson [24], can lead us to diagnosis and also help us to differentiate between elbow pain secondary to entrapment of the LABCN and other causes. It is crucial to avoid injecting the area close to the lateral epicondyle or the posterior interosseous nerve otherwise this may mislead us to the diagnosis of the cause of the elbow pain. The injection should be administered along the lateral margin of the biceps approximately 3 cm proximal to the elbow flexion crease. Last but not least, patients who present prolonged pain and paresthesia on the lateral forearm, which did not improve with general conservative treatment, are very likely to suffer from lateral antebrachial cutaneous neuropathy [1–4, 18, 23, 24].

Differential Diagnosis

Differential diagnosis may include lateral epicondylitis, cervical radiculopathy, radial tunnel and pronator teres syndromes, and biceps tendonitis. It is also equally important to differentiate between forearm paresthesia caused by disorders of the LABCN versus the superficial radial nerve. Mackinnon and Dellon, reported on the overlap pattern of the sensory distribution of the LABCN and the superficial branch of the radial nerve. A thorough medical history of the patient along with a detailed physical examination can be helpful in differentiating these conditions from lateral antebrachial cutaneous neuropathy [4, 16, 19].

Treatment

Conservative

Rest, ice, nonsteroidal anti-inflammatory medications, activity modification, and extension block splinting in 90° of elbow flexion, may be used. We can also employ local steroid injection lateral to the biceps tendon at the exit point of the lateral cutaneous nerve of the forearm, followed by splinting in flexion and supination for 7–10 days. Good results have also been reported with the use of ultrasound and transcutaneous electrical nerve stimulation (TENS) [1, 19, 22].

Operative

Under local, regional block or general anesthesia, the patient is positioned supine on the operating table with the entire extremity sterilely prepped and draped free on the hand table. A zig-zag, lazy "S" or longitudinal incision is made along the anterolateral margin of the biceps centered about 3 cm proximal to the elbow flexion crease, exposing the lateral edge of the biceps, where the LABCN is identified. After that the elbow is placed in full extension and pronation the lateral margin of the biceps tendon can be evaluated. A triangular wedge of tendon overlying the nerve is excised or sutured back as a reflected flap. The nerve can then be seen lying on the brachial fascia where it is typically flattened and constricted. At this site, the nerve should be meticulously released. As it is clearly shown in Fig. 22.1. The elbow is then taken through a full range of motion to confirm that the biceps tendon does not compress the nerve in any position. The wound is closed with a nonabsorbable interrupted suture, and the elbow is splinted in 90° of flexion in neutral rotation. The patient is removed from the splint the first or second day after surgery and returned to full activities at 2–3 weeks [1, 4, 19].

Conclusion

Lateral antebranchial cutaneous neuropathy is a relatively uncommon condition. However, it is a syndrome well defined with symptoms that involve pain and even paresthesia along the volar radial aspect of the distal forearm. There are several risk factors that can lead to entrapment of LABCN. These factors along with a thorough medical history and physical examination with good knowledge of the anatomic landmarks of the location of the nerve are adequate to help us recognize this condition. Electrodiagnostic studies can verify the diagnosis. Treatment of choice is the surgical release of the nerve at the site that it is compressed, which is usually between the biceps tendon and the branchialis fascia. In recurrent cases with no improvement after simple decompression and neurolysis and especially if there is an intractable neuroma, then a resection of the nerve and implantation of the proximal part in the brachialis or biceps muscles can provide good results.

References

1. Dailiana ZH, Roulot E, Le Viet D. Surgical treatment of compression of the lateral antebrachial cutaneous nerve. J Bone Joint Surg. 2000;82B:420–3.
2. Belzile E, Cloutier D. Entrapment of the lateral antebrachial cutaneous nerve exiting through the forearm fascia. J Hand Surg. 2001;26A:64–7.
3. Judge A, Fecho K. Lateral antebrachial cutaneous neuropathy as a result of positioning while under general anesthesia. Int Anesth Res Soc. 2010;110A:122–4.
4. Naam NH, Massoud HA. Painful entrapment of the lateral antebrachial cutaneous nerve at the elbow. J Hand Surg Am. 2004;29:1148–53.
5. Preston DC, Shapiro BE. Proximal neuropathies of the shoulder and arm. In: Electromyography and neuromuscular disorders. Philadelphia: Elsevier Saunders; 2013. p. 487–500.
6. Patel MR, Bassini L, Magill R. Compression neuropathy of the lateral antebracheal cutaneous nerve. Orthopedics. 1991;14:173–4.

7. Swain R. Musculocutaneous nerve entrapment: a case report. Clin J Sport Med. 1995;5:196–8.
8. Young AW, Redmond MD, Belandres PV. Isolated lesion of the lateral cutaneous nerve of the forearm. Arch Phys Med Rehabil. 1990;71:251–2.
9. Jablecki CK. Lateral antebrachial cutaneous neuropathy in a windsurfer. Muscle Nerve. 1999;22:944–5.
10. Davidson JJ, Bassett FH 3rd, Nunley JA 2nd. Musculocutaneous nerve entrapment revisited. J Shoulder Elb Surg. 1998;7:250–5.
11. Orthobullets [Internet]. Lateral antebrachial cut. Nerve; Updated 21 Oct 2016. Available from https://www.orthobullets.com/anatomy/10109/lateral-antebrachial-cut-nerve.
12. Beldner S, Zlotolow D, Melone CP, Agnes AM, Jones MH. Anatomy of the lateral antebrachial cutaneous ad superficial radial nerves in the forearm: a cadaver and clinical study. J Hand Surg Am. 2005;30(6):1226–30.
13. Rosen JE, Rokito AS, Khabie V, Zuckerman JD. Examination of the lateral antebrachial cutaneous nerve: an anatomic study in human cadavers. Am J Orthop. 1998;27:690–2.
14. Bourne MH, Wood MB, Carmichael SW. Locating the lateral antebrachial cutaneous nerve. J Hand Surg. 1987;12A:697–9.
15. Wongkerdsook W, Agthong S, Amarase C, Yotnuengnit P, Huanmanop T, Chentanez V. Anatomy of the lateral antebrachial cutaneous nerve in relation to the lateral epicondyle and cephalic vein. Clin Anat. 2010;24(1):56–61.
16. Mackinnon SE, Dellon AL. The overlap pattern of the lateral antebrachial cutaneous nerve and the superficial branch of the radial nerve. J Hand Surg. 1985;10A:522–6.
17. Davidovich ER, Nascimento OJ. Superficial radial nerve-lateral antebrachial cutaneous nerve anatomic variation. Brain Behav. 2013;4(1):70–4.
18. Felsenthal G, Mondell DL, Reischer MA, Mack RH. Forearm pain secondary to compression syndrome of the lateral cutaneous nerve of the forearm. Arch Phys Med Rehabil. 1984;65:139–41.
19. Allen DM, Nunley JA. Lateral antebrachial cutaneous neuropathy. Oper Tech Sports Med. 2001;9(4):222–4.
20. Patel C, Vishnubhakat S. Compression of lateral antebrachial cutaneous nerve in waitresses. J Clin Neuromuscul Dis. 2015;16(3):121–4.
21. Ramos JA. Venipuncture-related lateral antebrachial cutaneous nerve injury: what to know? Braz J Anesthesiol (English Edition). 2014;64(2):131–3.
22. Behl AR, Rettig AC, Rettig L. Lateral antebrachial cutaneous nerve compression after traumatic rupture of the long head of the biceps: a case series. J Shoulder Elb Surg. 2014;23(7):919–23.
23. Spindler HA, Felsenthal G. Sensory conduction in the musculocutaneous nerve. Arch Phys Med Rehabil. 1978;59:20–3.
24. Olson IA. The origin of the lateral cutaneous nerve of the forearm and its anesthesia for modified brachial plexus block. J Anat. 1969;105:381–2.

23 Wartenberg's Syndrome

Efstratios D. Athanaselis, Ioannis Antoniou, and Sokratis E. Varitimidis

Introduction

Wartenberg's syndrome or compression neuropathy of the superficial branch of the radial nerve (SBRN) is a rare neuropathy, which affects women more commonly than men with a ratio 4:1. Affected patients are usually between 40 and 70 years of age [1, 2].

SBRN compression neuropathy is a well-known and described syndrome. In 1932 Wartenberg published a series of five patients introducing the isolated neuropathy of the SBRN, called since then, "Wartenberg's syndrome" although first described by Stopford a decade before. By comparison with neuropathy of the lateral femoral cutaneous nerve (also known as meralgia paresthetica), Wartenberg named the syndrome "cheiralgia paresthetica" [3–5].

Moreover, the SBRN is the third most commonly damaged peripheral nerve, after spinal accessory and common peroneal nerves [6, 7].

Anatomy

The radial nerve emerges from the posterior compartment of the arm into the anterior compartment penetrating the lateral intermuscular septum approximately 10–12 cm proximal to the elbow. Approximately 6–10 cm distal to the lateral intermuscular septum and 3–4 cm proximal to the leading edge of supinator, it bifurcates into deep posterior interosseous nerve (PIN) and SBRN.

The PIN is a motor nerve that courses deep beneath the supinator muscle while the SBRN is a sensory nerve that travels in the forearm under the brachioradialis tendon and between the brachioradialis (BR) and extensor carpi radialis longus (ECRL) muscles lying laterally and posterior to the radial artery. It becomes subcutaneous piercing the fascia at the margin of the EPB in the distal one-third of the forearm, 7.5–9.5 cm (8.31 ± 1.14 cm) proximal to the radial styloid (RS) and it lies in the subcutaneous fat on the surface of the abductor pollicis longus (APL) and extensor pollicis brevis (EPB) muscles, near the radial vein [8–13] (Fig. 23.1).

The SBRN ends in two main branches. The lateral branch comes off 4–5 cm proximal to the RS (4.92 ± 1.44 cm) in a radial direction and innervates the radial aspect of the thumb. The main trunk of SBRN continues distally forming the medial branch. It ends up to three to five terminal branches which pass over the tendon of extensor pollicis longus (EPL) within 2–3 cm distally to the distal edge of the extensor retinaculum (2.69 ± 0.87 cm) and travel in an ulnar direction over the dorsum of the hand supplying the radial three digits (thumb, index, and middle

E. D. Athanaselis · I. Antoniou · S. E. Varitimidis (✉)
University Hospital of Larissa, Larissa, Greece

D. G. Sotereanos, L. K. Papatheodorou (eds.), *Compressive Neuropathies of the Upper Extremity*,
https://doi.org/10.1007/978-3-030-37289-7_23

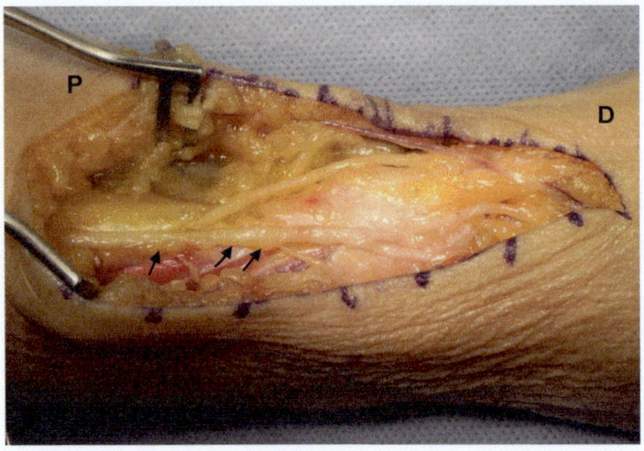

Fig. 23.1 Intra-operative photograph demonstrates the superficial branch of radial nerve (black arrows). (D, distal; P, proximal)

fingers). Therefore, the superficial radial nerve provides sensation to the dorsoradial hand, in particular to the dorsum of first and second web space and the dorsum of the thumb, index, and middle fingers proximal to the proximal interphalangeal joints with a few variations in the area of distribution [11, 12, 14].

However, anatomic variations of SBRN are not uncommon. Cadaveric dissection has shown that in 75% of cases SBRN and lateral antebrachial cutaneous nerve (LACN) have significant anatomical proximity and therefore, at least partial overlapping in sensory distribution [15, 16]. Moreover, such an overlapping may be present in the area of distribution of SBRN and dorsal cutaneous branch of ulnar nerve (DCBUN).

Pathophysiology

Compression neuropathy of SBRN can be the result either of intrinsic or extrinsic factors. The nerve can be compressed at the point it emerges from beneath the brachioradialis to the subcutaneous layer in the distal third of the forearm by the intervening fascia. It can also be compressed at any point along its course in the forearm by the relative motion of the brachioradialis and extensor carpi radialis longus (ECRL) during forearm rotation. Rare causes of pressure can be wrist ganglions or even exostosis in the area of the wrist [17, 18].

Extrinsic factors include compression from outside (i.e., wristbands, handcuffs, tight bracelet, wrist watch or wrist band) and injury of the dorsoradial aspect of the wrist [3–5, 11, 19–23].

Even mild pressure to the epineural vessels can provoke compression neuropathy via demyelinating conduction block and axon loss along the nerve. Subsequent oedema results in fibrosis increasing further the pressure on the nerve and affecting pain sensitivity. Excessive and prolonged compression may finally produce local intraneural sprouting and neuroma formation [11, 24–29].

Iatrogenic injuries include a long list of medical interventions that can cause SBRN injury, well documented in bibliography so far. For example, traction applied for reduction of fractures of the forearm can cause stretch injury to the nerve. Stab wounds for external fixator application, or incisions for De Quervain's operative treatment can also injure SBRN [30, 31]. Cannulation of the cephalic vein due to its proximity (80%) or intersection (68%) to SBRN [12, 13, 32, 33], harvesting of the radial artery in vascularized graft procedures [12, 34, 35], percutaneous fracture fixation with K-wires or external fixators (in up to 20% of cases) [36] and wrist arthroscopy [37, 38] are also included in the iatrogenic causes.

An interesting point is the possible involvement of SBRN in complex regional pain syndrome (CRPS), which was previously known as reflex sympathetic dystrophy (RSD). SBRN contains sympathetic fibers in a relatively high ratio and damage of these fibers due to nerve stretching in case of distal radius fractures and reduction manipulations, may explain the association between CRPS, and distal radius fractures [39–41].

Presentation and Differential Diagnosis

Vague pain with dysesthesias, paresthesia (tingling sensation) and numbness over the dorsoradial hand are typically reported by patients with SBRN neuropathy. Anatomical variations of ending branches of SBRN may result in considerable differences in distribution. Altered sensation in the dorsoradial aspect of the hand as compared with the contralateral, is present in 98% of cases [42, 43]. However, complete laceration of SBRN results in complete anesthesia in the area of nerve's distribution but even in such cases, pain and dysesthesias may be the main clinical problem. Formation of a painful neuroma is not uncommon.

The pain of Wartenberg's syndrome can be elicited by various provocative tests. A positive Tinel's sign over the course of the SBRN is the most common physical examination finding and can help in localization of the compression site which is usually in the area of brachioradialis tendon insertion. Tinel's sign can be elicited by repetitive wrist flexion, ulnar deviation and pronation. Finkelstein's test increases symptoms in the majority of patients, as well.

SBRN as a sensory nerve produces only sensory symptoms. Weakness of the PIN-innervated muscles in conjunction with SBRN sensory dysfunction suggests a more proximal lesion, above or at the level of radial nerve bifurcation.

Local anaesthetic injection can be a useful diagnostic test: resolution of the symptoms after an injection of 1–2 ml of fast-acting local anaesthetic (1% or 2% lidocaine) at the spot of greater tenderness is regarded as a positive test for compression neuropathy.

Pain is often localized in the region of 1st dorsal compartment and therefore, De Quervain's stenosing tenosynovitis can be wrongly diagnosed and even treated surgically. Patients with SBRN compression neuropathy tend to have symptoms at rest independently of wrist and thumb position while De Quervain's tenosynovitis pain is elicited by ulnar deviation of the hand and adduction of the thumb (Finkelstein's test) but not with pronation. Both of these conditions can of course be present simultaneously. In fact Wartenberg's syndrome is associated with De Quervain's disease in 20–50% of cases [43, 44].

Regional pain can be the result of LACN neuropathy as well. Provocative tests for SBRN neuropathy can be positive also in the case of lateral antebrachial cutaneous neuritis due to proximity of SBR and LAC nerves and distribution overlapping. Furthermore, both SBRN and LACN can be injured simultaneously due to their anatomical relationship [12].

Intersection syndrome is less frequent than De Quervain's disease. It was first described in the literature by Alfred-Armand-Louis-Marie Velpeau in 1841 and was named as "intersection syndrome" by James H. Dobyns in 1978. Pain, mild oedema and crepitus during flexion and extension of the wrist are the results of friction between first and second extensor compartments' tendons (APL, EPB and ECRL, ECRB). Tendons of the first dorsal compartment cross over the second compartment 4–6 cm proximal to Lister's tubercle. Repetitive flexion-extension of wrist (e.g. in rowers and heavy weight lifters) causes tendovaginitis of one or both compartments leading with chronicity in diffuse fibrosis and tears [45, 46].

Finally, Wartenberg's migrant sensory neuritis (WMSN) is a rare and exclusively sensory neuropathy of unknown etiology. As in SBRN compression neuropathy, sudden numbness often preceded by pain, is the main clinical finding but multiple cutaneous nerves can be involved [47–49].

Further Investigation

Electrodiagnostic Tests

Workup of SBRN compression neuropathy includes electrodiagnostic tests although these are often negative. Absent or prolonged distal radial sensory latency or decrease in the amplitude of the evoked response can be found, comparing side to side. Distal conduction may be normal while conduction in the forearm segment is impaired as segmental conduction velocity slowing is an expected finding in entrapment neuropathies. On the other hand, it is not uncommon for electrical abnormalities to be absent (up to 16%) [42, 43].

However, in all cases, stimulation of the radial nerve at the elbow evoked a recorded response over the LACN in the forearm indicating that it was also stimulated. Since the LACN is more superficial than SBRN, it is possible that "normal" radial sensory conduction studies in clinically involved patients may have actually recorded responses from a branch of LACN at the wrist rather than SBRN. Therefore, it is recommended that during all electrodiagnostic examinations for possible entrapment of the radial nerve in the forearm, musculocutaneous nerve (MCN) must be also stimulated at the elbow. In case of a recordable response from radial sensory nerve pickup electrodes, while MCN is stimulated, response is obviously from LACN [50].

Central lesions, as C6–C7 radiculopathy, do not affect radial sensory action potentials (SNAPs).

Ultrasound Examination

Ultrasonography (u/s) is a widely used and advantageous imaging technique for diagnosing hand pathology. Apart from its use in diagnosis of various dorsally sided problems of hand (e.g. De Quervain's disease, intersection syndrome, degenerative lesions of carpometacarpal joint of the thumb and tumor or tumor-like lesions) and in differential diagnosis among them, u/s can reveal an entrapment or injury of SBRN.

A high-end machine equipped with a broad band transducer of higher than 12 MHz frequency is essential for the ultrasound examination of SBRN along nearly all its course in longitudinal and transverse planes. Loss of normal fibrillary pattern with swelling and increased vascularity on colour flow imaging are usually the findings [51].

Magnetic Resonance Imaging

Magnetic resonance imaging can also be used in SBRN neuropathy revealing characteristic increase in signal intensity along the nerve with swelling in T2-weighted scans. However, MRI is rarely used for Wartenberg's syndrome diagnosis because it is a high-cost and time-consuming examination method adding very little to clinical and US evaluation of cheiralgia paresthetica.

Treatment

Wartenberg's syndrome is a compression neuropathy and can be treated conservatively at the early stages.

Spontaneous resolution of the symptoms is not uncommon as soon as any factor of external compression (e.g. wristwatch, bracelets, etc) is removed. Traction neurapraxia is usually resolved after a few weeks and splinting of the wrist and thumb can help.

As in every compression neuropathy, rest and activity modification can relieve muscle contraction and decrease the pressure on SBRN. Non-steroidal anti-inflammatory drugs help nerve inflammation to subside. Furthermore a long arm splint including wrist and elbow secures area immobilization and reduces brachioradialis pressure. Corticosteroid injections at the point of greater sensitivity along nerve's route can enhance anti-inflammatory action in situ, although there is no sufficient evidence to support this and moreover, they can cause skin atrophy [44].

Since effectiveness of conservative management (71%) is comparable to that of operative treatment (74%), surgical decompression is indicated only in cases that conservative management has failed and symptoms persist over 6 months [44]. Anatomical structures that are responsible for compression of SBRN must be removed. The nerve has to be released all along its length (Figs. 23.1, 23.2, and 23.3). A common site of pressure is the point where SBRN becomes subcutaneous in the distal third of forearm, piercing the fascia at the margin of the EPB, 8–9 cm proximal to the radial styloid. Post-traumatic or post-operative scar tissue formation is often a cause of compression and is surgically

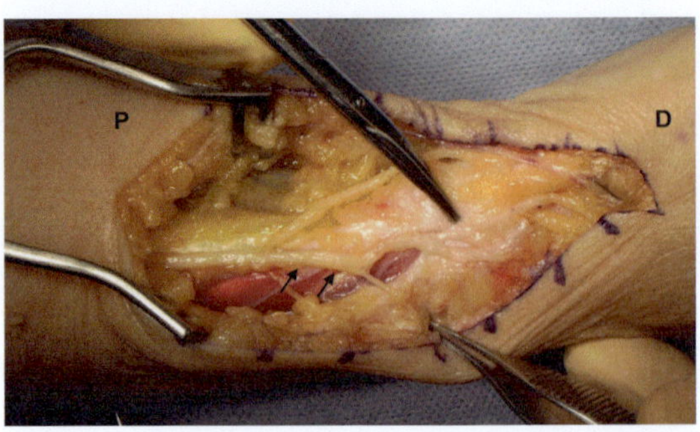

Fig. 23.2 Intra-operative photograph demonstrates the superficial branch of radial nerve (black arrows) during neurolysis. (D, distal; P, proximal)

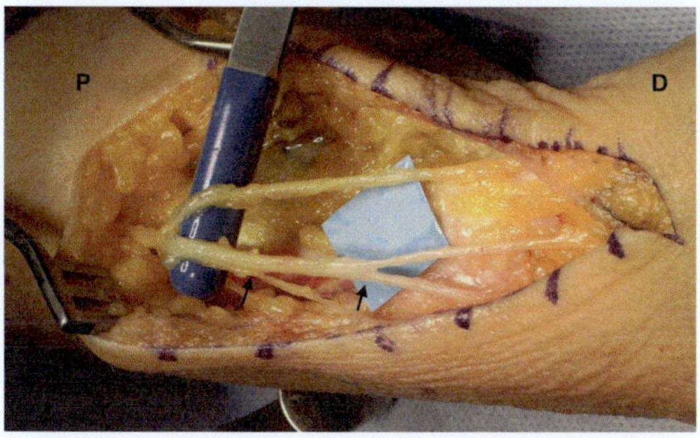

Fig. 23.3 Intra-operative photograph after neurolysis of the superficial branch of radial nerve along its length (black arrows). (D, distal; P, proximal)

treated by neurolysis. Longitudinal incision at the suspected area of compression, volarly to the point of positive Tinel's sign and meticulous surgical dissection are carried out minimizing the risk of new scar formation and LACN injury. Painful neuromas must be resected and the ends of nerve should be buried in healthy tissue (e.g. brachioradialis muscle). A short-arm thumb spica splint is applied post-operatively. Some surgeons prefer to do so in case of SBRN lacerations whereas others perform neurorraphy. Unfortunately, outcome of each procedure may be poor and symptoms often persist [52, 53]. In cases of recurrent Wartenberg's syndrome, revision neurolysis and nerve wrapping with autologous vein graft or synthetic nerve protectors can be performed to prevent further scarring around the nerve [54].

Meticulous intraoperative dissection, regardless of incision type, and care taken to identify SBRN branches, are essential in case of surgical approaches in dorsolateral aspect of the distal third of forearm such as De Quervain's tenosynovitis decompression and incisions for external fixators' pins application. Although there is not solid agreement in published studies, transverse skin incisions in the area are better to be avoided despite the cosmetic advantage. Some authors suggest that even cannulation of the cephalic vein should be avoided [11–13].

In any case, knowledge of nerve's anatomy is a prerequisite for minimizing the risk of iatrogenic SBRN injury.

References

1. Latinovic R, Gulliford MC, Hughes RA. Incidence of common compressive neuropathies in primary care. J Neurol Neurosurg Psychiatry. 2006;77:263–5.
2. Nordstrom DL, DeStefano F, Vierkant RA, Layde PM. Incidence of diagnosed carpal tunnel syndrome in a general population. Epidemiology. 1998;9:342–5.
3. Stopford J. Neuritis produced by a wristlet watch. Lancet. 1922;1:993–4.
4. Matzdorff P. Two rare cases of peripheral neuropathy. Klin Wochenschr. 1926;5:1187.
5. Wartenberg R. Cheiralgia parestetica [Isolated neuritis of the superficial radial nerve.]. Z Ger Neurol Psychiatr. 1932;141:145–55.
6. Kim DH, Kam AC, Chandika P, Tiel RL, Kline DG. Surgical management and outcome in patients with radial nerve lesions. J Neurosurg. 2001;95(4):584–94. Erratum in: J Neurosurg. 2002;96(1):162.
7. Kretschmer T, Antoniadis G, Braun V, Rath SA, Richter HP. Evaluation of iatrogenic lesions in 722 surgically treated cases of peripheral nerve trauma. J Neurosurg. 2001;94:905–12.
8. Thomas SJ, Yakin DE, Parry BR, Lubahn JD. The anatomical relationship between the posterior interosseous nerve and the supinator muscle. J Hand Surg. 2000;25A:936–41.
9. Abrams RA, Brown RA, Botte MJ. The superficial branch of the radial nerve: an anatomic study with surgical implications. J Hand Surg. 1992;17A:1037–41.
10. Abrams RA, Ziets RJ, Lieber RL, Botte MJ. Anatomy of the radial nerve motor branches in the forearm. J Hand Surg. 1997;22A:232–7.
11. Dang AC, Rodner CM. Unusual compression neuropathies of the forearm, part I: radial nerve. J Hand Surg Am. 2009;34(10):1906–14.
12. Robson AJ, See MS, Ellis H. Applied anatomy of the superficial branch of the radial nerve. Clin Anat. 2008;21:38–45.
13. Samarakoon LB, Lakmal KC, Thillainathan S, Bataduwaarachchi VR, Anthony DJ, Jayasekara RW. Anatomical relations of the superficial sensory branches of the radial nerve: a cadaveric study with clinical implications. Patient Saf Surg. 2011;5(1):28.
14. Mok D, Nikolis A, Harris PG. The cutaneous innervation of the dorsal hand: detailed anatomy with clinical implications. J Hand Surg [Am]. 2006;31:565–74.
15. Appleton AB. A case of abnormal distribution of the N. musculocutaneous with complete absence of the ramus cutaneous N. radialis. J Anat Physiol. 1911–1912;46:89.
16. Mackinnon SE, Dellon AL. The overlap pattern of the lateral antebrachial cutaneous nerve and the superficial branch of the radial nerve. J Hand Surg [Am]. 1985;10:522–6.
17. Margles SW. Palmar ganglion producing diminished sensation in the distribution of the radial digital nerve

of the thumb: a case not previously reported. Plast Reconstr Surg. 1994;93(7):1512–3.
18. Spinner RJ, Spinner M. Superficial radial nerve compression due to a scaphoid exostosis. J Hand Surg Br. 1996;21(6):781–2.
19. Grant AC, Cook AA. A prospective study of handcuff neuropathies. Muscle Nerve. 2000;23:933–8.
20. Bierman HR. Nerve compression due to a tight watchband. N Engl J Med. 1959;261:237–8.
21. Massey EW, Pleet AB. Handcuffs and cheiralgia paresthetica. Neurology. 1978;28:1312–3.
22. Stone DA, Laureno R. Handcuff neuropathies. Neurology. 1991;41:145–7.
23. Levin RA, Felsenthal G. Handcuff neuropathy: two unusual cases. Arch Phys Med Rehabil. 1984;65:41–3.
24. Bentley FH, Schlapp W. The effects of pressure on conduction in peripheral nerve. J Physiol. 1943;102:72–82.
25. Neary D, Ochoa J, Gilliatt RW. Sub-clinical entrapment neuropathy in man. J Neurol Sci. 1975;24:283–98.
26. Rydevik B, Lundborg G, Bagge U. Effects of graded compression on intraneural blood blow: an in vivo study on rabbit tibial nerve. J Hand Surg. 1981;6:3–12.
27. Rydevik B, Lundborg G. Permeability of intraneural microvessels and perineurium following acute, graded experimental nerve compression. Scand J Plast Reconstr Surg. 1977;11:179–87.
28. Spinner M, Spencer PS. Nerve compression lesions of the upper extremity: a clinical and experimental review. Clin Orthop Relat Res. 1974;104:46–67.
29. Werner CO. Lateral elbow pain and posterior interosseous nerve entrapment. Acta Orthop Scand Suppl. 1979;174:1–62; Spinner M, Spencer PS. Nerve compression lesions of the upper extremity: a clinical and experimental review. Clin Orthop Relat Res. 1974;104:46–67.
30. Belsole RJ. De Quervain's tenosynovitis—Diagnostic and operative complications. Orthopedics. 1981;4:899–903.
31. Braidwood AS. Superficial radial neuropathy. J Bone Joint Surg. 1975;57B:380–3.
32. Boeson MB, Hranchook A, Stoller J. Peripheral nerve injury from intravenous cannulation: a case report. AANA J. 2000;68(1):53–7.
33. Vialle R, Pietin-Vialle C, Cronier P, Brillu C, Villapadierna F, Mercier P. Anatomic relations between the cephalic vein and the sensory branches of the radial nerve: how can nerve lesions during vein puncture be prevented? Anesth Analg. 2001;93:1058–61.
34. Denton TA, Trento L, Cohen M, Kass RM, Blanche C, Raissi S, Cheng W, Fontana GP, Trento A. Radial artery harvesting for coronary bypass operations: neurologic complications and their potential mechanisms. J Thorac Cardiovasc Surg. 2001;121:951–6.
35. Grinsell D, Theile D. Radial nerve morbidity in radial artery free flaps: harvest of cephalic vein versus venae comitantes. ANZ J Surg. 2005;75:542–5.
36. Singh S, Trikha P, Twyman R. Superficial radial nerve damage due to Kirschner wiring of the radius. Injury. 2005;36:330–2.
37. Kiliç A, Kale A, Usta A, Bilgili F, Kabukçuoğlu Y, Sökücü S. Anatomic course of the superficial branch of the radial nerve in the wrist and its location in relation to wrist arthroscopy portals: a cadaveric study. Arthroscopy. 2009;25(11):1261–4.
38. Steinberg BD, Plancher KD, Idler RS. Percutaneous Kirschner wire fixation through the snuff box: an anatomic study. J Hand Surg [Am]. 1995;20:57–62.
39. Chakravarthy Marx S, Kumar P, Dhalapathy S, Anitha MC. Distribution of sympathetic fiber areas in the sensory nerves of forearm: an immunohistochemical study in cadavers. Romanian J Morphol Embryol. 2011;52(2):605–11.
40. Dürr W. Sudeck's disease after radius fracture. Langenbecks Arch Chir Suppl II Verh Dtsch Ges Chir. 1990:693–39.
41. Hove LM. Nerve entrapment and reflex sympathetic dystrophy after fractures of the distal radius. Scand J Plast Reconstr Surg Hand Surg. 1995;29(1):53–8.
42. Dellon AL, Mackinnon SE. Entrapment of the radial sensory nerve in the forearm. Hand Surg. 1986;11:199–205.
43. Dellon AL, Mackinnon SE. Radial sensory nerve entrapment. Arch Neurol. 1986;43:833–5.
44. Lanzetta M, Foucher G. Entrapment of the superficial branch of the radial nerve (Wartenberg's syndrome): a report of 52 cases. Int Orthop. 1993;17:342–5.
45. De Lima JE, Kim HJ, Albertotti F, Resnick D. Intersection syndrome: MR imaging with anatomic comparison of the distal forearm. Skelet Radiol. 2004;33:627–31.
46. De Maeseneer M, Marcelis S, Jager T, Girard C, Gest T, Jamadar D. Spectrum of normal and pathologic findings in the region of the first extensor compartment of the wrist: sonographic findings and correlations with dissections. J Ultrasound Med. 2009;28:779–86.
47. Nicolle MW, Barron JR, Watson BV, Hammond RR, Miller TA. Wartenberg's migrant sensory neuritis. Muscle Nerve. 2001;24:438–43.
48. Stork AC, van der Meulen MF, van der Pol WL, Vrancken AF, Franssen H, Notermans NC. Wartenberg's migrant sensory neuritis: a prospective follow-up study. J Neurol. 2010;257:1344–8.
49. Wartenberg R. Migrant sensory neuritis, a clinical study with review of literature. New York: Oxford University Press; 1958. p. 233–47.
50. Spindler HA, Dellon AL. Nerve conduction studies in the superficial radial nerve entrapment syndrome. Muscle Nerve. 1990;13:1–5.
51. Dębek A, Czyrny Z, Nowicki P. Sonography of pathological changes in the hand. J Ultrason. 2014;14:74–88.
52. Kline DG, Hudson AR. Nerve injuries. Philadelphia: WB Saunders; 1995.
53. Linscheid RL. Injuries to radial nerve at wrist. Arch Surg. 1965;91(6):942–6.
54. Xu J, Varitimidis SE, Fisher KJ, Tomaino MM, Sotereanos DG. The effect of wrapping scarred nerves with autogenous vein graft to treat recurrent chronic nerve compression. J Hand Surg Am. 2000;25(1):93–103.

Thoracic Outlet Syndrome

24

A. Lee Osterman and Matthew S. Wilson

There are few clinical entities in hand surgery and therapy that are more controversial and create as confusing a clinical picture as thoracic outlet syndrome (TOS). TOS is defined as compression of the neurovascular structures in the thoracic outlet [1]. An incomplete understanding of the anatomy and the lack of objective physical findings contribute to the confusion and controversy surrounding TOS. This entity remains the most difficult upper extremity compressive neuropathy to manage, given its elusive diagnosis and lack of consistent response to treatment. The following chapter provides a review of the history of this controversial entity and the relevant anatomy and highlights the current standards of diagnosis and recommended surgical treatment.

Anatomy

The thoracic outlet is the region from the intervertebral foramina to the coracoid process and contains the brachial plexus, subclavian artery, and vein [2]. There are three distinct anatomic areas where compression can occur: the interscalene triangle (or scalene interval), the costoclavicular space, and the subcoracoid space. Any condition, such as congenital variations, space-occupying lesions, inflammation, or fibrosis secondary to trauma, can narrow these spaces, resulting in compression neuropathy of the brachial plexus or arterial or venous compression.

The interscalene triangle is bordered anteriorly by the anterior scalene muscle, posteriorly by the middle scalene muscle, and inferiorly by the clavicle. The brachial plexus and subclavian artery pass through this space, and the subclavian vein passes anterior to it. The scalene muscles act as secondary respiratory muscles by causing elevation of the first rib during deep inspiration. Use of these muscles can cause neurovascular compression because of their intimate relationship with the brachial plexus and subclavian artery that pass between the anterior and middle scalene muscles. Abnormalities of the scalene muscles have been reported with overlapping insertions and variable fusions of the anterior and middle scalenes [3].The scalenus minimus is a supernumerary scalene muscle which originates from the transverse process of the C6–C7 vertebrae and inserts on the first rib and pleural fascia. It courses between the subclavian artery and lower brachial plexus. This anomalous muscle can narrow the scalene interval, resulting in neurovascular compression. It has been reported in 30–50% of cases of TOS [3]. Additional anomalous muscles

A. L. Osterman (✉)
Philadelphia Hand Center, King of Prussia, PA, USA

M. S. Wilson
Orthopaedic Hand Surgery, Thomas Jefferson University Hospital, Philadelphia Hand to Shoulder Center, Philadelphia, PA, USA

D. G. Sotereanos, L. K. Papatheodorou (eds.), *Compressive Neuropathies of the Upper Extremity*,
https://doi.org/10.1007/978-3-030-37289-7_24

reported to have a role in the development of TOS include the accessory middle scalene and subclavius posticus [4, 5].

The costoclavicular space or triangle is bordered anteriorly by the clavicle, costocoracoid ligament, and subclavius muscle; posteromedially by the first rib; and posterolaterally by the scapula [6, 7]. Compression of the subclavian vessel and brachial plexus can result from several causes: fracture callus or hematoma of the first rib or medial clavicle, poor posture with drooping shoulders, or congenital narrowing or abnormalities. Hypertrophy of the subclavius can result in compression of the subclavian vein, causing Paget–Schroetter syndrome, axillary-subclavian vein thrombosis [8]. The costoclavicular ligament is also implicated in compression of the subclavian vein [9].

The subcoracoid space is the least common site for entrapment of the three potential areas of compression [6]. The neurovascular bundle runs inferior to the coracoid and below the pectoralis minor, which inserts on the coracoid process. The pectoralis minor can impinge on the neurovascular bundle in hyperabduction of the extremity. Arm abduction stretches the neurovascular bundle around the coracoid and also tenses the pectoralis minor, which causes further compression. Wright [10] coined the term *hyperabduction syndrome* and described Wright's hyperabduction test. He described this in short, stocky men who repetitively extend their arms above their heads. Hyperabduction of the arm also moves the clavicle posteriorly and superiorly, narrowing the costoclavicular space.

Cervical ribs are one of the structures most commonly associated with TOS. Cervical ribs are present in 0.2–0.6% of individuals and bilateral in 50–80% [6]. They may be completely formed, but are more often incomplete and have a fibrous band or anlage connecting the bony tip of the cervical rib to the first rib. Wright [10] and Roos [9, 11] described nine types of fascial bands causing neurovascular compression. These fibrous bands frequently attach to the tip of a cervical rib, the transverse process of C7, or the first rib, and are commonly implicated in arterial compression. They can also result in compression of the brachial plexus, causing neurologic symptoms [12].

First rib anomalies can further narrow the thoracic outlet. These anomalies can include fusion of a cervical rib to the first rib, fusion of the first rib to the second rib, and abnormally positioned or bifid ribs. Fracture of the first rib can result in callus, which can cause compression of the neurovascular structures.

History

The history of TOS is rich with contributions from legendary surgeons: Galen, Vesalius, Halstead, Ochsner, DeBakey, and Adson. The history of TOS begins with Galen and Vesalius, with the recognition of cervical ribs. The diagnosis of cervical rib syndrome is first attributed to Willshire [13] in 1860. Surgical rib resection was first reported by Coote [14] in 1861 for cervical rib compression. First rib resection was originally reported by Murphy in 1910 [15].

The understanding of the pathogenesis of TOS has evolved over the last century. Adson and Coffey [16] reported on compression of the neurovascular structures by the scalene musculature. They recommended a new procedure, anterior scalenotomy, and removal of any abnormal tendinous insertions [16]. They subsequently described Adson's sign (discussed later). Ochsner et al. [17] reported on scalene muscle abnormalities and coined the term *scalenus anticus syndrome* in 1935. Scalenotomy subsequently became the most popular procedure for TOS; however, scalenotomy fell out of favor after a recurrence rate of 60% was noted [18]. Other pathologic factors were subsequently considered. Compression between the first rib and clavicle was implicated, with Falconer and Weddell [19] introducing the term *costoclavicular compression syndrome* in 1943. Gradually, attention became less focused on the scalene musculature and more on the contribution of the first rib. Roos [11] described a transaxillary approach to first rib resection in 1966. He reported a 93% improvement rate, and this subsequently became the preferred procedure for TOS. Roos focused the attention of surgeons back onto the brachial plexus compression rather than on the vascular compression and described many congenital bands causing TOS [9, 10]. Atasoy [8] combined Adson's work implicating the scalene interval as a site of compression and the work of Roos implicating the first rib. In 1996, Atasoy [8] reported combined transaxillary cervical rib resection and transcervical scalenectomy for complete decompression of the thoracic outlet.

The great number of surgeons who have contributed to this diagnostic entity, first focusing on vascular compression and later on neurologic compression, has led to a variety of nomenclature associated with TOS. This variety of nomenclature underscores the difficulty with diagnosis and its varied presentation. The greater entity of TOS has been called cervical rib syndrome, scalene anticus syndrome, subcoracoid–pectoralis minor syndrome, costoclavicular syndrome, first thoracic rib syndrome, scalenus medius syndrome, Paget–Schroetter syndrome, rucksack palsy, droopy shoulder syndrome, and hyperabduction syndrome. In this chapter, the encompassing term *thoracic outlet syndrome (TOS)*, as proposed by Peet et al. [20], is used.

Classification

Wilbourn [30] classified TOS into two main types, vascular and neurogenic (Table 24.1). The vascular type is much less common and represents fewer than 5% of TOS procedures performed. Vascular TOS is further subdivided into two subtypes, arterial TOS and venous TOS. Given the different subtypes, TOS can have a varied presentation. Compression of the subclavian vein and compression of the subclavian artery represent venous and arterial TOS, respectively, whereas compression of the brachial plexus results in neurogenic TOS. It is estimated that the brachial plexus is the most commonly compressed structure (90%), followed by the subclavian vein (6–7%) and subclavian artery (3–4%) [6, 22]. The vascular subtypes exhibit objective signs and symptoms of diagnosis, whereas the neurogenic types often do not. Thus, much controversy surrounding TOS relates to the neurogenic type.

Table 24.1 Classification of thoracic outlet syndrome

Vascular
Arterial thoracic outlet syndrome
Venous thoracic outlet syndrome
Neurogenic
True neurogenic thoracic outlet syndrome
Disputed neurogenic thoracic outlet syndrome

Arterial Thoracic Outlet Syndrome

Arterial TOS is the least common type, representing fewer than 1% of cases in a series of more than 2500 cases reported by Sanders et al. [23] Arterial TOS can be acute, chronic, or acute-on-chronic. Acute TOS is rapidly clinically evident and can result in limb-threatening ischemia. Signs and symptoms include pain, pallor, pulselessness, and paresthesias. Chronic or acute-on-chronic arterial TOS frequently presents with thromboembolic complications. Chronic arterial compression leads to intimal damage, arterial stenosis, thrombus formation, thromboembolic complications, and aneurysm formation. This is frequently diagnosed late. A history of unilateral Raynaud's disease should raise suspicion for a missed diagnosis of chronic arterial TOS. Likewise, a patient with neurologic compression as a result of TOS syndrome should be examined for signs of microembolic disease, including claudication, fingertip ulcerations, and cold intolerance. Arterial TOS is almost always caused by a bony anomaly causing compression [21]. Almost all patients have either a well-developed cervical rib or another bony anomaly causing compression [24, 25]. Dense fascial bands originating from a cervical rib or an elongated transverse process of C7 have specifically been implicated [26]. Additionally, a malunion of the clavicle or first rib may cause arterial compression [21]. These may result in compression of the subclavian artery, with positional changes seen with Adson's test and Wright's hyperabduction maneuver. The subclavian artery may be palpable superior to the clavicle, and a bruit may be present. If arterial TOS is encountered, a chest radiograph should be performed to evaluate for a cervical rib or another bony anomaly. The diagnosis of vascular TOS can be evaluated initially by noninvasive tests, such as duplex imaging, and confirmed with angiography. The treatment of acute arterial TOS is with urgent embolectomy. Treatment of chronic arterial TOS is with surgical decompression with arterial repair or reconstruction [21].

Venous Thoracic Outlet Syndrome

Venous TOS is occlusion of the subclavian vein in the thoracic outlet. It is more common than arterial TOS, but much less common than neurogenic TOS. It represents only 2–3% of all cases of TOS. As with arterial TOS, venous TOS can be acute or chronic. Acute venous TOS can occur because of a thrombus or can occur suddenly after sudden maximal arm use, termed *effort thrombosis* or *Paget–Schroetter syndrome*. Predisposing factors include the relationship of the vein to the subclavius tendon and costoclavicular ligament and the dimensions of the costoclavicular space. Occlusion of the subclavian vein typically occurs in muscular young men after strenuous exercise and is believed to be caused by impingement from the costoclavicular ligament. This may also occur with overhand athletes because of abduction of the arm, causing compression and occlusion of the subclavian vein [27]. Acute occlusion results in a sudden painful swelling of the arm, whereas a chronic occlusion presents more insidiously with swelling or cyanosis. The best test for diagnosis is dynamic venography [28]. If findings on static venography are normal, the arm may be abducted to 180°, showing pathologic compression in this position. Subclavian venous thrombosis most often occurs as a result of secondary causes, such as an underlying clotting abnormality or subclavian catheters. Extrinsic compression of the subclavian vein can also occur because of a tumor. Primary compression of the subclavian vein usually occurs in the costoclavicular space [28]. Treatment involves removing the clot with thrombolysis and subsequent correction of the underlying abnormality [28, 29]. If compression is caused by a congenitally tight costoclavicular space, this can be treated with surgical decompression by transaxillary first rib resection.

Neurogenic Thoracic Outlet Syndrome

Neurogenic TOS is by far the most common type, as classified by Wilbourn [30]. The most common etiology of neurogenic TOS is neck trauma in an individual with anatomic predisposition to narrowing at the thoracic outlet [31]. Hyperextension neck injuries result in scarring of the scalene muscles. Ochsner [17] described hypertrophy, degeneration, and fibrosis of the anterior scalene muscles. This is believed to result in neurologic compression. The second most common etiology of neurogenic TOS is repetitive stress injuries. Poor posture is also believed to play a role.

Wilbourn [30] subclassified neurogenic TOS into "true" neurogenic and "disputed" neurogenic types. "True" neurogenic TOS is exceedingly rare and shows objective signs of nerve compression, usually of the lower brachial plexus. Objective signs and symptoms include paresthesias in the lower plexus distribution, intrinsic wasting, decreased grip strength, and hypothenar atrophy. Patients typically have minimal pain, but do have objective findings of neurologic compression. "True" neurogenic TOS is almost always associated with a bony anomaly, such as a cervical rib causing nerve compression [30]. Paresthesias are the most common presenting symptom, characteristically involve the medial forearm and the fourth and fifth digits, and occur in up to 95% of individuals [32]. In a systematic review, Sanders et al., outlined the common symptomatology of neurogenic TOS which includes neck pain (88%), trapezius pain (92%), shoulder and/or arm pain (88%), supraclavicular pain (76%), chest pain (72%), occipital headache (76%) and paresthesias in all five finger (58%), digits IV and V (26%) or the radial digits (14%) [23].

Symptoms of "disputed" neurogenic TOS are more vague and can include shoulder pain, extremity weakness, headache, neck and scapular muscle spasm, arm dysesthesias, and paresthesias. Because of the preponderance of lower plexus involvement, paresthesias more commonly affect the medial forearm and fourth and fifth digits; however, they can also be vague, involving the entire arm. This vague presentation is characteristic of the disputed neurogenic type rather than the true neurogenic type. Patients may complain of a "dead arm" sensation, where the entire arm may "go to sleep." Patients may also note weakness and fatigue of the extremity, especially in the intrinsic musculature. Symptoms can be worsened with overhead activity and placing the arm in a hyperabducted position. Disputed neurogenic TOS may also cause vague vascular symptoms, such as swelling, cyanosis, and a cool hand.

Diagnosis

Because of the varied presentation of compression at the thoracic outlet, the diagnosis of TOS can be difficult. Additionally, the vast majority of patients with neurogenic TOS have the disputed type without objective findings or positive electrodiagnostic test results, making this diagnosis particularly challenging. The diagnosis is primarily clinical, with ancillary studies performed to rule out other diagnoses. Approximately 98% of symptoms are neurologic. It commonly presents between 20 and 40 years [1]. The incidence in women is three times that in men. The reasons for this are unclear, possibly related to an increased incidence of bony and soft tissue anomalies in the neck [33]. Interestingly, it is more common in patients with private health insurance and is rarely diagnosed in the Medicaid or worker's compensation population [34]. The incidence is increasing in the United States, but it is less prevalent in other countries, such as the United Kingdom.

TOS may occur simultaneously with carpal tunnel syndrome, cubital tunnel syndrome, or other compressive neuropathies, as a double-crush phenomenon. Proximal compression of the brachial plexus can result in increased susceptibility to compression in the carpal tunnel and cubital tunnel. Conversely, a reverse double-crush scenario is possible, with distal compression resulting in increased susceptibility to proximal compression because of altered proximal axoplasmic flow. Wood and Biondi [35] reported double-crush phenomena in 42% of cases of TOS. The most common double-crush associated with TOS was carpal tunnel syndrome, affecting 41 of 165 patients. Carpal tunnel is believed to occur in 20–45% of cases of TOS, and cubital tunnel syndrome is believed to occur in approximately 10% of cases [36]. These syndromes need to be excluded for the diagnosis of TOS to be made.

Initial workup should include a thorough and comprehensive physical examination, provocative tests, and diagnostic studies, such as cervical spine radiographs, chest radiographs, electrodiagnostic testing, and somatosensory evoked potentials (SSEPs).

Physical Examination

Because the diagnosis of TOS is frequently clinically based, with lack of objective confirmatory tests, the physical examination should be comprehensive. The physical examination should begin with the patient unclothed above the shoulders. The patient's shoulder posture should be assessed and the arms inspected for swelling. Tenderness in the neck, shoulder girdle, and clavicular fossa as well as Tinel's sign, scapular winging, and muscle spasm should be noted. A thorough physical examination of the upper extremity should be performed, including detailed muscle strength and sensation using Semmes–Weinstein monofilaments. Provocative tests should be conducted to rule out other conditions, such as carpal tunnel syndrome, cubital tunnel syndrome, cervical radiculopathy, tendonitis, and rotator cuff tears, starting distal and proceeding proximally. Only then should provocative tests for TOS be performed.

Adson's Test

Adson's test (or Adson's maneuver) is performed by placing the arm into extension and having the patient hyperextend the neck, turn the face toward the affected side, and take a deep breath, as originally described by Adson and Coffey [16] (Fig. 24.1a, b). The physician stands behind the patient and monitors for loss of radial pulse and reproduction of paresthesias. Inspiration tightens the accessory respiratory muscles, the scalenes, narrowing the scalene interval and causing compression of the brachial plexus and subclavian artery. A positive test result is classically described as obliteration of the radial pulse with inspiration. However, test results can be positive in normal, asymptomatic individuals, limiting the diagnostic value of the test [16]. Gergoudis et al. challenged the clinical utility of this test as they demonstrated that 51% of healthy volunteers had a diminished pulse with this maneuver [37]. Sanders and Hammond [28] believe that it has no clinical value for the diagnosis of TOS. Reproduction of the patient's symptoms should also be noted.

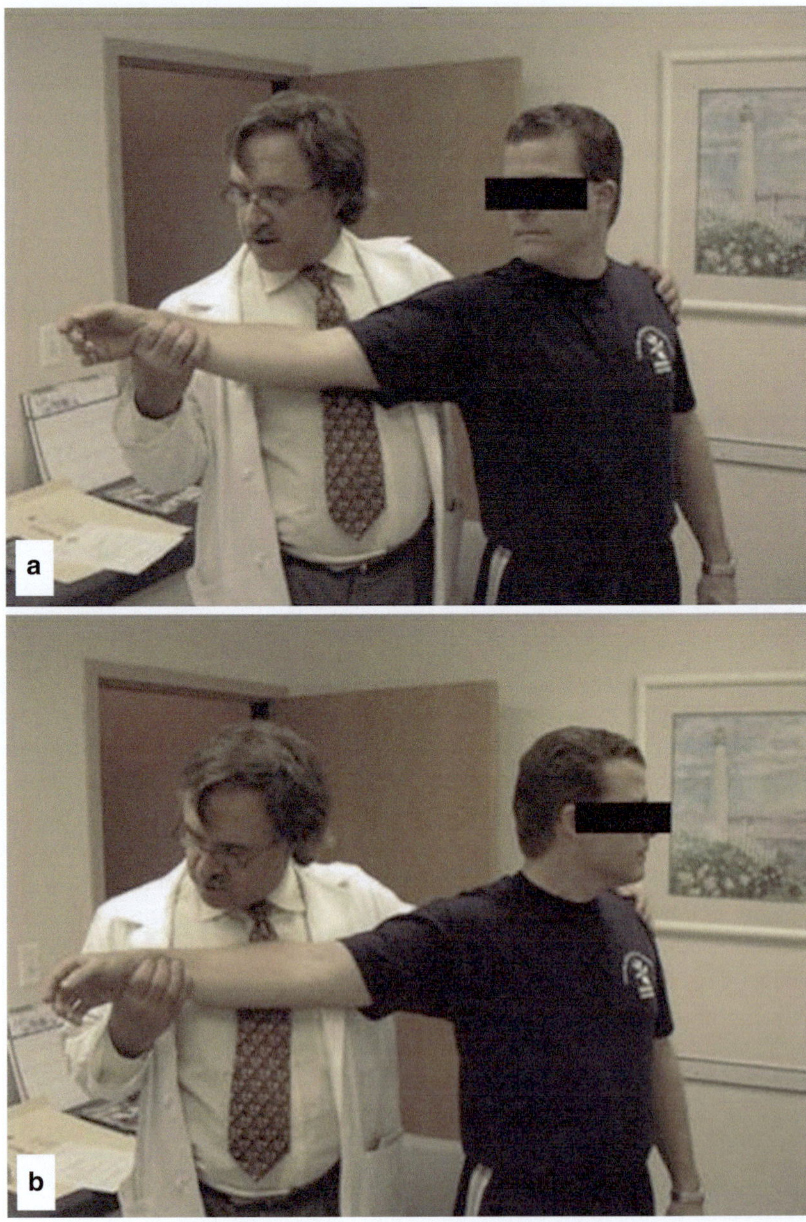

Fig. 24.1 (**a**) Adson's test is performed by having the patient place the arm at the side, hyperextend the neck, turn the face toward the affected side, and take a deep breath, as originally described by Adson. (**b**) A reverse Adson's test can follow the standard test by having the patient turn the head in the opposite direction. The examiner should look for pulse obliteration and reproduction of symptoms. Many patients can normally have a pulse diminution without symptoms

Wright's Hyperabduction Test

The arm is externally rotated and abducted to 180°, with the elbow flexed 90°, as the patient inhales deeply (Fig. 24.2). A positive test result shows a decrease in the pulse as the maneuver is performed. In Wright's [38] original description, a position of hyperabduction during sleep was noted to cause arm paresthesias. MacKinnon [39] modified the test by having the elbow extended, minimizing cubital tunnel compression. Some would consider reproduction of symptoms as a positive test result [16]. Hyperabduction causes compression in the subcoracoid region by the pectoralis minor muscle.

Roos' Test

Roos' test is also called the elevated arm stress test (Fig. 24.3) The arms are held in a position of 90° of abduction and externally rotated ("stick-up

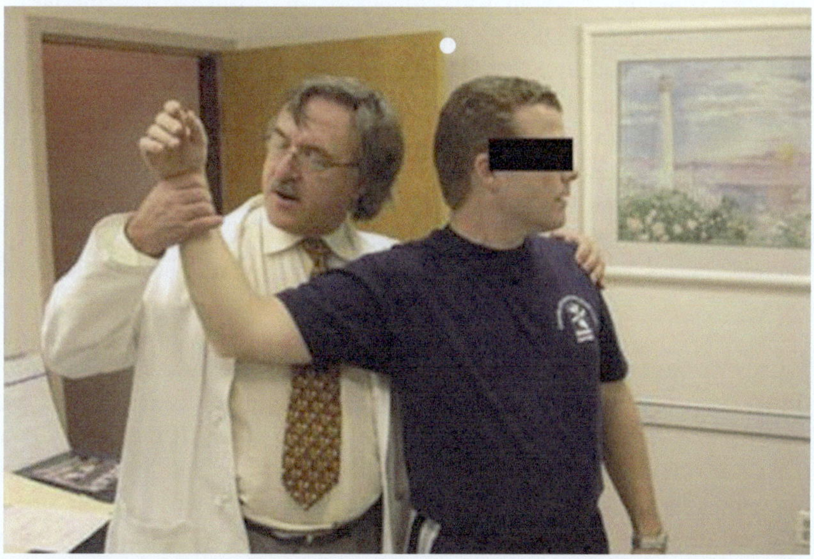

Fig. 24.2 Wright's hyperabduction test. The arm is externally rotated and abducted to 180°, with the elbow flexed 90°, as the patient inhales deeply. A positive result shows a decrease in the pulse as the maneuver is performed

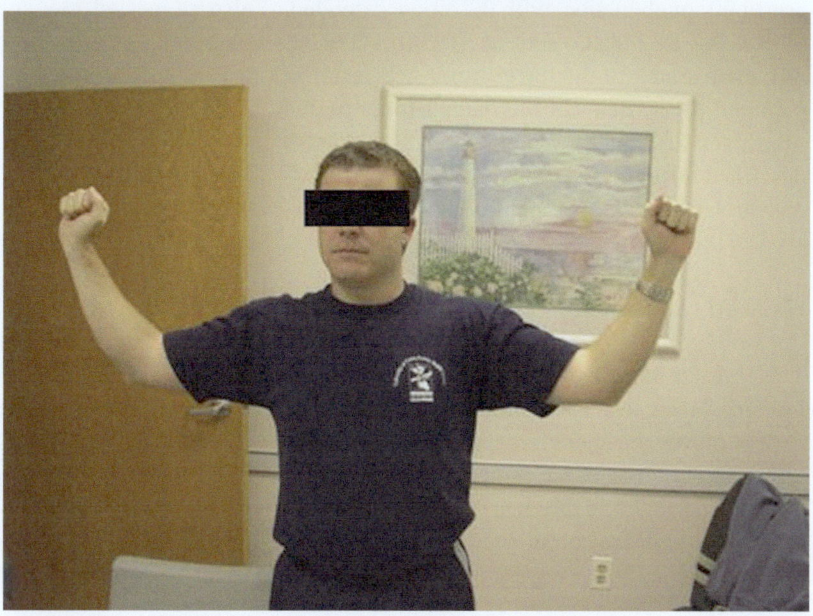

Fig. 24.3 The Roos' test or elevated arm stress test. The arms are held in a position of 90° of abduction and externally rotated ("stick-up position"). The patient then opens and closes the hands slowly for a period of 3 minutes. Reproduction of symptoms in the entire extremity or rapid fatigue of the extremity constitutes a positive result

position"). The patient then opens and closes the hands slowly for a period of 3 minutes. Reproduction of symptoms in the entire extremity or rapid fatigue of the extremity constitutes a positive test result. Patients with TOS typically cannot complete this test. The test is of the most diagnostic benefit when symptoms occur rapidly after elevation of the arm [22]. One study showed reproduction of symptoms in 94% of patients with neurogenic TOS [20]. Many authors [1, 2, 40] described this as the most reliable test for TOS. Aysin et al. evaluated 135 patient with neck and arm pain, 93 of whom had a diagnosis of TOS. The authors found that the Roos test had the highest sensitivity rate – 92% [41]. In contradistinction, the Roos test has a high false-positive rate as this maneuver can reproduce symptoms of other pathologies, including carpal tunnel syndrome, cubital tunnel syndrome and rotator cuff syndrome, and the results should be interpreted with caution.

Hunter's Test (Brachial Plexus Tension Test)

This test involves reproduction of the patient's symptoms by placing particular portions of the brachial plexus under maximal tension. Tension of the lower plexus is performed by placing the arm at 90° of abduction, with the elbow extended, the wrist extended, and the palm upward. Maximal stretch of the lower trunk will result in pain and paresthesias in the medial forearm and fourth and fifth digits. Whitenack et al. [26] also described different positions that result in maximal stretch of the upper and middle plexus.

Halsted Maneuver

The Halsted maneuver is also referred to as the military brace test or costoclavicular test. The patient moves the shoulders inferiorly and medially, protruding the chest, as in a military posture. This test narrows the thoracic outlet. Further narrowing can be accomplished by having the examiner apply downward traction to the arm, causing compression of the clavicle on the thoracic outlet.

Upper Limb Tension Test of Elvey

The upper limb tension test is performed in three positions. Position 1 is abduction of both arms to 90° with the elbow extended. Position 2 is position 1 plus dorsiflexion of the wrists. Position 3 is positions 1 and 2 plus tilting of the head to the contralateral side. A positive test result is indicated by pain and paresthesias radiating down the arm, with the strongest evidence of TOS indicated by a positive response in position 1. A recent study showed this to be a positive physical finding in 98% of a series of 50 patients with TOS [20].

A study of the false-positive rate with provocative physical examination testing in healthy subjects showed that outcomes of pulse alteration or paresthesias were unreliable [42]. When a positive outcome was defined as pain, Adson's test, the Halstead maneuver, and the supraclavicular pressure test (pressure over the supraclavicular fossa at the medial scalene muscle for 30 seconds) had reasonably low false-positive results. A positive outcome defined as discontinuation of the elevated arm stress test because of pain, or pain in the arm after multiple maneuvers, also had a low false-positive rate [43]. Others have also suggested low specificity of the diagnostic physical examination maneuvers discussed earlier.

Diagnostic Studies

Initial diagnostic studies for the evaluation of TOS are cervical spine radiographs, chest radiographs, electrodiagnostic testing, and SSEPs. Other studies include the use of duplex ultrasound, contrast arteriography, venography. MR neurography and brachial plexus imaging are considered emerging techniques for the diagnosis of neurogenic TOS [44]. There are tests that are useful for the diagnosis of vascular TOS and true neurogenic TOS; however, there are no "gold standard" diagnostic studies to confirm neurogenic TOS. The initial diagnostic studies are performed in disputed neurogenic TOS to rule out other entities. Cervical spine films evaluate for cervical disk disease, degenerative joint disease, or neural foramina narrowing, all of which can mimic TOS. Cervical spine films and chest radiographs should be evaluated for the presence of cervical ribs, an elongated C7 transverse process, and structural anomalies of the first rib and clavicle, which are commonly present in true neurogenic TOS. The C7 transverse process is elongated if it projects lateral to the plane of the T1 transverse process on the anteroposterior view. The apical lung segment should be evaluated on a chest radiograph to exclude a tumor. Pancoast tumor must be included in the differential diagnosis of a patient with paresthesias in the C8–T1 distribution.

If vascular compression is suspected, noninvasive tests, such as duplex ultrasonography, pulse volume recordings, and finger plethysmography can be used. If vascular compression is not suspected, these tests do not need to be included in the routine evaluation of neurogenic TOS. Vascular TOS can be further evaluated, with angiography and venography representing the "gold standard" for arterial and venous TOS, respectively. There are reports of the use of magnetic resonance angiography for the diagnosis of arterial TOS; however, evidence-based studies of CT angiography have recently been described, and this may become the imaging modality of choice [45]. Blum et al. recently demonstrated the utility of dynamic CT angiography suggesting that subclavian artery stenosis on dynamic CT angiography is strongly associated with TOS [46].

The best use for MRI is to exclude the diagnosis of cervical spine pathology rather than for the diagnosis of TOS. There are some case reports of MRI being used to identify compression of the brachial plexus [47, 48]; however, MRI is currently not the standard of care for the diagnosis of TOS. A recent blinded study performed to evaluate positional change in patients with TOS showed that MRA done in a provocative position, such as the Halsted maneuver, is more valuable in the diagnosis of TOS [49].

Electrodiagnostic Testing

Although patients with disputed neurogenic TOS have negative findings on electrodiagnostic testing, electromyography (EMG) and nerve conduction velocity (NCV) remain an important part of the initial evaluation of suspected TOS. EMG and NCV are performed to rule out sites of distal compression and to evaluate for possible double-crush syndrome. Because there are no gold standard tests for disputed neurogenic TOS, it is important to rule out other pathology, such as carpal tunnel syndrome and cubital tunnel syndrome, which can present with similar symptoms. Routine electrodiagnostic tests are not useful to confirm the presence of disputed neurogenic TOS [50]. However, they have utility for the diagnosis of true neurogenic TOS. True neurogenic TOS shows a reduction of the amplitude of ulnar and median compound nerve action potentials and a decreased or absent medial antebrachial cutaneous (MABC) sensory nerve action potential (SNAP) [51]. The advantage of electrodiagnostic testing is that, if the findings are positive, they can provide objective data for diagnosis. In patients with objective physical signs of nerve compression, such as intrinsic wasting, EMG and NCV show chronic denervation, reduced amplitude and prolongation of ulnar SSEP latency, delay in F wave latency, changes in median nerve motor action potential and ulnar nerve SNAP, and decreased MABC SNAP amplitude. A report of MABC SNAP in 16 patients showed decreased MABC SNAP amplitude in neurogenic TOS with lower plexus involvement, suggesting its possible use as an early diagnostic tool [52]. Tsao et al. reported on the electrodiagnostic features of 32 patients with surgically verified true neurogenic thoracic outlet syndrome and noted that there was uniform chronic axonal loss affecting the lower portion of the brachial plexus and disproportionately involved the T1 more than the C8 sensory and motor fibers. They found that upon testing the medial antebrachial cutaneous nerve and median motor nerve, combined conduction deficits were abnormal in 89% of patients with TOS [53]. Similarly, for suspected upper plexus lesions, the lateral antebrachial cutaneous nerve amplitude can be tested [54].

SSEPs are a measure of the electrical conduction of a distal sensation through the brachial plexus, nerve roots, spinal cord, and central nervous system. Several studies suggest that SSEPs are useful in the diagnosis of TOS in patients with objective signs of muscle wasting and weakness and are not useful in patients with only subjective signs of TOS [55–57]. They can be helpful in true neurogenic TOS, but there is no consensus in the literature as to their utility in disputed neurogenic TOS. Komanetsky et al. [58] reported 21 patients with TOS who were examined with SSEP monitoring. There was no significant difference in brachial plexus conduction time (interpeak latencies) between the TOS group and the control group. However, significant differences were noted with arm positioning, specifically, abduction and external rotation, suggesting that SSEPs are not helpful in the diagnosis of disputed TOS [58].

A final modality which has gained traction in the evaluation of patients with suspected TOS is anterior scalene blocks. The scalene muscle is injected with local anesthetic or botulinum toxin for both diagnostic and therapeutic purposes. Alleviation of symptoms will occur if the injected muscle is the site of compression. Braun et al. assessed the use of scalene blocks in patients with symptomatology consistent with TOS. Patients who underwent anterior scalene muscle blocks noted symptomatic and functional improvement after the blocks, with an increase in their work capacity in waist level push–pull tests, overhead bar push–pull tests, and extremity abduction stress test with repetitive hand gripping during static arm elevation [59]. Scalene blocks also appear to be prognostic in certain groups when it comes to predicting surgical outcome. Lum et al· found that a successful block correlated with a 14% higher rate of good surgical outcomes in patients older than 40 years [60].

Treatment

The first-line treatment is physical therapy. Most cases of TOS can be managed effectively with a therapy program, including a comprehensive program of postural modification, nerve gliding exercises, education, and strengthening [61].

Indications for surgery are straightforward for true neurogenic and vascular TOS. Patients with arterial compression or signs of arterial insufficiency should undergo urgent decompression, typically through a combined approach [62]. Indications for surgery in true neurogenic TOS include intrinsic wasting, frequently accompanied by objective EMG and NCV evidence of nerve compression [63]. Indications for disputed neurogenic classification are less clear. At a minimum, an extensive course of physical therapy should have been performed before surgical treatment. The patient should be evaluated for sites of distal compression and treated if necessary before contemplation of surgical treatment for TOS. MacKinnon and Patterson's [62] indications for surgery are failure of 3 months of supervised therapy and double-crush with failure of surgical management of the distal compression. However, others have developed differing surgical indications for disputed neurogenic TOS. Urschel [63] believed that it was mandatory to have prolongation of ulnar and median NCV across the thoracic outlet in addition to failure of conservative treatment before considering surgery.

There are two general surgical approaches to TOS. The first involves anterior scalenectomy, with or without brachial plexus neurolysis. The second involves removal of the first rib. In all cases, abnormal anatomy that may be causing compression should be addressed, such as a cervical rib or fibrous attachments to a cervical rib. Removal of the first rib can be accomplished through either a transaxillary approach or a supraclavicular approach. Each technique has proponents, and results are similar [64]. There is no consensus as to the best surgical approach or procedure for TOS.

Transaxillary Rib Resection

Transaxillary rib resection was first performed in 1966 by Roos [64], who popularized this approach. Proponents believe that it is a safer approach because dissection is not near the brachial plexus and axillary vessels. It also avoids the complication of long thoracic and phrenic nerve injuries and produces a more acceptable

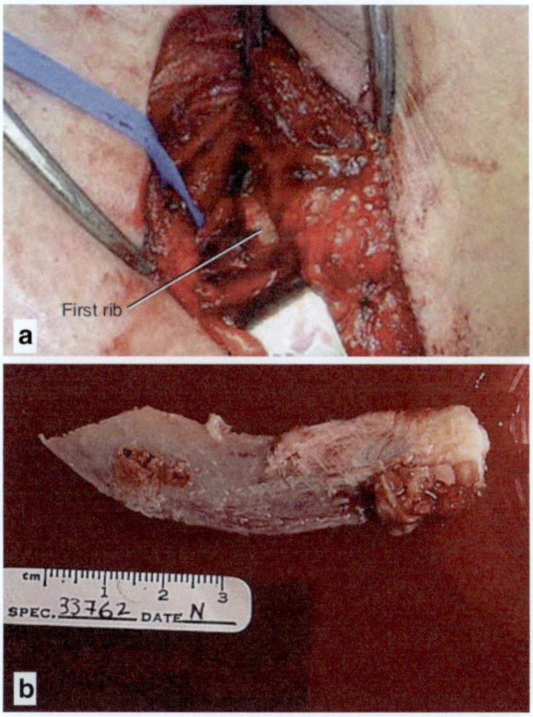

Fig. 24.4 (**a**) Visualization of the first rib. (**b**) Excised first rib

cosmetic result (Fig. 24.4a, b). Poor visualization of the posterior aspect of the first rib can result in a long residual first rib stump which is believed to play a role in recurrent TOS [65, 66]. For a successful outcome, the entire rib should be resected. Disadvantages of this approach include poor visualization of the posterior aspect of the first rib and lack of access to the brachial plexus (which frequently lies medial to the first rib) and congenital bands or cervical ribs. Formal exploration of the upper brachial plexus cannot be done through this approach.

Supraclavicular Rib Resection

The supraclavicular approach allows wider exposure of the brachial plexus and more direct access to the cervical ribs or fibrous bands causing compression. If anomalous first ribs or fibrous bands are present, they should be removed. This can be best accomplished through the supraclavicular approach. This approach also allows easier access to the brachial plexus and scalenes for scalenectomy and upper plexus neurolysis and is the approach favored by many neurosurgeons [67]. The disadvantage of the supraclavicular approach is a higher incidence of thoracic duct and phrenic nerve injuries. Phrenic nerve paralysis has been reported in up to 7% of cases [68].

An incision parallel to the clavicle is made approximately 2 cm above the clavicle and beginning 1 cm lateral to the midline (Fig. 24.5a–c).

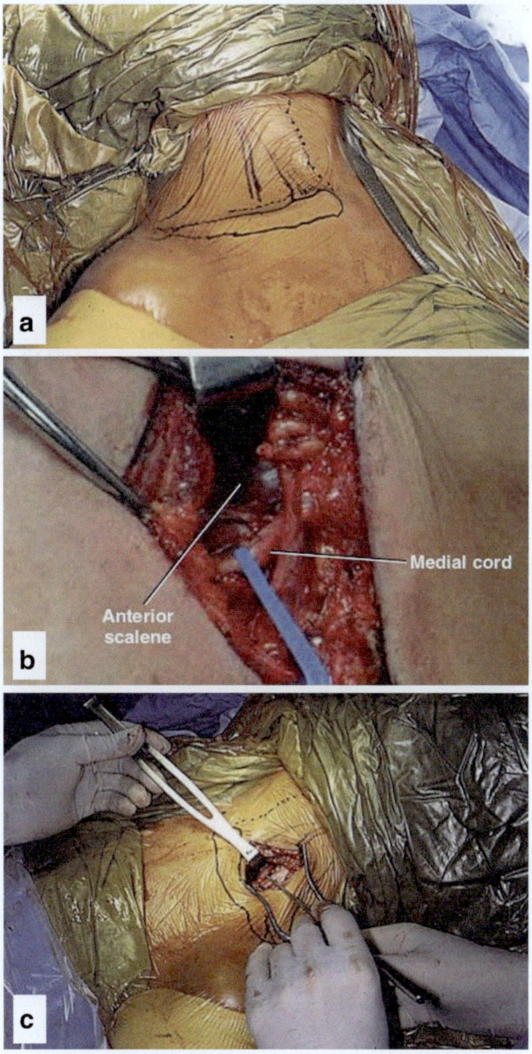

Fig. 24.5 (**a**) Supraclavicular approach allowing direct access to the brachial plexus and scalene. (**b**) View of the plexus emerging behind the anterior scalene. (**c**) After resection of the scalene, the artery and liberated plexus are evident

Supraclavicular nerves are identified, the platysma is incised, and the anterior scalene muscle is identified. The phrenic nerve is identified adjacent to the anterior scalene. The anterior scalene muscle is then divided at its insertion on the first rib. Neurolysis of the brachial plexus and middle scalenectomy can then be performed. This exposure can be used for isolated scalenectomy and brachial plexus neurolysis without first rib resection.

Anterior Scalenectomy and Brachial Plexus Neurolysis

Anterior scalenotomy was described by Adson and Coffey in 1927 [16]. This remained a popular operative treatment method until Clagett [69] reported a high failure rate with this procedure and recommended first rib resection instead. Anterior scalenectomy is reported to have a higher success rate than anterior scalenotomy, which does not involve removal of the anterior scalene muscle [70]. Anterior scalenectomy removes offending structures compressing the brachial plexus more effectively than scalenotomy alone. Also, middle scalenectomy can be performed easily, resulting in more complete decompression than scalenotomy alone. The reported failure rate of anterior scalenectomy alone is 12% [70]. Today, this procedure is most commonly used in conjunction with brachial plexus neurolysis. Combined neurolysis reportedly improves results [71]. It can also be performed as a combined approach with first rib resection and anterior scalenectomy.

Anterior scalenectomy involves a 5-cm incision superior and parallel to the clavicle. Dissection is carried through the platysma muscle. Then the clavicular head of the sternocleidomastoid is transected. The anterior scalene muscle is then identified. Structures at risk during this dissection include the thoracic duct and phrenic nerve. The anterior scalene muscle is then transected and removed in its entirety. Portions of the middle scalene muscle can also be removed if this muscle contributes to impingement of the brachial plexus. The complication rate is reported to be less than 2%, and includes brachial plexus injury, hemothorax, pneumothorax, phrenic nerve injury, lymphocele, and chylothorax [54]. Anterior scalenectomy can be performed with less morbidity than first rib resection.

Wehbé and Whitaker [72] described epineurectomy, which is excision of the epineurium and circumferential dissection of the affected nerves, with release of any offending structures. This technique involves a supraclavicular approach, with anterior scalenectomy, followed by extensive dissection of the brachial plexus and removal of the epineurium and any compressive structures. Wehbé and Whitaker [72] reported a 90% rate of alleviation of symptoms and a 10% recurrence rate [56]. Others recommend brachial plexus neurolysis only for revision surgery or in post-traumatic cases in which there is suspected scarring.

Combined Approach: Transaxillary Resection of the First Rib and Anterior and Middle Scalenectomy

This technique has been popularized by Atasoy, who recommended a combined approach for complete decompression of the thoracic outlet. First rib resection effectively decompresses the lower plexus, and scalenectomy decompresses the upper plexus. The first rib resection is performed first followed by immediate transcervical anterior and middle scalenectomy. The rationale that led to this surgical sequence is that scalenectomy is easier to perform once the distal insertions of the anterior and middle scalene muscles are released from the first rib. Results of this combined procedure show the lowest recurrence rate among various series of different operations for TOS [3, 68, 73]. To date, there are no randomized prospective trials involving a combined approach. This technique is also advocated for unsuccessful TOS surgery or recurrent TOS.

Treatment of Vascular Thoracic Outlet Syndrome

For patients with arterial compression, urgent surgical decompression is performed, followed by removal of an offending compressive structure, such as a cervical rib or fibrous bands. A combined approach is recommended. For patients with venous compression, thrombolysis is performed, followed by first rib resection. Percutaneous angioplasty can be performed at the same time as first rib resection to correct any residual subclavian vein stenosis [74].

Results

The results of most series show improvement in symptoms. Most patients show improvement after surgical treatment. However, a known percentage of patients do not improve with surgery in most series, and a small percentage of these patients have significant disability. Results are difficult to interpret because of the lack of a consensus about the diagnosis of TOS, lack of defined surgical indications, and lack of randomized prospective trials. Good to excellent results have been reported in 70–90% of patients in most reported studies [68, 69, 75]. Leffert and Perlmutter [76] reported 282 transaxillary first rib resections and noted an 85% improvement in pain. He also noted a high incidence of complications, with a 31% rate of intraoperative pneumothorax. Peek et al. looked at long-term follow-up of patients undergoing surgery for TOS. 51 of the 62 surgical procedures involved a first rib resection through a transaxillary approach. 54% of patients reported complete relief of symptoms while 96% noted improvement [77]. A review of 11 patients treated with brachial plexus neurolysis and scalenectomy without first rib resection showed that 82% had good outcomes, with return to normal everyday activity and either complete or significant relief of symptoms. The authors' conclusion was that microsurgical decompression through a supraclavicular approach without first rib resection is an effective treatment for TOS [78]. A series of 770 supraclavicular rib resections showed 59% excellent results and 27% good results, with a low incidence of complications [79]. Results with scalenectomy with first rib resection have not been conclusively proven to be better than those with anterior and middle scalenectomy alone [80, 81]. It is believed that removal of the first rib does not result in improvement; rather, improvement occurs because of the scalenectomy that is required to access the rib. Thus, some authors no longer perform first rib resection and instead perform anterior and middle scalenectomy alone [82]. Because there are few randomized comparative studies, there is no consensus as to the best surgical approach. A meta-analysis by Peek et al. found a mean improvement in the DASH score of 28.3 points after surgical treatment for TOS. Furthermore, an overall clinical success of ≥90% was found for vascular forms of TOS and was 60–80% for the NTOS patients [83].

Preoperative negative predictive factors include acute ischemia, sensory or motor deficit, and poorly systematized neurologic symptoms [84]. Psychological factors also play a significant role in the outcome of TOS surgery. Predictive factors associated with persistent disability include a history of major depression, unmarried status, and having less than a high school education [85]. A shorter duration of symptoms (<24 months) and the presence of a cervical rib may also imply an unfavorable surgical outcome [86].

Recurrent Thoracic Outlet Syndrome

True recurrent TOS occurs after a symptom-free interval following surgical intervention. If there was no improvement or symptom-free interval after surgery, the possibility of an incorrect diagnosis, secondary gain, or technical errors in surgery should be entertained. Pseudorecurrences are generally the result of technical errors including inadequate first rib removal, failure to remove a cervical rib, and inadvertent removal of the second rib instead of the first [87]. True recurrence assumes a correct diagnosis with successful treatment. Surgical decompression is reliable, but results tend to deteriorate over time [88]. True recurrence is usually caused by scar tissue surrounding the brachial plexus or caused by a residual first rib stump (>1 cm) causing further impingement [89]. In revision surgery, the supraclavicular approach is most commonly used because it provides excellent exposure to the brachial plexus for neurolysis. The complication rate associated with revision surgery is higher, and the success rate is lower [90].

Summary

TOS is compression of the neurovascular structures in the thoracic outlet. This condition is one of the most challenging upper extremity compressive neuropathies to manage, given the difficulty in diagnosis and lack of consistent response to treatment. The foundation of effective management is a thorough understanding of the anatomy of the thoracic outlet, the types and clinical presentation of TOS, and the physical examination procedures, diagnostic studies, and electrodiagnostic testing used. A course of therapy should always be tried as the first line of treatment before surgical intervention.

References

1. Rayan GM. Thoracic outlet syndrome. J Shoulder Elbow Surg. 1998;7:440–51.
2. Pratt NE. Neurovascular entrapment in the regions of the shoulder and posterior triangle of the neck. Phys Ther. 1986;66:1894.
3. Kirgis HD, Reed AF. Significant anatomic relations in the syndrome of the scalene muscles. Ann Surg. 1948;127:1182–201.
4. Paraskevas G, Ioannidis O, Papaziogas B, Natsis K, Spanidou S, Kitsoulis P. An accessory middle scalene muscle causing thoracic outlet syndrome. Folia Morphol (Warsz). 2007;66(3):194–7.
5. Forcada P, Rodriguez-Niedenfuhr M, Llusa M, Carrera A. Subclavius posticus muscle: supernumerary muscle as a potential cause for thoracic outlet syndrome. Clin Anat. 2001;14(1):55–7.
6. Atasoy E. Thoracic outlet syndrome anatomy. Hand Clin. 2004;20(1):7–14.
7. Ingesson EEU, Ribbe EB, Norgren LEH. Thoracic outlet syndrome: evaluation of a physiotherapeutical method. Manual Med. 1986;2:86–8.
8. Atasoy E. Thoracic outlet compression syndrome. Orthop Clin North Am. 1996;27:265–303.
9. Roos DB. Congenital anomalies associated with thoracic outlet syndrome: anatomy, symptoms, diagnosis and treatment. Am J Surg. 1976;132:771–8.
10. Wright IS. The neurovascular syndrome produced by hyperabduction of the arms: the immediate changes produced in 15 normal controls, and the effects on some persons of prolonged hyperabduction of the arms, as in sleeping, and certain occupations. Am Heart J. 1945;29:1.
11. Roos DB. The place for scalenotomy and first rib resection in thoracic outlet syndrome. Surgery. 1982;92:1077–85.
12. Troeng T. The anatomy of the thoracic outlet and the causes of thoracic outlet syndrome. Vasa. 1987;16:149–52.
13. Willshire WH. Supernumerary first rib: clinical records. Lancet. 1860;2:633.
14. Coote H. Pressure on the axillary vessels and nerve by an exostosis from cervical rib; interference with the circulation of the arm, removal of the rib and exostosis; recovery. Med Times Gaz. 1861;2:108.
15. Murphy T. Brachial neuritis caused by pressure of first rib. Aust Med J. 1910;15:582.
16. Adson AW, Coffey JR. Cervical rib: a method of anterior approach for relief of symptoms by division of the scalene anticus. Ann Surg. 1927;85:839.
17. Ochsner A, Gage M, Debakey M. Scalenus anticus (Naffziger's) syndrome. Am J Surg. 1935;28:696–9.
18. Raaf J. Surgery for cervical rib and scalenus anticus syndrome. JAMA. 1955;157:219.
19. Falconer MA, Weddell G. Costoclavicular compression of the subclavian artery and vein: relation to the scalenus anticus syndrome. Lancet. 1943;2:539.
20. Peet PM, Hendrickson JD, Anderson TD. Thoracic outlet syndrome: evaluation of a therapeutic exercise program. Proc Staff Meet Mayo Clin. 1956;31(9):281–7.
21. Patton GM. Arterial thoracic outlet syndrome. Hand Clin. 2004;20:107–11.
22. Oates SD, Daley RA. Thoracic outlet syndrome. Hand Clin. 1996;12:705–18.
23. Sanders RJ, Hammond SL, Rao NM. Diagnosis of thoracic outlet syndrome. J Vasc Surg. 2007;46(3):601–4.
24. Lindgren K. Thoracic outlet syndrome with special reference to the first rib. Ann Chir Gynaecol. 1993;82:218–30.
25. Judy KL, Heymann RL. Vascular complications of thoracic outlet syndrome. Am J Surg. 1972;123:521.
26. Whitenack SH, Hunter JM, Read RL. Thoracic outlet syndrome: a brachial plexopathy. In: Mackin EJ, Callahan AD, Skirven TM, et al., editors. Rehabilitation of the hand: surgery and therapy. 5th ed. St. Louis: Mosby; 2002. p. 703–31.
27. Douglas JR, Weiland AJ. Vascular pathology in the throwing athlete. Hand Clin. 2000;16:477–85.
28. Sanders RJ, Hammond SL. Venous thoracic outlet syndrome. Hand Clin. 2004;20:113–8.
29. Dale WA, Lewis MR. Management of thoracic outlet syndrome. Ann Surg. 1975;181:575.
30. Wilbourn AJ. The thoracic outlet syndrome is overdiagnosed. Arch Neurol. 1990;47:328–30.
31. Sanders RJ, Hammond SL. Etiology and pathology. Hand Clin. 2004;20(1):23–6.
32. Urschel HC Jr, Razzuk MA, Hyland JW, et al. Thoracic outlet syndrome masquerading as coronary

artery disease (pseudoangina). Ann Thorac Surg. 1973;16:239–48.
33. Roos DB. Thoracic outlet syndrome is underdiagnosed. Muscle Nerve. 1999;22(1):126–9.
34. Cherington M, Cherington C. Thoracic outlet syndrome: reimbursement patterns and patient profiles. Neurology. 1992;42:943–5.
35. Wood VE, Biondi J. Double-crush nerve compression in thoracic-outlet syndrome. J Bone Joint Surg Am. 1990;72:85–7.
36. Jones KJ. Thoracic outlet compression. In: Green D, Hotchkiss R, Pederson W, Wolfe S, editors. Green's operative hand surgery. 5th ed. Philadelphia: Elsevier; 2005. p. 1047–73.
37. Gergoudis R, Barnes RW. Thoracic outlet arterial compression: prevalence in normal persons. Angiology. 1980;31(8):538–41.
38. Wright IS. The neurovascular syndrome produced by hyperabduction of the arm. Am Heart J. 1945;29:1.
39. Mackinnon SE, Novak CB. Thoracic outlet syndrome. Curr Prob Surg. 2002;39:1070–145.
40. Brantigan CO, Roos DB. Diagnosis of thoracic outlet syndrome. Hand Clin. 2004;20(1):27–36.
41. Calis M, Mehmet A, Ayşin, D. Diagnostic values of clinical diagnostic tests in thoracic outlet syndrome. Türk Fiz Tıp Rehab Derg. 2010;56.
42. Warrens AN, Heaton JM. Thoracic outlet compression syndrome: the lack of reliability of its clinical assessment. Ann R Coll Surg Engl. 1987;69:203–4.
43. Plewa MC, Delinger M. The false-positive rate of thoracic outlet syndrome shoulder maneuvers in healthy subjects. Acad Emerg Med. 1998;5(4):337–42.
44. Baumer P, Kele H, Kretschmer T, et al. Thoracic outlet syndrome in 3T MR neurography-fibrous bands causing discernible lesions of the lower brachial plexus. Eur Radiol. 2014;24(3):756–61.
45. Remy-Jardin M, Remy J, Masson P, et al. Helical CT angiography of thoracic outlet syndrome: functional anatomy. Am J Roentgenol. 2000;174:1667–74.
46. Gillet R, Teixeira P, Meyer JB, Rauch A, Raymond A, Dap F, Blum A. Dynamic CT angiography for the diagnosis of patients with thoracic outlet syndrome: correlation with patient symptoms. J Cardiovasc Comput Tomogr. 2018;12(2):158–65.
47. Esposito MD, Arrington JA, Blackshear MN, et al. Thoracic outlet syndrome in a throwing athlete diagnosed with MRI and MRA. J Magn Reson Imaging. 1997;7:598–9.
48. Panegyres PK, Moore N, Gibson R, et al. Thoracic outlet syndromes and magnetic resonance imaging. Brain. 1993;116:823–41.
49. Demirbag D, Unlu E, Ozdemir F, et al. The relationship between magnetic resonance imaging findings and postural maneuver and physical examination tests in patients with thoracic outlet syndrome: results of a double-blind, controlled study. Arch Phys Med Rehabil. 2007;88(7):844–51.
50. Rousseff R, Tzvetanov P, Valkov I. Utility (or futility?) of electrodiagnosis in thoracic outlet syndrome. Electromyogr Clin Neurophysiol. 2005;45(3):131–3.
51. Le Forestier N, Moulonguet A, Maisonobe T, et al. True neurogenic thoracic outlet syndrome: electrophysiological diagnosis in six cases. Muscle Nerve. 1998;21(9):1129–34.
52. Seror P. Medial antebrachial cutaneous nerve conduction study, a new tool to demonstrate mild lower brachial plexus lesions: a report of 16 cases. Clin Neurophysiol. 2006;115(10):2316–22.
53. Tsao BE, Ferrante MA, Wilbourn AJ, Shields RW. Electrodiagnostic features of true neurogenic thoracic outlet syndrome. Muscle Nerve. 2014;49:724–7.
54. Ferrante M, Wilbourn A. The utility of various sensory nerve conduction responses in assessing brachial plexopathies. Muscle Nerve. 1995;18:879–89.
55. Yiannikas C, Walsh JC. Somatosensory evoked responses in the diagnosis of thoracic outlet syndrome. J Neurol Neurosurg Psychiatry. 1983;46:234–40.
56. Veilleux M, Stevens JC, Campbell JK. Somatosensory evoked potentials: lack of value for diagnosis of thoracic outlet syndrome. Muscle Nerve. 1988;11:571–5.
57. Synek VM. Diagnostic importance of somatosensory evoked potentials in the diagnosis of thoracic outlet syndrome. Clin Electroencephalogr. 1986;17:112–6.
58. Komanetsky RM, Novak CB, Mackinnon SE, et al. Somatosensory evoked potentials fail to diagnose thoracic outlet syndrome. J Hand Surg [Am]. 1996;21:662–6.
59. Braun RM, Shah KN, Rechnic M, Doehr S, Woods N. Quantitative assessment of scalene muscle block for the diagnosis of suspected thoracic outlet syndrome. J Hand Surg Am. 2015;40:2255–61.
60. Lum YW, Brooke BS, Likes K, Modi M, Grunebach H, Christo PJ, Freischlag JA. Impact of anterior scalene lidocaine blocks on predicting surgical success in older patients with neurogenic thoracic outlet syndrome. J Vasc Surg. 2012;55:1370–5.
61. Novak CB, Collins ED, Mackinnon SE. Outcome following conservative treatment management of thoracic outlet syndrome. J Hand Surg [Am]. 1995;20:542–8.
62. MacKinnon SE, Patterson GA. Supraclavicular first rib resection. Semin Thorac Cardiovasc Surg. 1996;8:208–13.
63. Urschel HC Jr. The transaxillary approach for treatment of thoracic outlet. Semin Thorac Cardiovasc Surg. 1996;8:214–20.
64. Roos DB. Transaxillary approach for first rib resection to relieve thoracic outlet syndrome. Ann Surg. 1966;163:354.
65. Urschel HC, Razzuk MA. Neurovascular compression in the thoracic outlet changing management over 50 years. Ann Surg. 1988;228:609–17.
66. Mingoli A, Feldhaus RJ, Farina C. Long-term outcome after transaxillary approach for thoracic outlet syndrome. Surgery. 1995;118:840–4.
67. Huang JH, Zager E. Thoracic outlet syndrome. Neurosurgery. 2004;55(4):897–902.
68. Sander RJ, Monsour JW, Gerber WF, et al. Scalenectomy versus first rib resection for treatment of thoracic outlet syndrome. Surgery. 1979;85:109–21.

69. Clagett OT. Presidential address: research and prosearch. J Thorac Cardiovasc Surg. 1962;44:153.
70. Sanders RJ. Results of the surgical treatment for thoracic outlet syndrome. Semin Thorac Cardiovasc Surg. 1996;8:221–8.
71. Mattson R. Surgical approach to anterior scalenectomy. Hand Clin. 2004;20(1):57–60.
72. Wehbe M, Whitaker ML. Epineurectomy for thoracic outlet syndrome. Hand Clin. 2004;20(1):83–6.
73. Cinà C, Whiteacre L, Edwards R, Maggisano R. Treatment of thoracic outlet syndrome with combined scalenectomy and transaxillary first rib resection. Cardiovasc Surg. 1994;2:514–8.
74. Schneider DB, Dimuzio PJ, Martin ND, et al. Combination treatment of venous thoracic outlet syndrome: open surgical decompression and intraoperative angioplasty. J Vasc Surg. 2005;42(3):599–603.
75. Sharp WJ, Nowak LR, Zamani T, et al. Long-term follow-up and patient satisfaction after surgery for thoracic outlet syndrome. Ann Vasc Surg. 2001;15(1):32–6.
76. Leffert RD, Perlmutter GS. Thoracic outlet syndrome: results of 282 transaxillary first rib resections. Clin Orthop Relat Res. 1999;368:66–79.
77. Peek J, Vos CG, Unlu C, Schreve MA, van de Mortel RHW, de Vries J-P. Long-term functional outcome of surgical treatment for thoracic outlet syndrome. Diagnostics. 2018;8:7.
78. Rochkind S, Shemesh M, Patish H, et al. Thoracic outlet syndrome: a multidisciplinary problem with a perspective for microsurgical management without rib resection. Acta Neurochir Suppl. 2007;100:145–7.
79. Hempel GK, Shutze WP, Anderson JF, Bukhari HI. 770 Consecutive supraclavicular first rib resections for thoracic outlet syndrome. Ann Vasc Surg. 1996;10:56–63.
80. Sanders RJ, Pearce WH. The treatment of thoracic outlet syndrome: a comparison of different operations. J Vasc Surg. 1989;10:626–34.
81. Sanders RJ, Monsour JW, Gerber FG, et al. Scalenectomy versus first rib resection for treatment of the thoracic outlet syndrome. Surgery. 1979;85:109–21.
82. Sanders RJ, Hammond SL. Supraclavicular first rib resection and total scalenectomy: technique and results. Hand Clin. 2004;20(1):61–70.
83. Peek J, Vos CG, Unlu C, van de Pavoordt HD, van den Akker PJ, de Vries JP. Outcome of surgical treatment for thoracic outlet syndrome: systematic review and meta-analysis. Ann Vasc Surg. 2017;40:303–26.
84. Degeorges R, Reynaud C, Becquemin JP. Thoracic outlet syndrome surgery: long-term functional results. Ann Vasc Surg. 2004;18(5):558–65. Epub 2004 Aug 6.
85. Axelrod DA, Proctor MC, Geisser ME, et al. Outcomes after surgery for thoracic outlet syndrome. J Vasc Surg. 2001;33(6):1220–5.
86. Yavuzer S, Atinkaya C, Tokat O. Clinical predictors ofsurgical outcome in patients with thoracic outlet syndrome operated on via transaxillary approach. Eur J Cardiothorac Surg. 2004;25(2):173–8.
87. Urschel HC Jr, Razzuk MA. The failed operation for thoracic outlet syndrome: the difficulty of diagnosis and management. Ann Thorac Surg. 1986;42:523–8.
88. Balci AE, Balci TA, Cakir O, et al. Surgical treatment of thoracic outlet syndrome: effect and results of surgery. Ann Thorac Surg. 2003;75(4):1091–6.
89. Mingoli A, Sapienza P, di Marzo L, Cavallaro A. Role of first rib stump length in recurrent neurogenic thoracic outlet syndrome. Am J Surg. 2005;190(1):156.
90. Cheng SWK, Stoney RJ. Supraclavicular reoperation for neurogenic thoracic outlet syndrome. J Vasc Surg. 1994;19:565–72.

Vein Wrapping of Peripheral Nerves: Surgical Technique

25

Loukia K. Papatheodorou and Dean G. Sotereanos

Introduction

Vein wrapping is a surgical technique used to treat scarred peripheral nerves serving as a barrier to prevent adhesion and scar tissue formation around the nerve. Cicatrix formation around peripheral nerves can occur after trauma and most commonly after failed surgical decompression for entrapment neuropathies [1–3]. Postoperative epineural scarring leads to mechanical constriction, nerve ischemia and loss of nerve gliding and subsequent traction to the nerve with motion of the adjacent joint. The result is a chronic neuropathy, called a "traction neuropathy" and the optimal treatment may involve a combination of procedures [2].

Most authors agree that after revision neurolysis of the scarred nerve, soft tissue coverage of the segment of scarred nerve is essential to prevent cicatrix reformation from contacting the epineurium. Therefore, a variety of supplementary techniques have been attempted to prevent adhesion to the nerve, ranging from interposition flaps (fat, muscle or free flaps) to nerve wrapping (vein wrapping, synthetic nerve protectors) [4–16]. However, many of these flaps require technically demanding dissection and do not always provide satisfactory results [7, 8]. Several experimental and clinical studies have shown good results of vein wrapping as adhesion barrier for recurrent entrapment neuropathies secondary to cicatrix of the nerve [12–21]. The ideal nerve wrapping material should prevent adhesions and inhibit cicatrix reformation around the previously scarred nerve, protecting the nerve from further compression and ameliorating nerve gliding during motion of the extremity.

Historical Perspective

Allograft vein wrapping of a scarred peripheral nerve with the use of allograft umbilical veins was used clinically before autologous vein wrapping with good results [10]. However, the autologous vein graft has been found to create fewer adhesions between the vein and the nerve compared with vein allografts. In an animal study, the investigators compared the femoral vein autografts with glutaraldehyde-preserved allografts and found that epineural scar formation in rat sciatic nerves wrapped with allograft vein was ten times more than in nerves wrapped with autograft vein [11].

Our group studied the effect of autologous vein wrapping of scarred peripheral nerve initially in two experimental studies and later in several clinical studies [12–21]. The safety of the procedure was studied first in an experimental study by wrapping with autologous vein graft of intact sciatic nerve in 30 rats [18]. No adverse

L. K. Papatheodorou (✉) · D. G. Sotereanos
Orthopaedic Specialists - UPMC,
University of Pittsburgh, Pittsburgh, PA, USA

D. G. Sotereanos, L. K. Papatheodorou (eds.), *Compressive Neuropathies of the Upper Extremity*,
https://doi.org/10.1007/978-3-030-37289-7_25

effects on the nerve were noted (no demyelinization, nerve degeneration or adhesion formation) [18]. Then, an experimental chronic nerve compression model was created in 100 rats [19]. The sciatic nerve was wrapped with autologous vein graft in 50 rats while the remaining 50 rats served as controls. Greater functional improvement of the sciatic nerves was found in the vein-wrapping group than in the control group [19]. Based on the electrophysiologic testing, the latency was significantly shorter in the vein-wrapping group than in the control group [19]. Moreover, histologic examination showed marked nerve degeneration and scar tissue developed around the nerve in the control group but not in the vein-wrapping group [19]. These experimental studies showed that the autologous vein wrapping could prevent scar formation around the nerve and improve the nerve functional recovery of chronic compressed nerves.

Furthermore, the inhibition of scar formation around the nerve with the autologous vein wrapping technique has been verified by human histopathologic analysis [20, 21]. Biopsies obtained from re-exploration of autologous vein-grafted nerves showed no adhesions between the intima of the vein and the nerve [20, 21]. Additionally, neovascularization of the vein graft and structural transformation of the vein endothelium was also noted in biopsy specimen [21].

Although the mechanism still remains uncertain, the autologous vein wrapping technique appears to prevent extrinsic epineurial scar formation and to preserve or restore intrinsic epineurial vascularity. It is suggested that locally produced molecules from either the nerve or the autologous vein graft or both may be responsible for the neovascularization and structural transformation of the endothelium of the vein graft, contributing to the nerve functional recovery [21].

A most recent experimental study using a rodent chronic nerve compression model further confirmed this hypothesis [22]. 90 rats were randomly divided into three groups. In the sham group, exposure of the right sciatic nerve was performed in 30 rats. In the control group, chronic constriction injury of the right sciatic nerve was produced in 30 rats. In the vein-wrapping group, the chronic constriction injury of the right sciatic nerve was followed by autologous vein wrapping in 30 rats. In this study, significantly higher concentrations of vascular endothelial growth factor (VEGF) and hepatocyte growth factor (HGF) in the ligated sciatic nerves were noted in the vein-wrapping group rather than in the other groups [22]. These findings suggest that these neurotrophic factors may play a mechanistic role in the neovascularization and structural changes observed in vein graft. Additionally, the results of the qualitative histologic analysis suggested that the vein wrapping can prevent nerve degeneration and scar tissue formation, while it can regenerate the myelin sheaths improving the nerve functional recovery [22]. Moreover, immunohistochemistry results indicated that the vein wrapping prevented upregulation of markers of inflammation and nerve damage caused by chronic constriction injury [22]. Thus, these findings suggest that vein wrapping can reduce inflammation and nerve damage.

Indications

The use of the autologous vein graft wrapping technique is indicated mainly for treatment of significant epineurial scarring. This technique is recommended in patients with recurrent entrapment neuropathies with at least two previous operations, which failed to resolve the symptoms. Recalcitrant carpal and cubital tunnel syndromes are the most common indications. In addition, vein wrapping can also be applied in recurrent radial tunnel syndrome and in patients with significant post-traumatic nerve scarring or neuroma formation.

Although the nerve scarring can be suspected preoperatively, based on the symptoms or electrodiagnostic findings, it is important that it be confirmed intraoperatively. Patients usually present with recurrent symptoms after an adequate surgical decompression. It must be noted that recurrent symptoms occur after a distinct symptom free period following previous surgery. The persistence of symptoms after previous surgical decompression is mostly correlated with incomplete nerve decompression or release. Severe pain worsening with activities is the chief complaint of patients. Paresthesia and numbness are also common symptoms. Abnormal two-point discrimination and positive Tinel's sign are noted in most patients. Presence of muscular atrophies is highly indicative of severe intrinsic scarring of the nerve. Electrodiagnostic findings usually include decreased electrical amplitude and sensory conduction after stimulation of the nerve, while muscle denervation is less often.

The autologous vein wrapping technique is not recommended in patients with chronic lower extremity venous insufficiency. Before revision surgery, a consultation by a vascular surgeon is recommended in patients with peripheral vascular disease or deep venous thrombosis history. In patients with coronary heart disease, the saphenous vein is a major source of vein grafts for reconstructive cardiac surgery and that should be taken into consideration.

Surgical Technique

The patient is positioned supine with the affected arm placed on an arm table. General anesthesia is used for the autologous saphenous vein wrapping technique because of the need to have two operating fields (one in the upper extremity for the nerve exploration and another in the lower extremity for the harvesting the saphenous vein graft). This procedure involves revision decompression with neurolysis of the affected nerve in the upper extremity, harvesting the greater saphenous vein from the ipsilateral or contralateral lower extremity, preparing the vein graft properly and then wrapping the autologous vein graft around the compressed nerve segment.

Under tourniquet control, the affected nerve is surgically explored at the upper extremity using the pre-existing incision, which is extended both proximally and distally. The compressed nerve should be identified in an unscarred healthy environment both proximally and distally and then dissected towards the scarred section. The nerve is lysed from the surrounding scar tissue and completely freed of any adhesions. If excessive scarring or lack of epineural vascularity of the nerve is noted, an internal neurolysis is performed under the microscope. After the completion of the revision decompression of the nerve, it is important to measure the length of the segment of the nerve that has to be vein wrapped. The required length of the vein graft is four to five times the scarred length of the nerve. A vein graft length of 25–30 cm is usually needed.

The greater saphenous vein harvesting is initiated only after confirmation of the severe scarred nerve intraoperatively (Fig. 25.1). The ipsilateral or contralateral lower extremity can be used for harvesting of the greater saphenous vein graft. To minimize the length of the incision and the morbidity of the donor site, a vein stripper is used to harvest the vein graft (Fig. 25.2a, b). Under tourniquet control at the lower extremity, a small

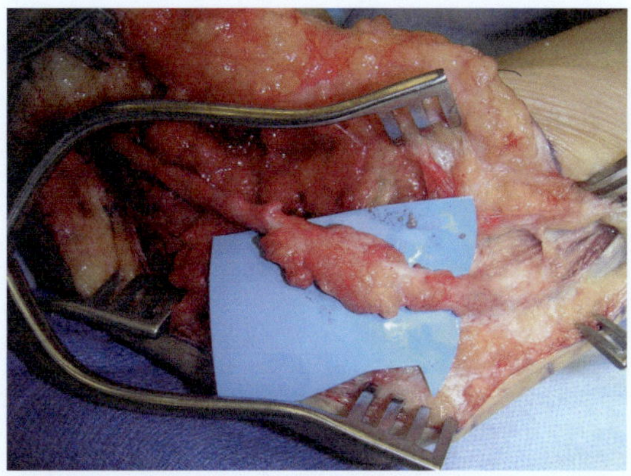

Fig. 25.1 Intra-operative photograph of revision ulnar nerve decompression. Note the excessive scar formation around the ulnar nerve

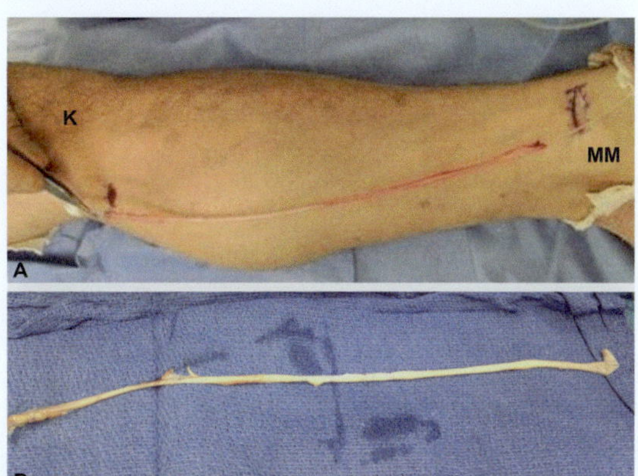

Fig. 25.2 (**a**) Harvesting of greater saphenous vein graft in the lower extremity using a vein stripper (K: knee, MM: medial malleolus). (**b**) Greater saphenous vein graft

incision is made 1 cm anterior to the medial malleolus. The greater saphenous vein is identified and is ligated distally. Attention must be paid to avoid injury to the associated saphenous nerve. A small longitudinal phlebotomy is made at the distal end of the vein graft. The vein stripper is introduced through the phlebotomy and is advanced proximally within the vein to the predetermined length. As the vein stripper guide is advanced proximally, it can be palpated through the skin. A second incision is made over the stripper guide proximally and the vein is ligated proximally. The vein stripper guide is advanced out of the vein through a second longitudinal phlebotomy at the proximal end of the vein graft (Fig. 25.2a, b). The saphenous vein graft is retrieved by slowly pulling out the stripper (Fig. 25.2a, b). The leg tourniquet is deflated, hemostasis is obtained and the skin is closed. Alternatively, the saphenous vein graft can be harvested through a continuous incision or interrupted incisions and dissection without the use of a vein stripper.

The saphenous vein graft is incised and opened longitudinally at a site table (Fig. 25.3a). Upon completion of the saphenous vein graft preparation, the vein graft is circumferentially wrapped around the scarred segment of the exposed affected nerve from distal to proximal (Figs. 25.3b and 25.4). Care is taken to wrap the vein graft with the intima of the vein against the nerve. One of the ends of the vein graft is tacked distal to the scarred segment of the nerve on a tissue that is not mobile. Each loop of the vein graft is loosely stitched to adjacent loop with a 7-0 prolene stitch (Fig. 25.4). During the wrapping procedure, attention is paid to ensure that each wrap is not too snug, to avoid potential constriction of the nerve. The other end of the vein graft is tacked proximal to the scarred segment of the nerve on unscarred tissue. The entire segment of the scarred affected nerve must be completely covered with the autologous saphenous vein graft to prevent recurrence (Figs. 25.5 and 25.6). The arm tourniquet is deflated and meticulous hemo-

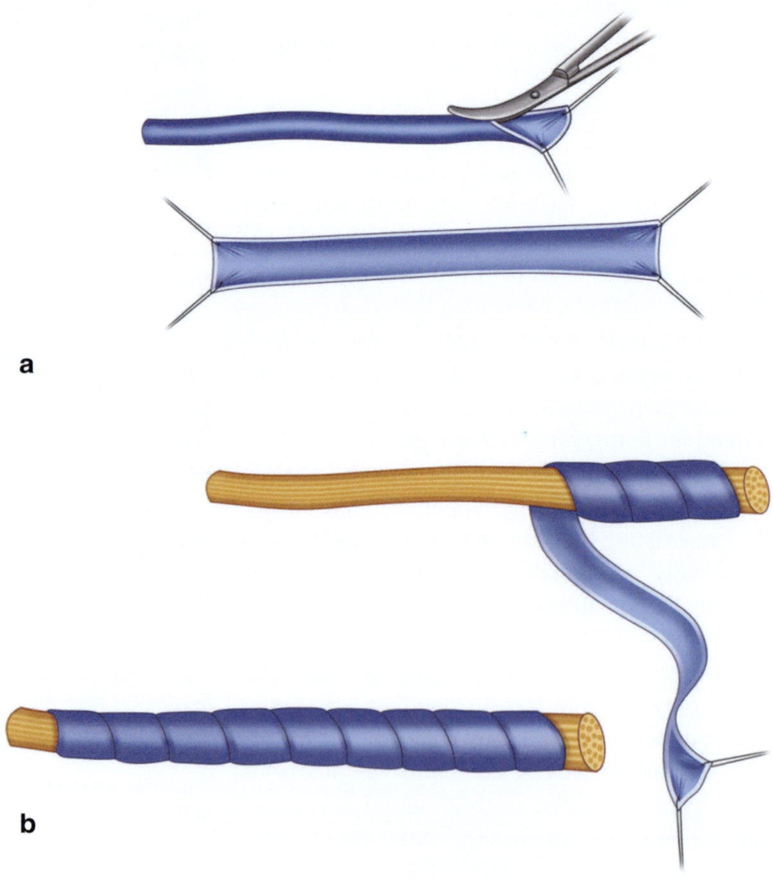

Fig. 25.3 Schematic of vein wrapping technique. (**a**) The saphenous vein graft is split longitudinally and is open to create a rectangle. (**b**) The saphenous vein graft is then wrapped around the scarred segment of the nerve with its intima against the nerve

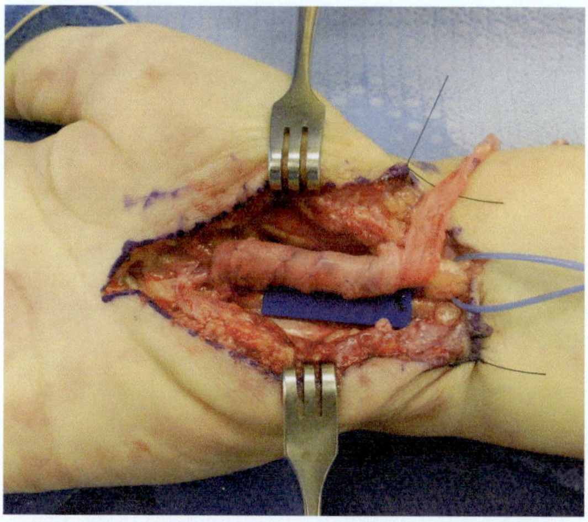

Fig. 25.4 Intra-operative photograph. The autologous saphenous vein graft is wrapped around the scarred segment of the median nerve in a distal to proximal direction with its intima against the nerve. Each ring of the wrapped vein is tacked to the adjacent rings with a 7-0 prolene stitch

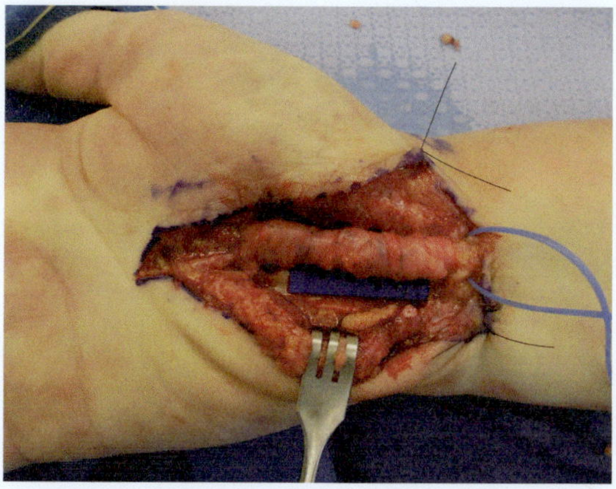

Fig. 25.5 Intra-operative photograph. The autologous saphenous vein graft is covering the entire scarred segment of the median nerve at the wrist

stasis is obtained. The wound is irrigated followed by routine wound closure.

Postoperatively, for recurrent carpal tunnel cases the wrist is immobilized in slight extension for 2 weeks and active and passive range of motion exercises follow. In recurrent cubital tunnel cases, the elbow is not immobilized to allow early mobilization with active range of motion exercises. In traumatic cases, immobilization is individualized with a trend toward early mobilization to prevent postoperative adhesions and microtraction of the nerve.

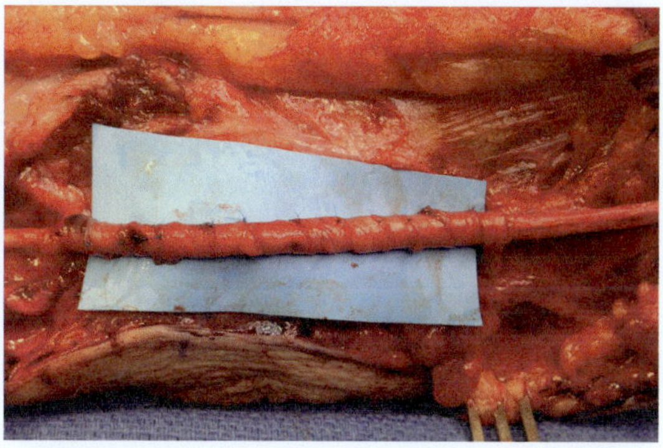

Fig. 25.6 Intra-operative photograph. The autologous saphenous vein graft is covering the entire scarred segment of the ulnar nerve at the elbow

Additionally, scar massage, desensitization and strengthening exercises can also be initiated, if required. Heavy lifting is to be avoided for 6 weeks after surgery.

Outcomes

Several clinical studies have shown that the autologous vein wrapping is an effective supplementary technique for treating recurrent entrapment neuropathies [12–17]. After autologous vein wrapping of the previously scarred nerve, significant pain reduction and improvement in sensation have been reported in the majority of patients with recalcitrant carpal or cubital tunnel syndrome. Grip strength and two-point discrimination also were improved postoperatively. Electrodiagnostic studies revealed improvement of findings postoperatively in several patients, although they did not return to normal values. No complications due to the saphenous vein graft harvesting were noted other than transient leg swelling at the donor site, which resolved in approximately 6 months.

Since the original clinical studies, the senior author (D.G.S.) has noted consistently good results with the autologous vein wrapping technique in more than one hundred patients with recurrent carpal or cubital tunnel syndrome and severe post-traumatic nerve scarring.

Based on the senior author's (D.G.S.) clinical experience, repeated peripheral nerve decompression should always be performed in combination with an ancillary technique to enhance scar-free nerve functional recovery. For patients with recurrent carpal or cubital tunnel syndrome, multiple operations and excessive scarring of the nerve, we perform revision decompression with repeated neurolysis of the nerve (external as well as possible internal) and autologous vein wrapping around the scarred segment of the nerve. Additionally, coverage with hypothenar fat pad flap is performed in patients with recurrent carpal tunnel syndrome and minimal medial epicondylectomy can be performed, if it is indicated, in patients with recurrent cubital tunnel syndrome.

In summary, the autologous vein wrapping technique can be used as an adhesion barrier for treatment of scarred peripheral nerves. Both experimental and clinical studies demonstrated that autologous vein wrapping is an efficacious/excellent adjuvant procedure for the treatment of recurrent entrapment neuropathies secondary to scarring of the nerve. Even though the mechanism still remains uncertain, the autologous vein wrapping technique can prevent adhesion around the nerve, improve the gliding of the nerve during motion of the extremity and promote the functional recovery of the nerve.

References

1. Stutz N, Gohritz A, van Schoonhoven J, Lanz U. Revision surgery after carpal tunnel release-analysis of the pathology in 200 cases during a 2 year period. J Hand Surg Br. 2006;31:68–71.
2. Hunter JM. Recurrent carpal tunnel syndrome, epineural fibrous fixation, and traction neuropathy. Hand Clin. 1991;7:491–504.
3. Rogers MR, Bergfield TG, Aulicino PL. The failed ulnar nerve transposition. Etiology and treatment. Clin Orthop Relat Res. 1991;269:193–200.
4. Mathoulin C, Bahm J, Roukoz S. Pedicled hypothenar fat pad flap for median nerve coverage in recalcitrant carpal tunnel syndrome. Hand Surg. 2000;5:33–40.
5. Strickland JW, Idler RS, Lourie GM, Plancher KD. The hypothenar fat pad flap for management of recalcitrant carpal tunnel syndrome. J Hand Surg Am. 1996;21:840–8.
6. Zancolli EA, Angrigiani C. Posterior interosseous island forearm flap. J Hand Surg Br. 1988;13:130–5.
7. Dellon AL, Mackinnon SE. The pronator quadratus muscle flap. J Hand Surg Am. 1984;9:423–7.
8. Rose EH, Norris MS, Kowalski TA, Lucas A, Flegler EJ. Palmaris brevis turnover flap as an adjunct to internal neurolysis of the chronically scarred median nerve in recurrent carpal tunnel syndrome. J Hand Surg Am. 1991;16:191–201.
9. Papatheodorou LK, Williams BG, Sotereanos DG. Preliminary results of recurrent cubital tunnel syndrome treated with neurolysis and porcine extracellular matrix nerve wrap. J Hand Surg Am. 2015;40:987–92.
10. Masear VR, Colgin S. The treatment of epineural scarring with allograft vein wrapping. Hand Clin. 1996;12:773–9.
11. Ruch DS, Spinner RM, Koman LA, Challa VR, O'Farrell D, Levin LS. The histologic effect of barrier vein wrapping of peripheral nerves. J Reconstr Microsurg. 1996;12:291–5.
12. Sotereanos DG, Giannakopoulos PN, Mitsionis GI, Xu J, Herndon JH. Vein graft wrapping for the treatment of recurrent compression of the median nerve. Microsurgery. 1995;16(11):752–6.
13. Varitimidis SE, Riano F, Vardakas DG, Sotereanos DG. Recurrent compressive neuropathy of the median nerve at the wrist: treatment with autogenous saphenous vein wrapping. J Hand Surg Br. 2000;25:271–5.
14. Varitimidis SE, Vardakas DG, Goebel F, Sotereanos DG. Treatment of recurrent compressive neuropathy of peripheral nerves in the upper extremity with an autologous vein insulator. J Hand Surg Am. 2001;26:296–302.
15. Varitimidis SE, Riano F, Sotereanos DG. Recalcitrant post-surgical neuropathy of the ulnar nerve at the elbow: treatment with autogenous saphenous vein wrapping. J Reconstr Microsurg. 2000;16:273–7.
16. Kokkalis ZT, Jain S, Sotereanos DG. Vein wrapping at cubital tunnel for ulnar nerve problems. J Shoulder Elbow Surg. 2010;19(2 Suppl):91–7.
17. Sotereanos DG, Xu J. Vein wrapping for the treatment of recurrent carpal tunnel syndrome. Tech Hand Up Extrem Surg. 1997;1:35–40.
18. Xu J, Sotereanos DG, Moller AR, Jacobsohn J, Tomaino MM, Fischer KJ, et al. Nerve wrapping with vein grafts in a rat model: a safe technique for the treatment of recurrent chronic compressive neuropathy. J Reconstr Microsurg. 1998;14:323–30.
19. Xu J, Varitimidis SE, Fisher KJ, Tomaino MM, Sotereanos DG. The effect of wrapping scarred nerves with autogenous vein graft to treat recurrent chronic nerve compression. J Hand Surg Am. 2000;25:93–103.
20. Vardakas DG, Varitimidis SE, Sotereanos DG. Findings of exploration of a vein-wrapped ulnar nerve: report of a case. J Hand Surg Am. 2001;26:60–3.
21. Chou KH, Papadimitriou NG, Sarris I, Sotereanos DG. Neovascularization and other histopathologic findings in an autogenous saphenous vein wrap used for recalcitrant carpal tunnel syndrome: a case report. J Hand Surg Am. 2003;28:262–6.
22. Murakami K, Kuniyoshi K, Iwakura N, Matsuura Y, Suzuki T, Takahashi K, et al. Vein wrapping for chronic nerve constriction injury in a rat model: study showing increases in VEGF and HGF production and prevention of pain-associated behaviors and nerve damage. J Bone Joint Surg Am. 2014;96:859–67.

Cervical Radiculopathy Mimicking Carpal Tunnel Syndrome

26

Gurpreet Surinder Gandhoke
and Raymond F. Sekula

Epidemiology

Cervical Radiculopathy

The annual incidence of cervical radiculopathy is reported to be 107.3 per 100,000 men and 63.5 per 100,000 women [1]. Risk factors for cervical radiculopathy include white race, cigarette smoking, and prior lumbar radiculopathy [2]. Other proposed factors include lifting heavy objects, driving equipment that vibrates, and playing golf. The incidence of trauma preceding the onset of cervical radiculopathy is relatively low.

Carpal Tunnel Syndrome

The sex-specific annual incidences of carpal tunnel syndrome have been reported as 505.6 per 100,000 person-years in women and 139.1 per 100,000 person years in men in the general population [3].

G. S. Gandhoke
Marion Bloch Neuroscience Inst, Saint Luke's Hospital of Kansas City, Kansas, MO, USA

R. F. Sekula (✉)
Department of Neurological Surgery, University of Pittsburgh Medical Center (UPMC) Presbyterian, Pittsburgh, PA, USA
e-mail: sekularf@upmc.edu

Etiology

Cervical Radiculopathy

A combination of mechanical compression, chemical irritation is attributed to be the cause of cervical radiculopathy. A compromise of the neural foramen opening due to disc extrusion, uncal hypertrophy, osteophyte formation, ligament hypertrophy limits the mobility of the nerve root. Space occupying lesions like tumors, infection and trauma can also contribute to cervical root irritation [4]. Inflammatory cytokines released from herniated discs are responsible for the radicular pain [5].

Carpal Tunnel Syndrome

Most cases of carpal tunnel syndrome are idiopathic. Secondary causes include space occupying lesions (tumors, hypertrophic synovial tissue, fracture callus, and osteophytes), metabolic and physiologic conditions (pregnancy, hypothyroidism, and rheumatoid arthritis), infections, neuropathies (associated with diabetes mellitus or alcoholism), and familial disorders. Repetitive activities requiring wrist extension or flexion, obesity, rapid dieting, shorter height, hysterectomy without oophorectomy, and recent menopause have also been reported risk factors for the development of carpal tunnel syndrome [6].

D. G. Sotereanos, L. K. Papatheodorou (eds.), *Compressive Neuropathies of the Upper Extremity*,
https://doi.org/10.1007/978-3-030-37289-7_26

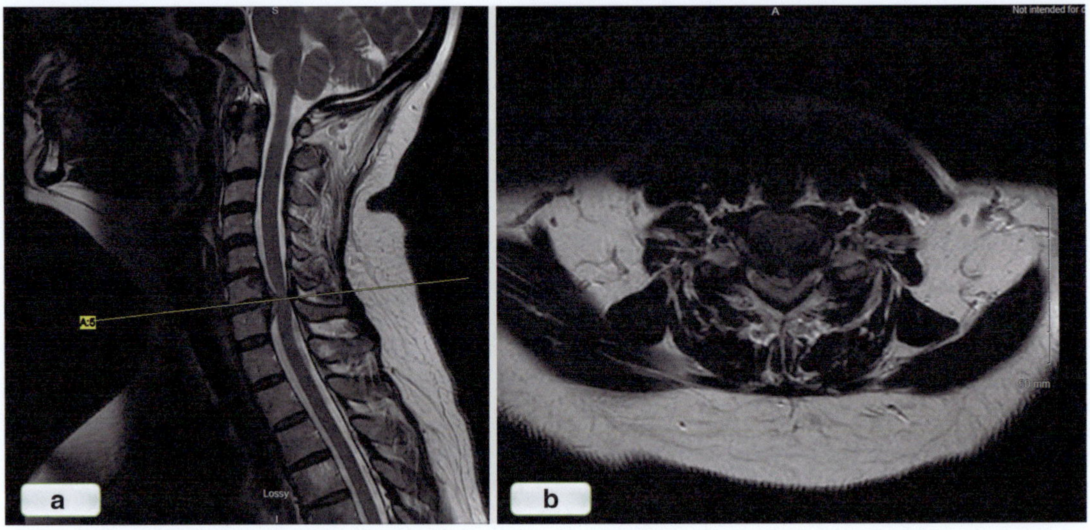

Fig. 26.1 (**a**, **b**) Sagittal and axial T2-weighted MRI, respectively, with line passing through the level of disc herniation

Diagnosis

Cervical Radiculopathy

Patient history and physical examination in addition to a thorough understanding of the innervations of each cervical root is crucial in locating the pathology. Axial neck pain, shoulder pathology, cardiac disease, brachial plexitis, tennis elbow and carpal tunnel syndrome can all confound the diagnosis. In addition, cervical radicular symptoms may not follow typical dermatomal distribution due to variability in cervical dermatomes [7, 8]. Most patients experience axial neck, trapezius and intrascapular pain. It is common for patients with cervical radiculopathy to have temporary relief of their symptoms when they hold their arms above their head, this decreases stretch of the affected nerve root [9]. Provocative maneuvers like the Spurling's sign can elicit symptoms by narrowing the neural foramen. Other provocative tests include the shoulder abduction test, the Valsalva. These tests are more reliable in providing accurate diagnosis as a group than as any single test in isolation [10]. Cervical radiographs are obtained to study the sagittal alignment and to look for the presence of instability, but are often of limited utility, and a MRI of the cervical spine is, most often, the diagnostic test of choice.

Figure 26.1a, b depicting sagittal and axial T2 weighted MRI respectively with line passing through the level of disc herniation. Correlating the patients clinical symptoms with the MRI findings is critical, due to the high rate of false positive MRI findings in the asymptomatic patient [11]. CT may be used to determine the osseous contribution (e.g., to rule out ossified posterior longitudinal ligament disease.

Figure 26.2a, b depicting sagittal and axial computerized tomography images respectively, revealing a severe case of ossified posterior longitudinal ligament causing central canal stenosis.

Carpal Tunnel Syndrome

Classic symptoms include numbness, tingling, numbness, burning and pain in at least two of the three digits supplied by the median nerve (the thumb and the index and middle fingers). Symptoms can resolve within 6 months in about one-third of patients, particularly younger patients, and a poor prognosis is predicted by the presence of bilateral symptoms and a positive Phalen test. The severity of symptoms and signs does not often corelate well the extent of nerve compression [12].

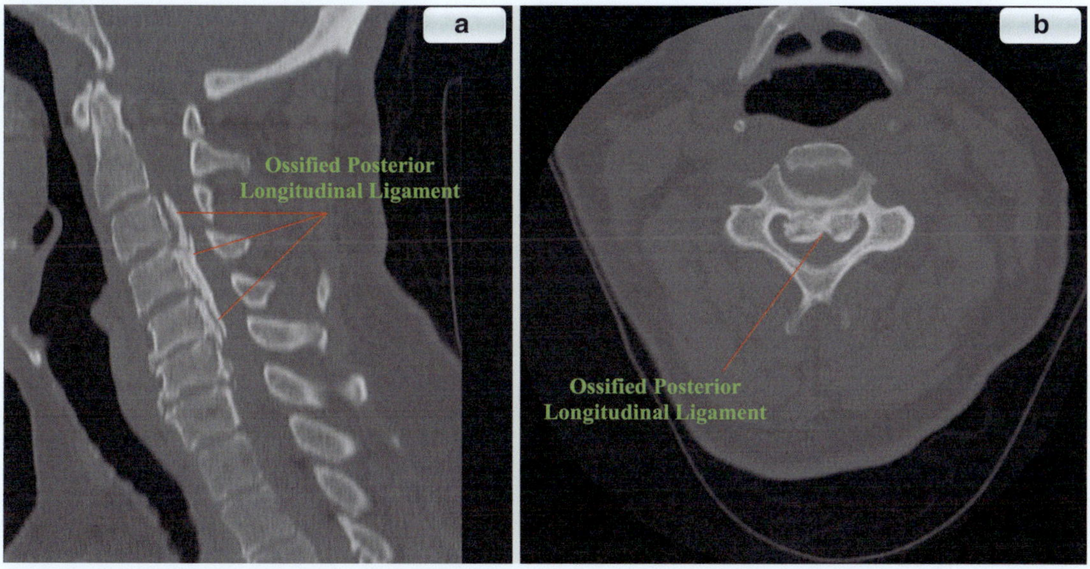

Fig. 26.2 (**a**, **b**) Sagittal and axial computerized tomography images, respectively, revealing a severe case of ossified posterior longitudinal ligament causing central canal stenosis

Table 26.1 Depicts important electrophysiological differences between carpal tunnel syndrome and cervical radiculopathy

Diagnosis	Nerve conduction study	Electromyography
Radiculopathy	Usually sensory normal Motor may be abnormal	Fibrillations of muscles at rest supplied by spinal nerve root (take about 3–4 weeks to manifest, after the compression) Denervation of the ipsilateral paraspinal muscles- Posterior rami (sensory) innervate the paraspinal muscles.
Neuropathy	Conduction delay often at site of compression	Absence of denervation in posterior myotomes (paraspinal muscles). EMG usually normal

Electrodiagnostic Studies

Table 26.1 depicts important electrophysiological differences between carpal tunnel syndrome and cervical radiculopathy.

In a study on EMG for the diagnosis of cervical radiculopathy, the affected level was accurately identified in 57%, 10% had non-specific findings, while 33% had a normal EMG [13]. An EMG can thus be used as an adjunct only.

Treatment

Cervical Radiculopathy

Nonoperative treatment should be attempted in all patients except in the event of a progressive neurological deficit. This may involve nonsteroidal anti-inflammatories, short courses of opioid narcotics or oral steroids. Cervical range of motion and strengthening exercises along with neck traction has been shown to improve neck disability index, arm pain at 6 months and 1 year [14]. There are data, which supports epidural steroid injections in the treatment of cervical radiculopathy, with upwards of 60% patients benefitting from long-term symptomatic relief without untoward complications [15, 16]. For cervical radiculopathy in the absence of myelopathy, surgery is recommended in patients who have root-related dysfunction for at least 6 weeks, have concordant root compression on advanced imaging, and who have failed nonoperative treatments. In addition surgical decompression should be considered in patients with less than 6 weeks of symptoms, but who have significant or progressive motor weakness [8]. The anterior cervical discectomy and fusion, anterior cervical arthroplasty, and the posterior cervical lamino foraminotomy are surgical options in the treatment of cervical radiculopathy.

Carpal Tunnel Syndrome

Surgery may improve clinical outcomes compared with wrist splints. There is insufficient evidence to know if surgery is as effective as local corticosteroid injections in treating carpal tunnel syndrome. Both endoscopic and open carpal tunnel release are options and the evidence does not clearly point to any one of the two surgical options being more effective [15].

Discussion

Our algorithm (Fig. 26.3) will aid the reader in making the proper diagnosis when one is uncertain of a diagnosis of cervical radiculopathy or carpal tunnel syndrome or both (i.e., double crush syndrome). The following key points will help the reader decipher a clinically challenging case of trying to differentiate the two pathologies. A few points to consider include:

- The reported incidence of concurrent cervical radiculopathy and carpal tunnel syndrome is high [17–19].
- Men are more susceptible to cervical radiculopathy and women are more susceptible to carpal tunnel syndrome [1, 3, 20–23].
- Higher incidence of carpal tunnel syndrome in women compared to men [17, 21–23].

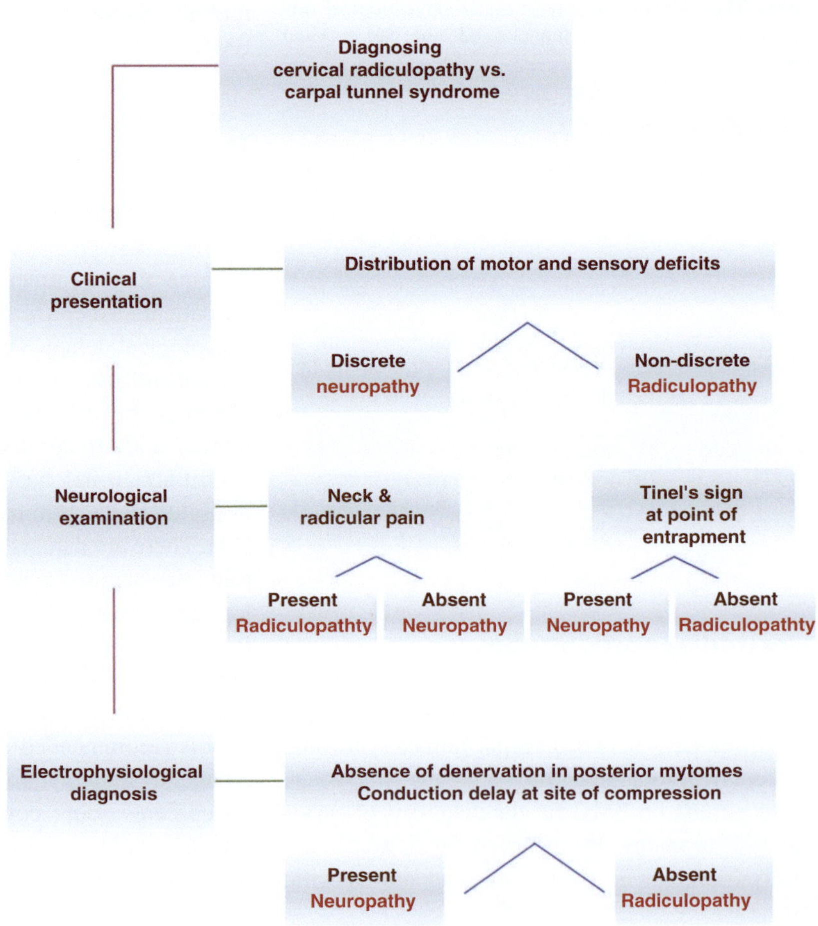

Fig. 26.3 Proposed algorithm to aid diagnosis in a case of cervical radiculopathy mimicking as carpal tunnel syndrome

- The age group in women most likely to suffer from only carpal tunnel syndrome is the sixth decade. For men, the age range was from sixth to the eight decades [3, 17].
- A cervical root lesion causes more profound motor deficit as compared to carpal tunnel syndrome [17].
- Neck and upper back pain are highest in patients with only cervical radiculopathy, and lowest in patients with only carpal tunnel syndrome [17].
- Positive Tinel's and Phalen's sign decreases from carpal tunnel syndrome to double crush syndrome to cervical radiculopathy [17].
- Symptoms of cervical radiculopathy cause more intolerable symptoms leading to more clinical visits [17].

The Double Crush Hypothesis

According to the "double-crush syndrome" hypothesis, the peripheral nerves are more sensitive to pressure, and a proximal nerve lesion makes the distal segment of the nerve more susceptible to anatomic deterioration by causing interruption in the axoplasmic conduction due to compression. Okmen et al. [24] performed a prospective cross-sectional observational study on 40 patients with chronic cervical radiculopathy. They compared both affected cervical nerve roots of the affected side to the unaffected side with high-resolution ultrasound. Ulnar and median nerve cross sectional areas were measured. They found that cervical radiculopathy does not have any effect on the peripheral nerves. This refutes the hypothesis of the double-crush syndrome. Morgan et al. [25] have also questioned the credibility of this hypothesis of the double crush syndrome and based on their finding of 69 out of 12,376 cases of carpal tunnel syndrome and ulnar neuropathy at the elbow satisfying the pathophysiologic and one of the anatomic requirements of the double crush syndrome, conclude that a cervical root lesion can seldom serve as the proximal lesion with these entrapment neuropathies in the double crush syndrome.

There is thus, no clear-cut electro-diagnostic evidence to differentiate a pure carpal tunnel syndrome from a double crush syndrome. The median motor distal latency and the sensory nerve conduction velocity (palm to wrist) is not significantly different between these pathologies [17]. Therefore, in cases with no clear-cut electrodiagnostic evidence, we recommend to proceed first with carpal tunnel release. If the symptoms persist postoperatively then surgical treatment for cervical radiculopathy is recommended.

Conclusion

Based on the above algorithm, the diagnosis of cervical radiculopathy and carpal tunnel syndrome can be simplified. Anatomical and Physiological studies have refuted the hypothesis of the double crush syndrome and blaming a cervical root compression for an increased likelihood of a peripheral neuropathy may not be accurate.

References

1. Radhakrishnan K, Litchy WJ, O'Fallon WM, Kurland LT. Epidemiology of cervical radiculopathy. A population-based study from Rochester, Minnesota, 1976 through 1990. Brain. 1994;117(Pt 2):325–35.
2. Roth D, Mukai A, Thomas P, Hudgins TH, Alleva JT. Cervical radiculopathy. Dis Mon. 2009;55(12):737–56.
3. Mondelli M, Giannini F, Giacchi M. Carpal tunnel syndrome incidence in a general population. Neurology. 2002;58(2):289–94.
4. Shelerud RA, Paynter KS. Rarer causes of radiculopathy: spinal tumors, infections, and other unusual causes. Phys Med Rehabil Clin N Am. 2002;13(3):645–96.
5. Kang JD, Georgescu HI, McIntyre-Larkin L, Stefanovic-Racic M, Evans CH. Herniated cervical intervertebral discs spontaneously produce matrix metalloproteinases, nitric oxide, interleukin-6, and prostaglandin E2. Spine. 1995;20(22):2373–8.
6. Akelman E, Weiss AP. Carpal tunnel syndrome. Etiology and endoscopic treatment. Orthop Clin North Am. 1995;26(4):769–78.
7. Lee MW, McPhee RW, Stringer MD. An evidence-based approach to human dermatomes. Clin Anat. 2008;21(5):363–73.

8. Woods BI, Hilibrand AS. Cervical radiculopathy: epidemiology, etiology, diagnosis, and treatment. J Spinal Disord Tech. 2015;28(5):E251–9.
9. Fast A, Parikh S, Marin EL. The shoulder abduction relief sign in cervical radiculopathy. Arch Phys Med Rehabil. 1989;70(5):402–3.
10. Wainner RS, Fritz JM, Irrgang JJ, Boninger ML, Delitto A, Allison S. Reliability and diagnostic accuracy of the clinical examination and patient self-report measures for cervical radiculopathy. Spine. 2003;28(1):52–62.
11. Matsumoto M, Fujimura Y, Suzuki N, Toyama Y, Shiga H. Cervical curvature in acute whiplash injuries: prospective comparative study with asymptomatic subjects. Injury. 1998;29(10):775–8.
12. Lo SF, Chou LW, Meng NH, Chen FF, Juan TT, Ho WC, et al. Clinical characteristics and electrodiagnostic features in patients with carpal tunnel syndrome, double crush syndrome, and cervical radiculopathy. Rheumatol Int. 2012;32(5):1257–63.
13. Ashworth NL. Carpal tunnel syndrome. London: BMJ Publishing Group; 2016, 2 p.
14. Partanen J, Partanen K, Oikarinen H, Niemitukia L, Hernesniemi J. Preoperative electroneuromyography and myelography in cervical root compression. Electromyogr Clin Neurophysiol. 1991;31(1):21–6.
15. Fritz JM, Thackeray A, Brennan GP, Childs JD. Exercise only, exercise with mechanical traction, or exercise with over-door traction for patients with cervical radiculopathy, with or without consideration of status on a previously described subgrouping rule: a randomized clinical trial. J Orthop Sports Phys Ther. 2014;44(2):45–57.
16. Rathmell JP, Aprill C, Bogduk N. Cervical transforaminal injection of steroids. Anesthesiology. 2004;100(6):1595–600.
17. Bush K, Hillier S. Outcome of cervical radiculopathy treated with periradicular/epidural corticosteroid injections: a prospective study with independent clinical review. Eur Spine J. 1996;5(5):319–25.
18. Flak M, Durmala J, Czernicki K, Dobosiewicz K. Double crush syndrome evaluation in the median nerve in clinical, radiological and electrophysiological examination. Stud Health Technol Inform. 2006;123:435–41.
19. Richardson JK, Forman GM, Riley B. An electrophysiological exploration of the double crush hypothesis. Muscle Nerve. 1999;22(1):71–7.
20. Salemi G, Savettieri G, Meneghini F, Di Benedetto ME, Ragonese P, Morgante L, et al. Prevalence of cervical spondylotic radiculopathy: a door-to-door survey in a Sicilian municipality. Acta Neurol Scand. 1996;93(2–3):184–8.
21. Bongers FJ, Schellevis FG, van den Bosch WJ, van der Zee J. Carpal tunnel syndrome in general practice (1987 and 2001): incidence and the role of occupational and non-occupational factors. Br J Gen Pract. 2007;57(534):36–9.
22. de Krom MC, Knipschild PG, Kester AD, Thijs CT, Boekkooi PF, Spaans F. Carpal tunnel syndrome: prevalence in the general population. J Clin Epidemiol. 1992;45(4):373–6.
23. Atroshi I, Gummesson C, Johnsson R, Ornstein E, Ranstam J, Rosen I. Prevalence of carpal tunnel syndrome in a general population. JAMA. 1999;282(2):153–8.
24. Metin Okmen B, Okmen K, Altan L. Investigation of the effect of cervical radiculopathy on peripheral nerves of the upper extremity with high-resolution ultrasonography. Spine. 2018;43(14):E798–803.
25. Morgan G, Wilbourn AJ. Cervical radiculopathy and coexisting distal entrapment neuropathies: double-crush syndromes? Neurology. 1998;50(1):78–83.

Suprascapular Neuropathy

27

Christopher M. Treat and Christopher C. Schmidt

Introduction

Shoulder pain and weakness is one of the most common complaints seen in an orthopedic practice and may result from a myriad of etiologies. One etiology that is relatively uncommon and often overlooked is suprascapular neuropathy. This condition was first described by Kopell and Thompson in 1959 and has largely been considered a diagnosis of exclusion [1, 2]. However, due to technological improvements, suprascapular neuropathy has become much more recognized as a source of shoulder disability and pain. Multiple etiologies of suprascapular nerve pathology include shoulder fractures and dislocations, massive rotator cuff tears, dynamic compression as seen in overhead athletes, idiopathic, and ganglion cysts [3–8]. The nerve is vulnerable to injury at any point along its course but injury seems to occur at either the scapular spine, suprascapular notch, and/or spinoglenoid notch [6–8]. For instance, supraspinatus and infraspinatus muscle retraction following a massive rotator cuff tear tethers the nerve against the scapular spine causing a stretch injury; rotator cuff repair is reported to indirectly relieve the symptoms, in part, by resolving the neuropathy [8, 9]. Furthermore, due to the its indirect course through the notches and around the spine, extreme shoulder motion can alter the nerve's tension causing a dynamic stretch injury [6–12]. Idiopathic compression typically occurs at the suprascapular and/or spinoglenoid notches. The presenting symptoms and clinical findings depend on the location of the nerve pathology. Injury of the nerve at the suprascapular notch affects the supraspinatus and infraspinatus muscles leading to weakness in shoulder abduction and external rotation, while a lesion at the spinoglenoid notch only affects the infraspinatus muscle resulting in a sole loss of external rotation strength. Treatment options conservative and operative interventions. This chapter will focus diagnosis and treatment of suprascapular nerve compression or stretch injury occurring at the suprascapular and/or spinoglenoid notches.

Anatomy

The suprascapular nerve is a mixed motor and sensory nerve arising from the upper trunk of the brachial plexus (Fig. 27.1). It receives contributions predominately from C5 and C6 fibers with approximately 22% of individuals also receiving

C. M. Treat
Hillcrest Medical Center, Tulsa, OK, USA

C. C. Schmidt (✉)
Department of Orthopaedic Surgery, University of Pittsburgh Medical Center, Pittsburgh, PA, USA
e-mail: schmidtc96@comcast.net

D. G. Sotereanos, L. K. Papatheodorou (eds.), *Compressive Neuropathies of the Upper Extremity*,
https://doi.org/10.1007/978-3-030-37289-7_27

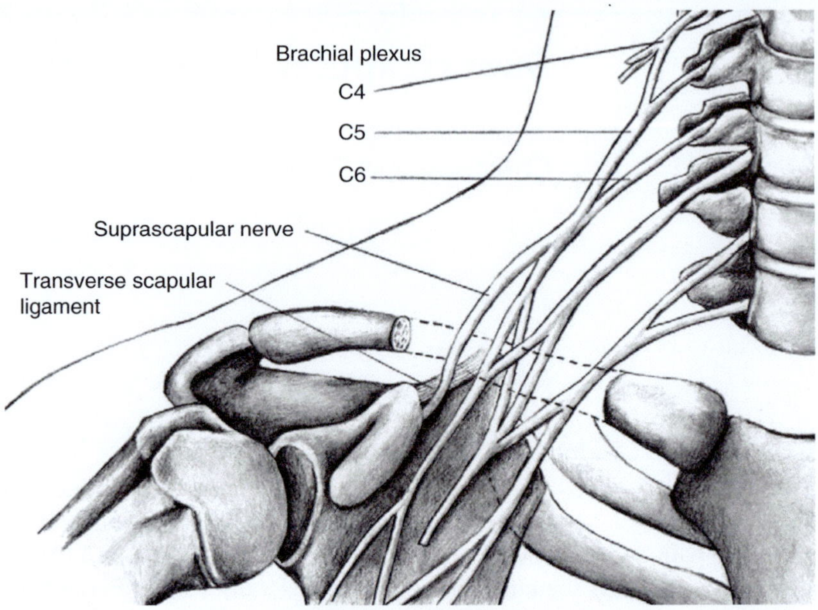

Fig. 27.1 The origin of the suprascapular nerve from the upper trunk of the brachial plexus. (Reprinted with permissions from Boykin et al. [35])

contributions from C4 [13, 14]. It has largely been considered a motor nerve innervating the supraspinatus and infraspinatus muscles; but, it also has sensory fibers. Studies have shown that the suprascapular nerve provides sensation to the posterior shoulder capsule, acromioclavicular joint, subacromial bursa, coracohumeral, and coracoclavicular ligaments [11, 15]. Further, cadaveric studies have found that as many as 15% of the population has a cutaneous branch of the suprascapular nerve supplying the proximal lateral arm [3, 13].

The circuitous course of the suprascapular nerve around the scapular spine and fixation points at the suprascapular and spinoglenoid notches makes it vulnerable to injury (Figs. 27.2, and 27.3) [6–8]. The suprascapular nerve originates at the Erb's point, located on the surface of the scaleneus medius approximately 2–3 cm above the clavicle [3, 6, 11, 14, 15]. The nerve then passes deep to the inferior belly of the omohyoid, which is a key landmark for identification [15–17]. The suprascapular nerve runs posteriorly through the suprascapular notch, beneath the transverse scapular ligament where it bifurcates into two motor branches approximately 1 cm from the supracapular notch (Fig. 27.4) [2, 6, 17]. A medial branch innervates the supraspinatus muscle and a lateral branch descends around the lateral margin of the scapular spine and passes beneath the spinoglenoid ligament at

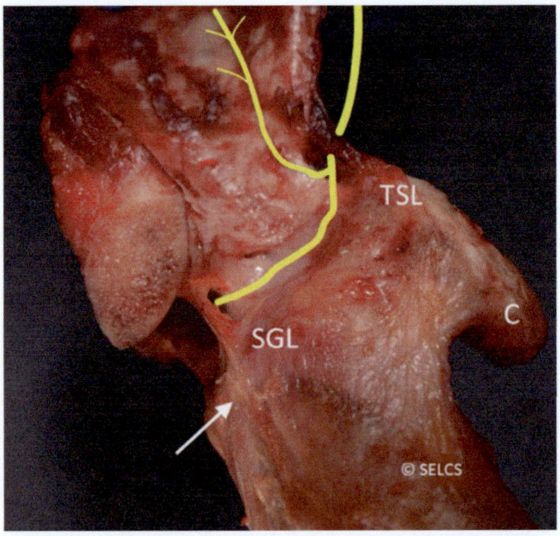

Fig. 27.2 A cadaveric specimen following removal of the acromion demonstrating the spinoglenoid ligament (SGL); the transverse scapular ligament (TSL), the coracoid process (C) as well as the course of the supraspinatus nerve traversing beneath the transverse scapular ligament and spinoglenoid ligament (yellow). Note the insertion of the spinoglenoid ligament to the posterior capsule (Arrow)

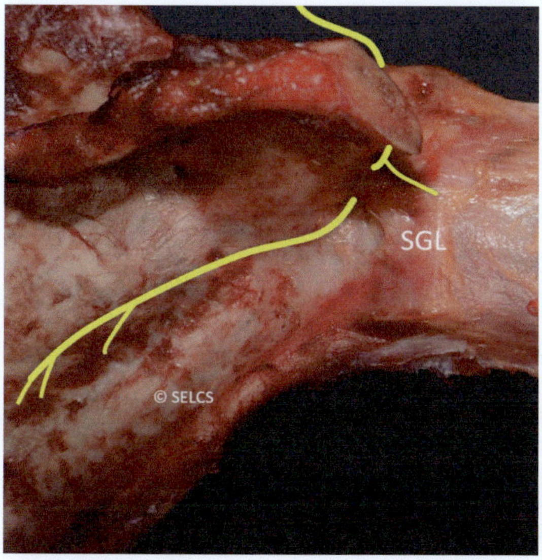

Fig. 27.3 A cadaveric specimen demonstrating the suprascapular nerve (yellow) coursing beneath the spinoglenoid ligament (SGL) at the spinoglenoid notch

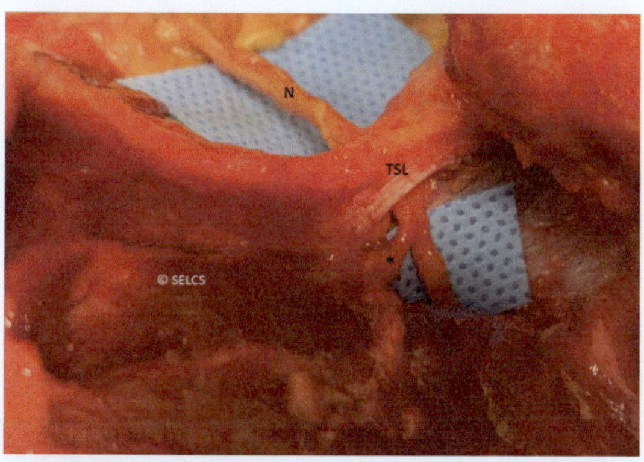

Fig. 27.4 A cadaveric specimen demonstrating the suprascapular nerve (N) coursing beneath the transverse scapular ligament (TSL). Note the motor branch of the suprascapular nerve to the supraspinatus muscle (Asterisk ∗)

the spinoglenoid notch to supply motor innervation to the infraspinatous muscle (Figs. 27.2 and 27.3) [2, 6, 17–19].

The suprascapular notch is a bony depression about the medial aspect of the scapula that is located approximately 4.5 (±0.5 cm) from the posterolateral acromion (Fig. 27.5) [20]. It is

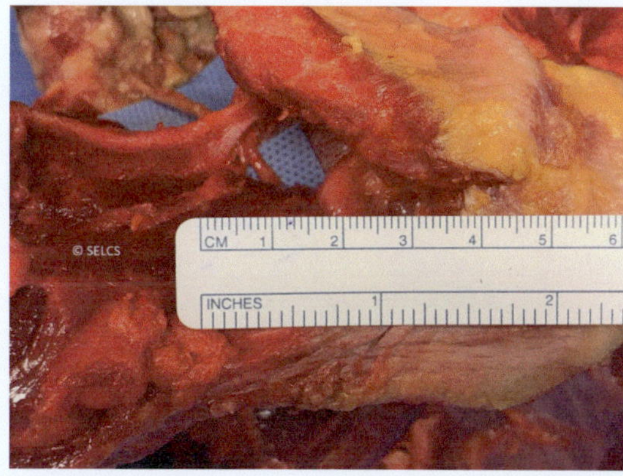

Fig. 27.5 A cadaveric specimen showing the location and orientation of the suprascapular notch which is located approximately 4.5 (±0.5 cm) from the posterolateral acromion [2, 16]. The suprascapular notch is oriented 45° counter-clockwise from the coronal plane (the ruler is parallel to the coronal plane)

oriented 45° counterclockwise from the coronal plane (Fig. 27.5; the ruler is parallel to the coronal plane). It is bordered medially by the scapula, laterally by the by the base of the coracoid, and superiorly by the transverse scapular ligament. Several anatomic variations of the suprascapular notch have been described and cadaveric studies have demonstrated six types of scapulae (Fig. 27.6) [21, 22]. In type I the entire superior border of the scapula shows a depression (8% of specimens). Type II is wide, blunted, and V-shaped notch (31%). In type III the notch is U-shaped. This is the most common type of notch (48%). In type IV, the notch is V-shaped (3%). The type V notch is like the type III but has partial ossification of the transverse scapular ligament. In type VI the transverse scapular ligament is completely ossified [21, 22]. Partial or complete ossification of the transverse scapular ligament occurs in 25% of the cases [23].

The spinoglenoid notch is a depression at the lateral base of the scapular spine located 1.8–2.1 cm medial to the glenoid rim and bordered superiorly by the spinoglenoid ligament (Figs. 27.2 and 27.3) [16, 24]. The spinoglenoid

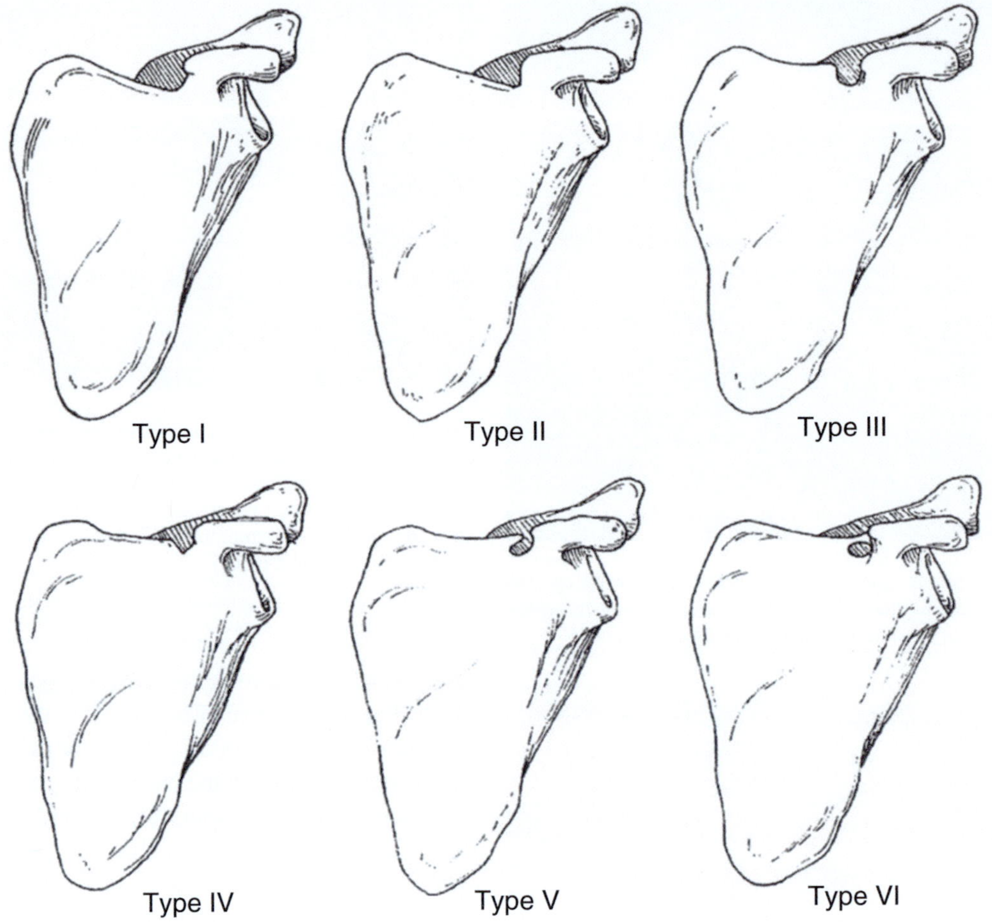

Fig. 27.6 Classification of abnormalities of the suprascapular notch described by Rengachary [21]. (Adapted with permission from Rengachary et al. [21])

ligament originates on the spine of the scapula and inserts on the superior margin of the glenoid neck and superoposterior joint capsule (Figs. 27.2 and 27.3) [3, 5, 25]. This ligament represents a possible dynamic etiology for suprascapular neuropathy because of its insertion into the posterior glenohumeral joint capsule [3, 5, 25]. Cross arm adduction and internal rotation can tighten the spinoglenoid ligament through its capsular attachments causing a dynamic neuropraxia [3, 5, 7, 25, 26].

The suprascapular artery is a branch of the thyrocervical trunk and typically runs superficial to the transverse scapular ligament, whereas the suprascapular nerve runs beneath the transverse scapular ligament. However, a subligamentous suprascapular artery has been reported in literature in 3% of the surgical patients (Fig. 27.7) [63].

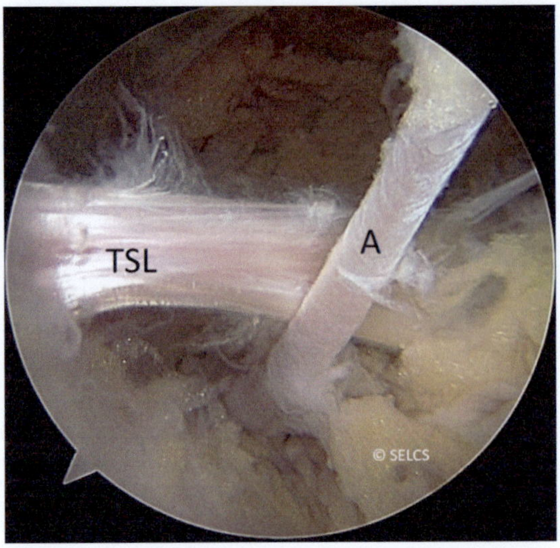

Fig. 27.7 An arthroscopic view showing the transverse scapular ligament (TSL) and a subligamentous suprascapular artery (A)

Clinical Presentation and Exam

The clinical presentation depends largely on the location of the nerve injury and presence or absence of a ganglion cyst.

Suprascapular Notch Compression

Patients with suprascapular neuropathy due to compression of the transverse scapular ligament typically present with symptoms of pain and weakness [23]. Pain is often moderate to severe, located around the posterolateral shoulder and exacerbated with overhead motions [5, 27]. The pain fibers are located proximal in the nerve so transverse scapular ligament compression, as opposed to spinoglenoid compression, is typically more painful [2, 28]. There may be significant weakness of abduction and external rotation due to denervation of the supraspinatus and infraspinatus muscles. It is thought that compression at this level is the result of anatomic variations of either the notch or the transverse scapular ligament [15, 29]. Clinical findings are loss of shoulder motion and strength in positions of abduction and external rotation. In severe cases, atrophy of both the supraspinatus and infraspinatus fossae is often seen (Fig. 27.8). The suprascapular nerve stretch test is useful in diagnosing compression at the suprascapular notch (Fig. 27.9) [30]. The test is performed with the clinician standing behind the patient. One hand is used to laterally rotate the head away from the affected shoulder while the other hand is used to gently retract the shoulder. A positive test cause pain in the posterior shoulder [30].

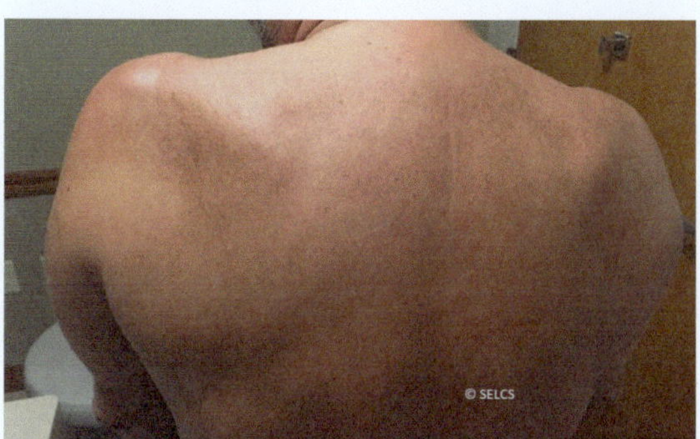

Fig. 27.8 Clinical photograph demonstrating atrophy of the supraspinatus and infraspinatus of a left shoulder with suprascapular nerve compression at the transverse scapular ligament

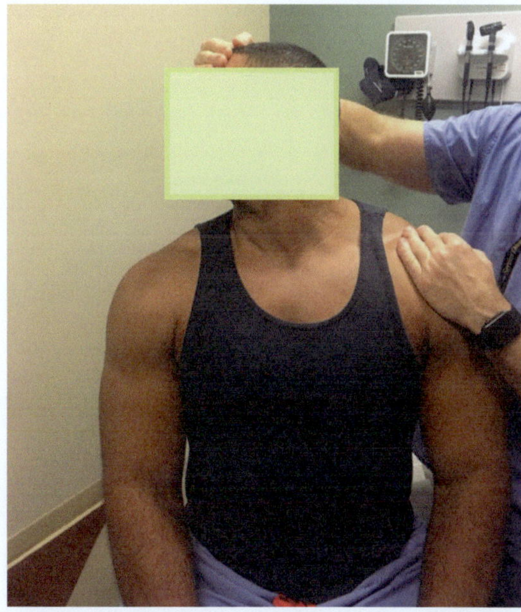

Fig. 27.9 A provocative test for suprascapular neuropathy. A clinical photograph demonstrating the suprascapular nerve stretch test described by Lafosse et al. for compression at the transverse scapular ligament. The clinician is behind the patient. One hand is used to laterally rotate the head away from the affected shoulder while the other hand is used to gently retract the shoulder. A positive test will result in posterior shoulder pain [13]

Spinoglenoid Notch Compression

Patients with entrapment of the suprascapular nerve at the spinoglenoid notch typically do not complain of severe pain because the nerve at this level is composed of pure motor neurons [2, 17, 28, 29]. Young athletes and manual laborers participating in overhead sports and repetitive overhead work present with a dull shoulder ache and subtle external rotational weakness in 0° of abduction [13, 17, 23, 29, 31]. Shoulder external rotation in 90° of abduction and abduction strength are preserved due to the compensatory actions of the supraspinatus, teres minor and serratus anterior muscles [2, 6, 7, 18, 32, 33]. The cross-arm adduction test is useful

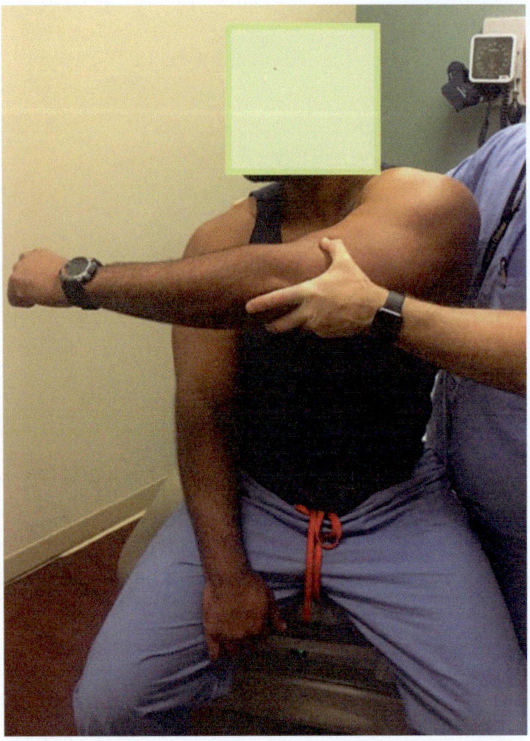

Fig. 27.10 A provocative test for suprascapular neuropathy. A clinical photograph demonstrating the cross-arm adduction test for spinoglenoid ligament compression a positive will result in posterior shoulder pain

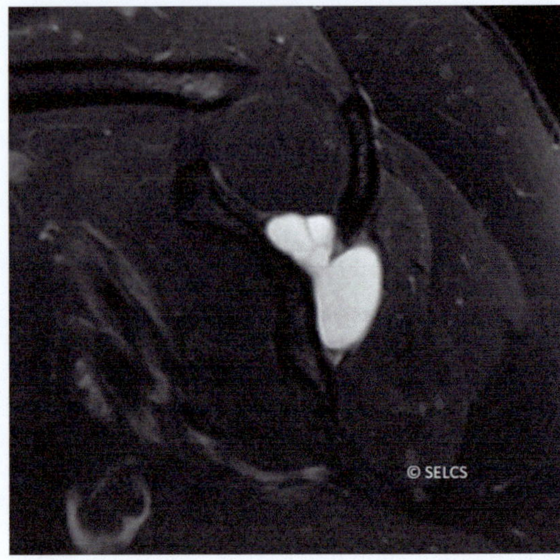

Fig. 27.11 MRI reveals a large ganglion cyst with proven EMG nerve compression at both the suprascapular and spinoglenoid notches

in diagnosing spinoglenoid pathology [12, 23, 28, 34]. The test is performed by forward flexing the arm to 90° and adducting the arm; pain provocation is a positive test (Fig. 27.10). Cadaveric studies have shown that shoulder adduction and internal rotation tightens the inferior portion of the spinoglenoid ligament due to its fibrous interaction with the posterior capsule (Figs. 27.2 and 27.3) [12, 23, 28, 34]. Caution should be taken when solely attributing a positive test to nerve compression because the test is also positive with acromioclavicular joint arthritis.

Spinoglenoid Notch and/or Suprascapular Notch Due to Ganglion Cyst

Ganglion cysts typically occur behind the superoposterior labrum and are believed to be due to labral tears forming one-way valves (Fig. 27.11) [10, 29]. These patients can present with pain, weakness, and atrophy of the supraspinatus and/or infraspinatus muscles [4, 15, 29]. The pain can be a result of the mass effect of the cyst or the labral lesion. The motor loss depends largely on the size and location of the ganglion cyst. Typically, the ganglion cyst causes nerve compression near the spinoglenoid notch resulting in infraspinatus weakness, but a large cyst can affect both the suprascapular and spinoglenoid regions producing denervation in both the supra- and infraspinatus muscles [3, 10, 28].

Diagnostic Tests

Radiological Imaging

The Stryker notch view allows for visualization of the suprascapular notch. This view is obtained by placing the hand on top of the head and x-ray beam angled 10° cephalad (Fig. 27.12a, b) [35, 36]. We had found this helpful in determining if the transverse scapular ligament is ossified. If the notch cannot be adequate visualized on plain radiographs, a scapular CT scan (<1 mm cuts) is ordered preoperatively to determine the need to remove bone during decompression.

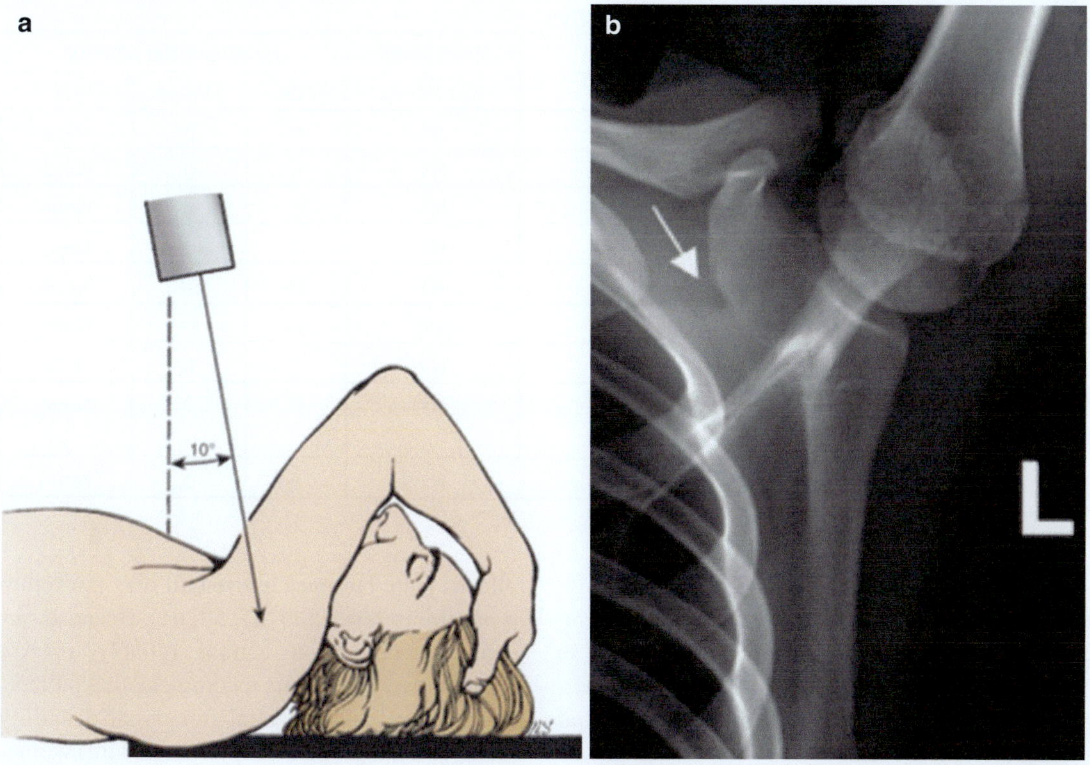

Fig. 27.12 (**a**, **b**) Stryker notch view; position for the Stryker notch view. The patient is supine with the cassette posterior to the shoulder. The humerus is flexed approximately 120°, placing the hand on top of the head. The angle of the x-ray tube is 10° superior. (**b**) A Stryker notch radiograph of the left shoulder, made with the beam aimed 15° cephalad to provide visualization of the suprascapular notch (arrow) [36]

MRI is the advanced imaging modality of choice for diagnosing suprascapular neuropathy. This modality allows assessment for soft tissue lesions and concomitant intra-articular pathology such as labral and rotator tears [10]. MRI is highly sensitive and specific in demonstrating the presence of and size of the ganglion with a sensitivity and specificity of up to 95% reported in the literature (Fig. 27.11) [10, 12, 23]. Typical MRI findings of ganglion cysts include homogeneity, low signal on T1-weighted images, and high signal on T2-weighted images. The T2-weighted oblique sagittal view allows for visualization of the suprascapular nerve as it courses through the supraspinatus fossa, around the spinoglenoid notch and into the infraspinatus fossa [2, 10]. In addition, supra- and/or infraspinatus muscle edema is a reliable sign of suprascapular nerve compression [37, 38].

Nerve Conduction Velocity (NCV) and Electromyography (EMG)

NCV and EMG studies are useful in diagnosing, locating, determining the severity of the neuropathy. They also help to rule out upper trunk plexopathy and cervical radiculopathy Their sensitivity and specificity varies from 74% to 91%; however, similar to carpal tunnel syndrome, suprascapular nerve compression may occur even in the setting of a negative NCV/EMG [4, 9, 28, 34]. EMG findings of significant denervation are denervation increased insertional activity, fibrillations, spontaneous, positive sharp waves [10, 39]. The usual latency or nerve conduction velocity ranges from 1.7 to 3.7 ms for the supraspinatus. A value greater than 2.7 ms indicates an abnormality [23]. A latency value greater than 3.3 ms (range 2.4–4.2 ms) indicates compression of the infraspinatus [23]. The stimulation point is

Needle EMG examination:

Muscle	Insertional	Spontaneous activity		
	Insertional	Fibs	+Wave	Other 1
Biceps brachii.L	N1	0	0	None
Deltoid.L	N1	0	0	None
Triceps brachii.L	N1	0	0	None
Rhomboid major.L	N1	0	0	None
Supraspinatus.L	N1	3+	3+	None
Infraspinatus.L	Inc	4+	4+	None
Trapezius.L	N1	0	0	None
Sternocleidomastoid.L	N1	0	0	None
C5 paraspinal.L	N1	0	0	None

Fig. 27.13 EMG findings of denervation are observed in both the supraspinatus and infraspinatus muscles

performed at Erb's point [23]. In patients with compression at the transverse scapular ligament, EMG findings of denervation are observed in both the supraspinatus and infraspinatus muscles, while in patients with dynamic spinoglenoid compression, the EMG findings would reveal denervation of the infraspinatus and normal findings in the supraspinatus (Fig. 27.13) [6, 23].

Diagnostic Injections

A diagnostic injection of 1% lidocaine over the suprascapular notch can be a useful test to diagnosis neuropathy [9, 23, 24]. Plancher et al. [23] describes a technique for the suprascapular nerve injection at the suprascapular notch using a 25-guage, 1.5 in needle. The needle is placed into the suprascapular notch from a posterosuperior injection approximately 3 cm medial to the Neviaser portal aiming anteriorly [23]. Pain relief after injection is an indication of pathology [9, 23, 24].

Treatment

There is no high-level evidence-based studies to guide treatment recommendations for suprascapular neuropathy. The process of treatment recommendations requires shared decision making between the doctor and patient. Patients need to understand that surgical decompression usually relieves pain, but muscle strength may not return to pre-injury levels [45–47, 52, 61]. Because surgical decompression cannot reliably reverse strength loss, the authors recommend that patients presenting with substantial functional disability due to either significant supra- and/or infraspinatus muscle weakness and/or atrophy, EMG evidence of denervation, or failure of 3–6 months of symptom duration are best treated with surgical decompression [4, 6, 8, 10].

Nonoperative treatment can be effective management for cases of suprascapular neuropathy without physical signs atrophy and EMG evidence of significant denervation. Nonoperative treatment includes NSAIDs, activity modificaitons, physical therapy for shoulder motion and strengthening exercises and corticosteroid injecitons. It is recommended to instruct patients to avoid overhead activites. Good to excellent results have been demonstrated with non-operative treatment; albeit it may take 6–12 months for maximal improvement [4, 10]. If patients fail to improve after 6 months of non-operative treatment, operative treatment is recommended [4, 10].

The method of surgical treatment depends on the etiology and location of the compression. A number of methods have been described and for the sake of brevity this chapter will describe our preferred techniques. This includes open decompression at the transverse scapular notch and/or spinoglenoid notch, arthroscopic transverse scapular notch decompression, arthroscopic labral repair with or with decompression of the ganglion cyst, and arthroscopic spinoglenoid ligament release.

Open Decompression of the Suprascapular Notch and Spinoglenoid Notch

The posterior approach provides the needed exposure to decompress the suprascapular nerve from just proximal to the transverse scapular ligament to the infraspinatus muscle. A 10–12 cm skin incision is made parallel and 1–2 cm superior to the scapular spine. The trapezius is sharply elevated off the scapular spine and lifted superiorly to expose the supraspinatus muscle (Fig. 27.14). The supraspinatus muscle is then identified and retracted posteriorly with a wide hand held retractor. Blunt dissection is then performed and the suprascapular ligament and notch is palpated. A Kittner (blunt) dissector is used to clean the surrounding soft tissues to expose the transverse scapular ligament. Care should be taken to avoid injury to the suprascapular artery and vein immediately superficial to the ligament. The transverse scapular ligament is then sharply released while protecting the suprascapular nerve, which lies below (Fig. 27.15). The trapezius is then reattached to the scapular spine with transosseous sutures (0 strong absorbable stitch) [45–50].

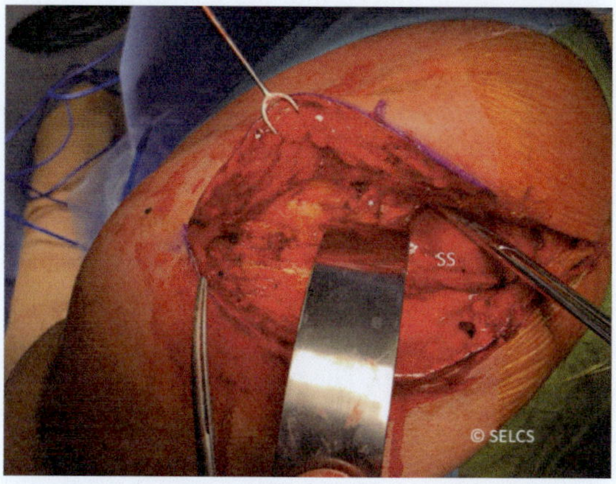

Fig. 27.14 A cadaveric specimen showing the open approach; The trapezius has been elevated and a deep retractor is used to retract the supraspinatus muscle (SS) inferiorly to expose the suprascapular notch and transverse scapular ligament (Asterisk ∗)

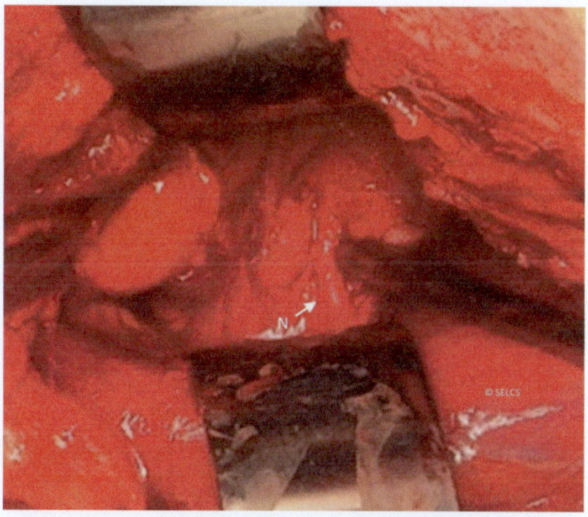

Fig. 27.15 A cadaveric specimen with magnification of the suprascapular notch after release of the transverse scapular ligament demonstrating the suprascapular nerve (N)

The spinoglenoid notch is decompressed by detaching the posterior deltoid inferiorly from the scapular spine to visualize the infraspinatus muscle [47]. The infraspinatus muscle is retracted posteriorly to expose the spinoglenoid ligament, suprascapular nerve running around the scapular spine, and posterosuperior gangion cysts (Figs. 27.16 and 27.17). The posterior deltoid is then reattached to the scapular spine through transosseous sutures (0 strong absorbable stitch).

Arthroscopic Technique for Decompression of the Suprascapular Notch

Arthroscopic techniques for suprascapular nerve decompression have also been associated with favorable results in the literature. The reported advantages of the arthroscopic approach include faster rehabilitation, decreased postoperative morbidity, and improved visualization of neurovascular structures and associated intra-articular pathology [6]. However, this

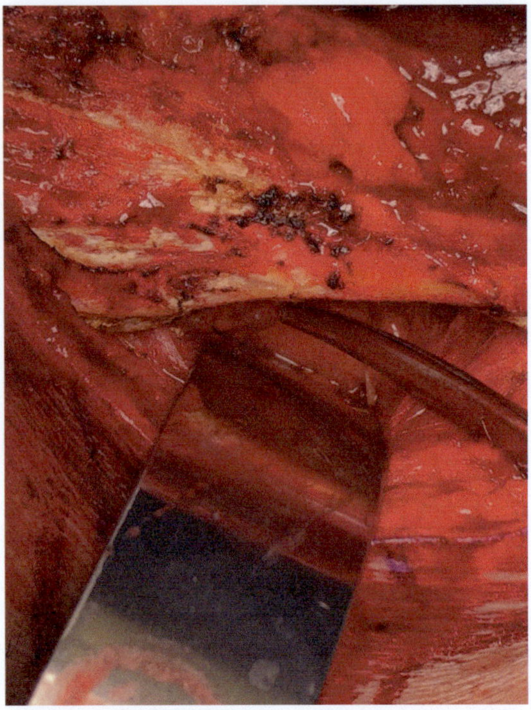

Fig. 27.16 A cadaveric specimen. The posterior deltoid has been detached from the scapular spine and a deep retractor is used to retract the infraspinatus inferiorly to expose the spinoglenoid notch. Note the ganglion cyst at the tip of the Kelly

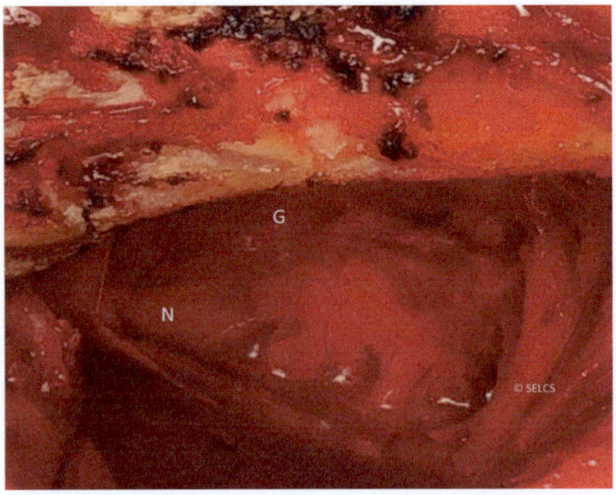

Fig. 27.17 A cadaveric specimen demonstrating a close-up view of a ganglion cyst (G) in the spinoglenoid notch. Note the close proximity of the suprascapular nerve (N) to the ganglion cyst

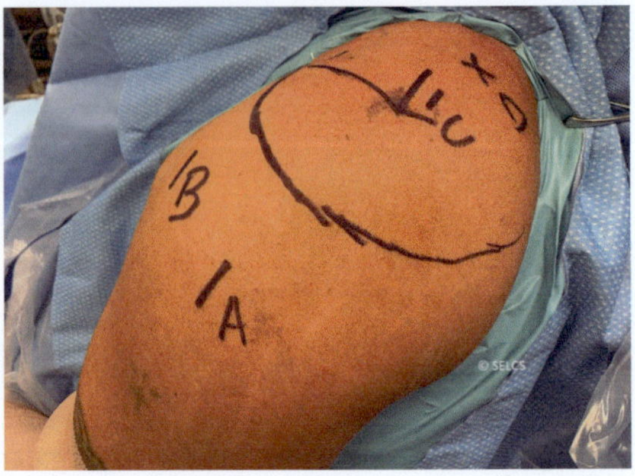

Fig. 27.18 Arthroscopic suprascapular nerve decompression. Arthroscopic portals for suprascapular nerve decompression. (A) posterolateral portal; (B) anterolateral portal; (C) Nevasier portal; (D) suprascapular nerve portal as described by Lafosse et al. this portal is approximately 7 cm from the lateral border of the acromion

approach requires a thorough understanding of anatomy and can be technically challenging. A variety of arthroscopic techniques have been described in the literature [40, 50, 51]. The senior authors preferred arthroscopic approach utilizes four portals (Fig. 27.18); a lateral portal (A), an anterolateral portal (B), a Neviaser portal (C) and a suprascapular nerve portal as described by Lafosse et al. (D) [30, 40]. The arthroscope is placed into the lateral portal (A); the portal is in line with the posterior clavicle. An arthroscopic shaver is placed into the anterolateral portal (B) and the bursa is removed to expose the coracoacromial ligament. The coracoacromial ligament (CAL) is followed anterior to the supraspinatus muscle to the base of the coracoid. A Wissinger rod is placed through Neviasser portal (C) to aid in dissection with the goal to identify the coracoclavicular (CC) ligaments (Fig. 27.19). The transverse scapular ligament is identified as the medial continuity of the conoid ligament above the suprascapular notch (Figs. 27.19 and 27.20). Care must be taken to identify the suprascapular artery. In the case where the artery is accidently injured then it can be coagulated as long as the artery is above the ligament. Next, the Lafosse suprascapular nerve

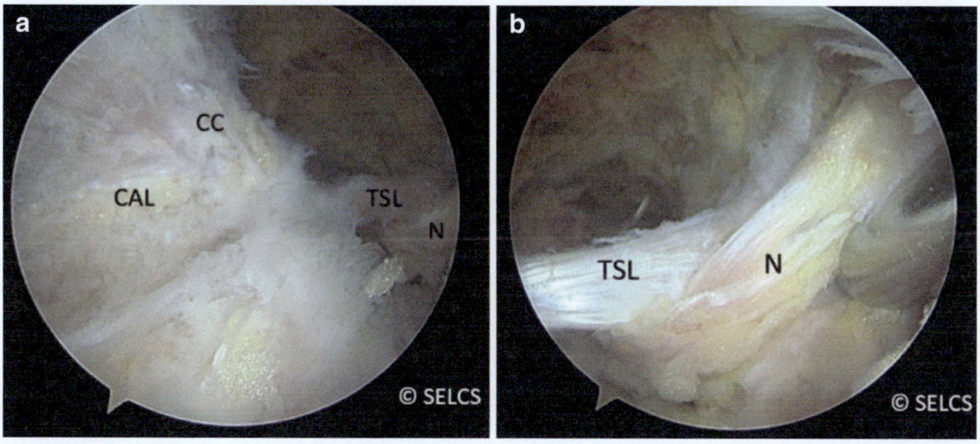

Fig. 27.19 (**a**) An arthroscopic view showing the coracoacromial ligament; (CAL) Coracoclavicular ligaments; (CC) transverse scapular ligament; (TSL) and suprascapular nerve (N). (**b**) An arthroscopic view showing the suprascapular nerve (N) coursing beneath the transverse scapular ligament (TSL)

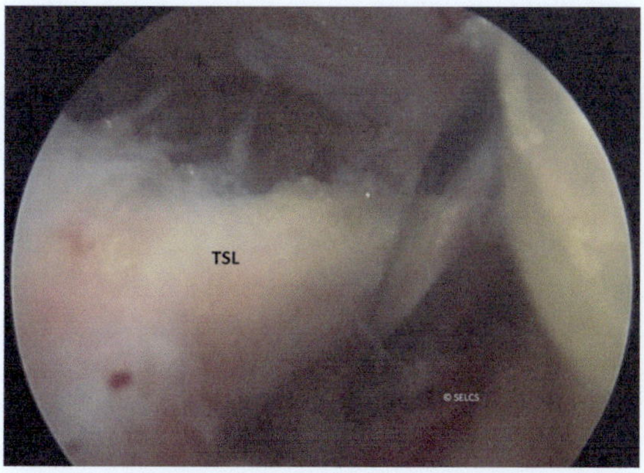

Fig. 27.20 An arthroscopic view showing a probe placed through the Lafosse portal protecting the suprascapular nerve in preparation for arthroscopic release. Note the transverse scapular ligament (TSL)

portal (D) is created and a probe is inserted to protect and move the nerve medially while arthroscopic scissors are inserted through the Neviaser portal (C) to release the transverse scapular ligament and decompress the nerve (Fig. 27.21). After transecting the transverse scapular ligament, the decompression is assessed with gentle manipulation of the suprascapular nerve (Fig. 27.22). If there is residual compression of the nerve, usually resulting from bony hypertrophy within the suprascapular notch, a notchplasty should be performed along the lateral border of the suprascapular notch with a bur [11, 30, 40].

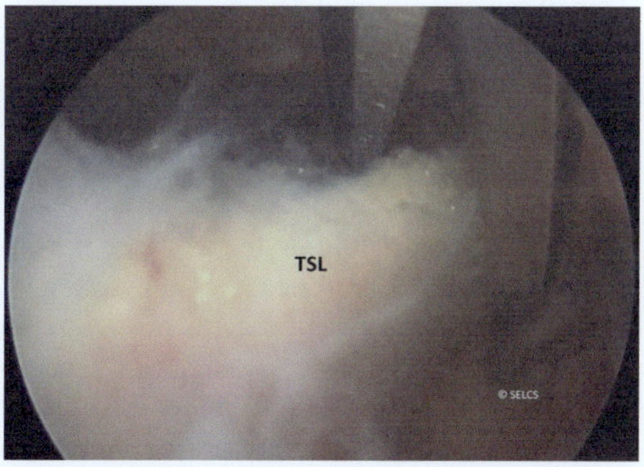

Fig. 27.21 An arthroscopic view showing the release of the transverse scapular ligament (TSL) with arthroscopic scissors

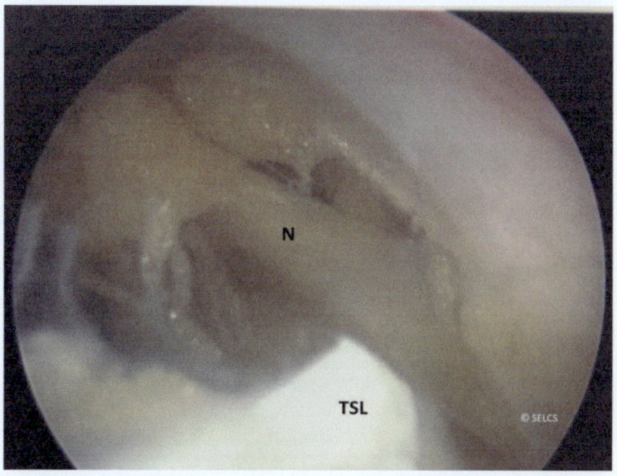

Fig. 27.22 An arthroscopic view showing adequate release of the transverse scapular ligament (TSL); note the suprascapular nerve (N)

Arthroscopic Labral Repair with and without Ganglion Decompression

Several techniques have been described arthroscopic decompression of ganglion cyst with and without labral repair. Labral repair appears to be optional. Decompression can be performed through the labral tear or a capsulotomy can be made at a precise location determined by the preoperative MRI [29, 58]. Care should be taken to avoid injuring the suprascapular nerve which lies on average 3.0 cm from the supraglenoid tubercle at the suprascapular notch and 2.5 cm from the supraglenoid tubercle at the base of the scapular spine; therefore, the safe zone in the posterior aspect of the glenoid lies within 2 cm of the glenoid rim [20].

Arthroscopic Spinoglenoid Ligament Release

Plancher et al. [23, 53] described a 2-portal technique for arthroscopic release of the spinoglenoid ligament. The patient may be positioned in either the lateral decubitus position or the beach chair position. If the beach chair position is utilized, then the hemithorax should be draped up to the spine to ensure adequate exposure. The posterolateral (working) portal is located approximately 4-cm medial to the most posterior lateral aspect of the acromion. This position allows direct access to the spinoglenoid ligament. The medial (viewing) portal is located along the scapular spine approximately 4-cm medial to the lateral portal. The authors note that the spinoglenoid notch was located approximately 1–2 cm inferior to the posterolateral portal. A probe was inserted through the posterolateral portal and the neurovascular structures and spinoglenoid ligament were identified. At this point, a cutting device is placed through the posterolateral portal and the spinoglenoid ligament was released under direct visualization. A probe is then utilized to assess for adequate decompression. If it is determined to be inadequate, then a third portal can be established between the medial and posterolateral portals and blunt switching stick allowed for extended retraction of the infraspinatus muscle [23, 53].

Results

Multiple studies have showed good results with open and arthroscopic decompression of the suprascapular nerve at the suprascapular notch (Tables 27.1 and 27.2). The studies on open repair are retrospective cohorts without a control group [12, 49, 54, 55]. The postoperative strength improvement is based on manual muscle testing and not a dynameter. Collectively, the studies show high rates (91–96%) of complete pain relief,

Table 27.1 Publications reporting outcomes after open suprascapular nerve decompression at the suprascapular notch

Author	Year	No. of shoulders	Location of decompression	Outcome
Kim [47]	2005	31	SSN	90% improved to grade 4 or 5 supraspinatus power, 10% improved to grade 3; 32% improved to grade 4 or above infraspinatus power, 45% to grade 2 or 3 and 23% improved to grade 1. Preoperative pain universally improved with decompression
Fabre [46]	1999	35	SSN	31 of 35 (88%) reported good to excellent results, 2 of 35 (5.7%) fair results, and 1 of 35 (2.8%) poor results. Constant score improved from 47% to 77%
Post [42]	1993	26	SSN	25 of 26 (96%) of patients had good to excellent results, complete pain relief and normal shoulder function. 1 of 26 (3.8%) of patients had a fair result.
Callahan [33]	1991	23	SSN	21 of 23 (91%) of patients had complete pain relief 2 of 23 (8.6%) of patients had minimal residual shoulder pain but felt markedly improved.

Table 27.2 Publications reporting outcomes after arthroscopic suprascapular nerve decompression at the suprascapular notch

Author	Year	No. of shoulders	Location of decompression	Outcome
Garcia [57]	2015	10	SSN	All patients reported pain relief. The UCLA score increased from 11.7 to 26.1 points, the SF-36 questionnaire score was 122.9 and the raw pain score was 88%.
Arriaza [56]	2013	4	SSN	All patients reported complete pain relief at 2 weeks postoperatively. Pre-injury level was achieved at a mean of 7 ± 1 months. At final follow up, UCLA scores improved 12 points, qDASH scores improved 20 points
Lafosse [40]	2007	10	SSN	All patients had improvements in their postoperative EMG findings, pain and function

improvements in relative Constant score from 47% to 77%, and partial to complete strength return [12, 49, 54, 55]. Complete strength return is not certain and it most likely related to severity of the neuropathy prior to surgery. The lack of return of complete strength is best shown by Kim who reported on 31 patients that were treated with open decompression of the suprascapular nerve and found that at a mean of 18 month follow up, 90% of patients improved to grade 4 or 5 supraspinatus power and 10% improved to grade 3 supraspinatus power [55]. The authors also found that 32% of patients improved to grade 4 or above infraspinatus power, 45% to grade 2 or 3, and the remainder improved to grade 1 [55].

Several arthroscopic studies have shown good to excellent results with arthroscopic decompression of the suprascapular nerve at the suprascapular notch (Table 27.2). Lafosse et al. [40] reported on ten patients who were treated with arthroscopic decompression and found that at a mean of 15 month follow up, all patients had improvements in their postoperative electromyographic findings, pain and function [40]. Arriaza et al. [56] reported on four elite swimmers who underwent arthroscopic suprascapular nerve decompression at the suprascapular notch. The authors found that at a mean follow up of 18.5 months all patients showed marked improvement. All four patients reported complete pain relief at 2 weeks postoperatively and achieved their pre-injury level at a mean of 7 months [56]. Garcia et al. [57] reported on nine patients (ten shoulders) who underwent arthroscopic suprascapular nerve decompression at the suprascapular notch and found that at a mean follow up of 16.6 months all patients had pain relief, the UCLA scores increased from 11.7 to 26.1 points, the SF-36 Questionnaire score was 122.9 and the raw pain score was 88% [57].

Multiple studies have showed good to excellent results with both open and arthroscopic suprascapular nerve decompression at the spinoglenoid notch (Table 27.3). Mall et al. [42] reported on 29 patients that underwent open suprascapular nerve decompression at the spinoglenoid notch and found that at a mean of 4.3 year follow up 19 patients regained full external rotation strength (66%), 9 patients (31%) improved to 4/5 strength, and 1 patient (3%) had external rotation strength of 3/5, and of the 29 shoulders, 23 (79%) showed improved external rotation within 1 week of surgery. In addition, all cases showed improved external rotation strength by at least 1 full strength grade. They also found that the mean ASES score improved to 75 (range, 60–100) [45]. Ferretti et al. [43] reported on three patients who underwent open decompression at the spinoglenoid notch and found that at a mean of 2 year follow up all three patients had returned to sport at their pre-injury level and one of three patients demonstrated a notable reduction in atrophy [43]. Fehrman et al. [44] reported on six patients who underwent open posterior ganglion excision from the spinoglenoid notch and found that all patients reported an improvement in their pain. Two of the six patients had persistent infraspinatus atrophy with an external rotation strength deficit of 30% and 40% respectively [44].

Table 27.3 Publications reporting outcomes after open suprascapular nerve decompression at the spinoglenoid notch

Author	Year	No. of shoulders	Location of decompression	Outcome
Mall [42]	2013	29	SGN	66% regained full ER strength, 31% improved to 4/5, 3% had ER strength of 3/5. Mean ASES score improved to 75
Fabre [54]	1999	35	SGN (2)	31 of 35 (88%) reported good to excellent results, 2 of 35 (5.7%) fair results, and 1 of 35 (2.8%) poor results. Constant score improved from 47% to 77%
Ferretti [43]	1998	3	SGN	All patients returned to sport at their pre-injury level. One of three patients had a notable reduction in atrophy
Fehrman [44]	1995	6	SGN	All patient reported improvement in pain. Two of six patients residual infraspinatus atrophy.

Table 27.4 Publications reporting outcomes after arthroscopic suprascapular nerve decompression at the spinoglenoid notch

Author	Year	No. of shoulders	Location of decompression	Outcome
Hashiguchi [59]	2016	6	SGN	All patients showed excellent improvement in pain and muscle strength at the final follow-up examination. The mean constant score was improved from 60.5 points preoperatively to 97.2 points postoperatively. The mean VAS score decreased from 4.5 on the day of the surgery to 2.5 within 1 week postoperatively. Postoperative MRI showed disappearance or reduction of the spinoglenoid cyst in four and two patients, respectively. There were no complications
Kim [41]	2012	28	SGN	The mean VAS and constant and Rowe scores improved significantly compared to preoperative score, however no statistically significant difference between SLAP repair alone and SLAP repair and cyst decompression.
Shah [4]	2011	24	SGN and/or SSN	Statistically significant improvement in VAS *(17/24, 71%)* ASES *(18/24, 85%)* and SSV *(17/24, 71%)* scores.
Abboud [58]	2006	18	SGN	Found improvements in postop ASES & Penn shoulder scores for all outcomes measured including pain, satisfaction, and function
Westerheide [60]	2006	14	SGN	14 of 14 patients had improvement in pain and improved external rotation strength. The average SST score improved from 4.3 to 11.5 postoperatively.

Several studies have published there results after arthroscopic suprascapular nerve decompression at the spinoglenoid notch (Table 27.4). Shah et al. [4] reported on 27 patients who underwent arthroscopic supracapular nerve decompression at the suprascapular and/or spinoglenoid notch. Twenty-four patients had a positive preoperative EMG and all patients had an intact rotator cuff by MRI or CT scan. The authors found that at a mean follow up of 22.5 months 75% and 71% of patients had statistically significant improvement in ASES and SSV scores, respectively. 71% of patient reported that they would have surgery again [4]. Abboud et al. [58] retrospectively evaluated 18 patients who underwent arthroscopic decompression of a spinoglenoid cyst. Nine patients had decompression alone, and nine had decompression with labral repair and found improvements in postoperative ASES and Pennsylvania shoulder scores for all outcomes measured including pain, satisfaction, and function. However, the authors found no difference in outcomes when comparing the group that had an isolated decompression with the group that had decompression and labral repair [58]. Hashiguchi et al. [59] reported on six patients who underwent arthroscopic treatment of a SLAP lesion with associated spinoglenoid cyst and found at that at a mean follow up of 63.7 months all patients had excellent improvements in pain and muscle strength. The mean constant score improved from 60.5 points preoperatively to 97.2 points postoperatively. The mean visual analog scale (VAS) score decreased from 4.5 on the day of surgery to 2.5 within 1 week postoperatively. Westerheide et al. [60] reported on 14 patients who underwent arthroscopic treatment for suprascapular nerve neuropathy secondary to a spinoglenoid ganglion cyst. At a mean follow up of 51 months the authors found that all patients had improved external rotation strength and improved pain. In addition, the average Simple Shoulder Test (SST) score improved from 4.3 to 11.5 postoperatively [60].

An area of controversy exists in the literature regarding the management of patients with labral tears causing ganglion cysts. The debate is whether to perform cyst decompression and SLAP repair or simply perform a SLAP repair alone. There are no high-level of evidence studies to determine the appropriate treatment guidelines. Several studies show no difference in outcomes between the two groups and report high patient satisfaction. Kim et al. [41] compared outcomes in SLAP repair alone with SLAP repair with cyst decompression and found no difference in mean VAS scores and Constant and Rowe scores [41]. Schroder et al. [61] reported on 42 patients who underwent only arthroscopic labral repair for spinoglenoid cyst with concomitant labral tear and found high patient satisfaction [61]. However, one poorly controlled retrospective study reported improved external rotation strength in patients who underwent cyst decompression compared to patients who had SLAP repair alone [62]. Abboud et al. [58] retrospectively compared outcomes in nine patients with decompression alone and nine patients with decompression along with labral repair and found no difference in outcomes [58]. Because there is only low-level evidence guiding treatment, we recommend arthroscopic labral repair, cyst decompression and/or spinoglenoid release for patients with either substantial preoperative weakness, atrophy, or EMG evidence of denervation.

Conclusion

Suprascapular neuropathy has become a much more recognized source of shoulder pain and disability. Diagnosis and treatment demands a thorough understanding of the suprascapular nerve and scapular anatomy. Surgical and nonsurgical options have been described with both demonstrating good results. However, there are no high-level studies to guide treatment recommendations. Because surgical decompression does not always restore preinjury motor strength, the authors recommend that patients presenting with substantial functional disability due to either supra- and/or infraspinatus muscle weakness and/or atrophy, EMG evidence of denervation, or failure of 3–6 months of symptom duration are best treated with surgical decompression [6, 9]. Open and arthroscopic suprascapular nerve decompressions are equal efficacious in alleviating pain and improving patient reported outcomes.

References

1. Thompson WA, Kopell HP. Peripheral entrapment neuropathies of the upper extremity. N Engl J Med. 1959;260:1261–5.
2. Bhatia DN, de Beer JF, van Rooyen KS, du Toit DF. Arthroscopic suprascapular nerve decompression at the suprascapular notch. Arthroscopy. 2006;22(9):1009–13.
3. Ebraheim NA, Whitehead JL, Alla SR, Moral MZ, Castillo S, McCollough AL, Yeasting RA, Liu J. The suprascapular nerve and its articular branch to the acromioclavicular joint: an anatomic study. J Shoulder Elbow Surg. 2011;20(2):e13–7. https://doi.org/10.1016/j.jse.2010.09.004. Epub 2010 Dec 30. PubMed PMID: 21194975.
4. Shah AA, Butler RB, Sung SY, Wells JH, Higgins LD, Warner JJ. Clinical outcomes of suprascapular nerve decompression. J Shoulder Elbow Surg. 2011;20(6):975–82. https://doi.org/10.1016/j.jse.2010.10.032. Epub 2011 Feb 1. PubMed PMID: 21277808.
5. Vigasio A, Marcoccio I. Hourglass-like constriction of the suprascapular nerve: a contraindication for minimally invasive surgery. J Shoulder Elbow Surg. 2018;27(2):e29–37. https://doi.org/10.1016/j.jse.2017.08.021. Epub 2017 Nov 6. PubMed PMID: 29102255.
6. Hama H, Ueba Y, Moringa T, Suzuki K, Kuroki H, Yamamuro T. A new strategy for treatment of supra-

scapular entrapment neuropathy in athletes: shaving of the base of the scapular spine. J Shoulder Elbow Surg. 1992;1:253–60.
7. Gosk J, Urban M, Rutowski R. Entrapment of the suprascapular nerve: anatomy, etiology, diagnosis, treatment. Ortop Traumatol Rehabil. 2007;9:68–74.
8. Mallon WJ, Wilson RJ, Basamania CJ. The association of supra- scapular neuropathy with massive rotator cuff tears: a preliminary report. J Shoulder Elbow Surg. 2006;15:395–8.
9. Costouros JG, Porramatikul M, Lie DT, Warner JJ. Reversal of suprascapular neuropathy following arthroscopic repair of massive supraspinatus and infraspinatus rotator cuff tears. Arthroscopy. 2007;23:1152–61. https://doi.org/10.1016/j.arthro.2007.06.014.
10. Piasecki DP, Romeo AA, Bach BR Jr, Nicholson GP. Suprascapular neuropathy. J Am Acad Orthop Surg. 2009;17(11):665–76. Review. PubMed PMID: 19880677.
11. Moen TC, Babatunde OM, Hsu SH, Ahmad CS, Levine WN. Suprascapular neuropathy: what does the literature show? J Shoulder Elbow Surg. 2012;21(6):835–46. https://doi.org/10.1016/j.jse.2011.11.033. Epub 2012 Mar 23. Review. Erratum in: J Shoulder Elbow Surg. 2012;21(10):1442. PubMed PMID: 22445163.
12. Callahan JD, Scully TB, Shapiro SA, Worth RM. Suprascapular nerve entrapment. A series of 27 cases. J Neurosurg. 1991;74:893–6.
13. Black KP, Lombardo JA. Suprascapular nerve injuries with isolated paralysis of the infraspinatus. Am J Sports Med. 1990;18:225–8.
14. Drez D Jr. Suprascapular neuropathy in the differential diagnosis of rotator cuff injuries. Am J Sports Med. 1976;4:43–5.
15. Joshi J, Singla A. Suprascapular nerve block. In: Pain procedures in clinical practice. 3rd ed. London: Elsevier Health Sciences; 2011. p. 255–9.
16. Budeyri A, Krishnan S. Open and arthroscopic suprascapular nerve decompression. In: Operative techniques: shoulder and elbow surgery. 2nd ed. Philadelphia: Wolters Kluwer; 2016. p. 370–9.
17. Romeo AA, Ghodadra NS, Salata MJ, Provencher MT. Arthroscopic suprascapular nerve decompression: indications and surgical technique. J Shoulder Elbow Surg. 2010;19(2 Suppl):118–23. https://doi.org/10.1016/j.jse.2010.01.006. PubMed PMID: 20188277.
18. Miller RH, Azar FM, Throckmorton TW. Shoulder and elbow injuries. In: Campbells operative orthopaedics. 13th ed. Elsevier, Inc; 2017; p. 2298–345.
19. Ferretti A, Cerullo G, Russo G. Suprascapular neuropathy in volleyball players. J Bone Joint Surg Am. 1987;69:260–3.
20. Bigliani LU, Dalsey RM, McCann PD, April EW. An anatomical study of the suprascapular nerve. Arthroscopy. 1990;6:301–5. https://doi.org/10.1016/0749-8063(90)90060Q.
21. Rengachary SS, Burr D, Lucas S, et al. Suprascapular nerve entrapment neuropathy: a clinical, anatomical and comparative study. Part 2: anatomical study. Neurosurgery. 1979;5(4):447–51.
22. Warner JP, Krushell RJ, Masquelet A, Gerber C. Anatomy and relationships of the suprascapular nerve: anatomical constraints to mobilization of the supraspinatus and infraspinatus muscles in the management of massive rotator-cuff tears. J Bone Joint Surg Am. 1992;74(1):36–45. PubMed PMID: 1734012.
23. Plancher KD, Petterson SC. Posterior Shoulder pain and arthroscopic decompression of the suprascapular nerve at the transverse scapular ligament. Oper Tech Sports Med. 2014;22(1):58–72.
24. Barber FA. Suprascapular nerve block for shoulder arthroscopy. Arthroscopy. 2005;21:1015. https://doi.org/10.1016/j.arthro.2005.05.033.
25. Barwood SA, Burkhart SS, Lo IK. Arthroscopic suprascapular nerve release at the suprascapular notch in a cadaveric model: an anatomic approach. Arthroscopy. 2007;23(2):221–5. PubMed PMID: 17276231.
26. Demirhan M, Imhoff AB, Debski RE, Patel PR, Fu FH, Woo SLY. The spinoglenoid ligament and its relationship to the suprascapular nerve. J Shoulder Elbow Surg. 1998;7:238–43.
27. Houtz C, McCulloch PC. Suprascapular vascular anomalies as a cause of suprascapular nerve compression. Orthopedics. 2013;36(1):42–5. https://doi.org/10.3928/01477447-20121217-07. PubMed PMID: 23276335.
28. Momaya AM, Kwapisz A, Choate WS, Kissenberth MJ, Tolan SJ, Lonergan KT, Hawkins RJ, Tokish JM. Clinical outcomes of suprascapular nerve decompression: a systematic review. J Shoulder Elbow Surg. 2018;27(1):172–80. https://doi.org/10.1016/j.jse.2017.09.025. Review. PubMed PMID: 29221575.
29. Lichtenberg S, Magosch P, Habermeyer P. Compression of the suprascapular nerve by a ganglion cyst of the spinoglenoid notch: the arthroscopic solution. Knee Surg Sports Traumatol Arthrosc. 2004;12:72–9.
30. Lafosse L, Piper K, Lanz U. Arthroscopic suprascapular nerve release: indications and technique. J Shoulder Elbow Surg. 2011;20(2 Suppl):S9–13. https://doi.org/10.1016/j.jse.2010.12.003. Review. PubMed PMID: 21281924.
31. Cummins CA, Bowen M, Anderson K, Messer T. Suprascapular nerve entrapment at the spinoglenoid notch in a professional baseball pitcher. Am J Sports Med. 1999;27:810–2.
32. Freehill MT, Shi LL, Tompson JD, Warner JJ. Suprascapular neuropathy: diagnosis and management. Phys Sportsmed. 2012;40(1):72–83. https://doi.org/10.3810/psm.2012.02.1953. Review. PubMed PMID: 22508253.
33. Walch G, Boulahia A, Calderone S, Robinson AH. The "dropping" and 'hornblowers' signs in evaluation of rotator-cuff tears. J Bone Joint Surg Br. 1998;80:624–8.
34. Gerber C, Blumenthal S, Curt A, Werner CML. Effect of selective experimental suprascapular nerve block

on adduction and external rotation strength of the shoulder. J Shoulder Elbow Surg. 2007;16:815–20. https://doi.org/10.1016/j.jse.2007.02.120.
35. Boykin RE, Friedman DJ, Higgins LD, Warner JJ. Suprascapular neuropathy. J Bone Joint Surg Am. 2010;92(13):2348–64. https://doi.org/10.2106/JBJS.I.01743. Review. PubMed PMID: 20926731.
36. Jensen KL, Tirman P, Rockwood CA. Radiographic evaluation of shoulder problems. In: Rockwood and matsens the shoulder. 5th ed. Philadelphia: Elsevier; 2018. p. 135–68.
37. Yanny S, Toms AP. MR patterns of denervation around the shoulder. AJR Am J Roentgenol. 2010;195(2):W157–63. https://doi.org/10.2214/AJR.09.4127. Review. PubMed PMID: 20651176.
38. Neto N, Nunnes P. Spectrum of MRI features of ganglion and synovial cysts. Insights Imaging. 2016;7(2):179–86.
39. Shi LL, Freehill MT, Yannopoulos P, Warner JJ. Suprascapular nerve: is it important in cuff pathology? Adv Orthop. 2012;2012:516985. https://doi.org/10.1155/2012/516985. Epub 2012 Nov 1. PubMed PMID: 23193484; PubMed Central PMCID: PMC3501891.
40. Lafosse L, Tomasi A, Corbett S, Baier G, Williems K, Gobezie R. Arthroscopic release of suprascapular nerve entrapment at the suprascapular notch: technique and preliminary results. Arthroscopy. 2007;23:34–42. https://doi.org/10.1016/j.arthro.2006.10.003.
41. Kim DS, Park HK, Park JH, Yoon WS. Ganglion cyst of the spinoglenoid notch: comparison between SLAP repair alone and SLAP repair with cyst decompresion. J Shoulder Elbow Surg. 2012;21:1456–63. https://doi.org/10.1016/j.jse.2012.01.013.
42. Mall NA, Hammond JE, Lenart BA, Enriquez DJ, Twigg SL, Nicholson GP. Suprascapular nerve entrapment isolated to the spinoglenoid notch: surgical technique and results of open decompression. J Shoulder Elbow Surg. 2013;22(11):e1–8. https://doi.org/10.1016/j.jse.2013.03.009. Epub 2013 May 8. PubMed PMID: 23664748.
43. Ferretti A, De Carli A, Fontana M. Injury of the suprascapular nerve at the spinoglenoid notch: the natural history of infraspinatus atrophy in volleyball players. Am J Sports Med. 1998;26:759–63.
44. Fehrman DA, Orwin JF, Jennings RM. Suprascapular nerve entrapment by ganglion cysts: a report of six cases with arthroscopic findings and review of the literature. Arthroscopy. 1995;11(6):727–34. Review. PubMed PMID: 8679037.
45. Elzinga KE, Curran MW, Morhart MJ, Chan KM, Olson JL. Open anterior release of the superior transverse scapular ligament for decompression of the suprascapular nerve during brachial plexus surgery. J Hand Surg Am. 2016;41(7):e211–5. https://doi.org/10.1016/j.jhsa.2016.03.005. Epub 2016 Apr 22. PubMed PMID: 27113908.
46. Prasad GL. An all-anterior approach for quadruple nerve transfer for upper trunk brachial plexus injuries. World Neurosurg. 2018;120:e651–9. https://doi.org/10.1016/j.wneu.2018.08.139. Epub 2018 Aug 27. PubMed PMID: 30165220.
47. Steinmann S, Elhassan B. Nerve problems related to the shoulder. In: Rockwood and matsens the shoulder. 5th ed. Elsevier, Inc; 2009. p. 1093–122.
48. Post M. Diagnosis and treatment of suprascapular nerve entrapment. Clin Orthop Relat Res. 1999;368:92–100.
49. Post M, Grinbiat E. Suprascapular nerve entrapment: diagnosis and results of treatment. J Shoulder Elbow Surg. 1993;2:190–7.
50. Post M, Mayer J. Suprascapular nerve entrapment: diagnosis and treatment. Clin Orthop Relat Res. 1987;223:126–36.
51. Romeo AA, Rotenberg DD, Bach BR Jr. Suprascapular neuropathy. J Am Acad Orthop Surg. 1999;7(6):358–67. PubMed PMID: 11497489.
52. Lafosse L, Tomasi A. Technique for endoscopic release of suprascapular nerve entrapment at the suprascapular notch. Tech Shoulder Elbow Surg. 2006;7:1–6. https://doi.org/10.1087/00132589-200603000-00001.
53. Plancher KD, Luke TA, Peterson RK, Yacoubian SV. Posterior shoulder pain: a dynamic study of the spinoglenoid ligament and treatment with arthroscopic release of the scapular tunnel. Arthroscopy. 2007;23:991–8. https://doi.org/10.1016/j.arthro.2007.03.098. PMid: 17868839.
54. Fabre T, Piton C, Leclouerec G, Gervais-Delion F, Durandeau A. Entrapment of the suprascapular nerve. J Bone Joint Surg Br. 1999;81:414–9.
55. Kim DH, Murovic JA, Tiel RL, Kline DG. Management and outcomes of 42 surgical suprascapular nerve injuries and entrapment. Neurosurgery. 2005;57:120–7.
56. Arriaza R, Ballesteros J, López-Vidriero E. Suprascapular neuropathy as a cause of swimmer's shoulder: results after arthroscopic treatment in 4 patients. Am J Sports Med. 2013;41(4):887–93. https://doi.org/10.1177/0363546513477383. Epub 2013 Feb 28. PubMed PMID: 23449835.
57. Garcia Júnior JC, Paccola AM, Tonoli C, Zabeu JL, Garcia JP. Arthroscopic release of the suprascapular nerve: surgical technique and evaluation of clinical cases. Rev Bras Ortop. 2015;46(4):403–7. https://doi.org/10.1016/S2255-4971(15)30252-4. eCollection 2011 Jul-Aug. PubMed PMID: 27027028; PubMed Central PMCID: PMC4799278.
58. Abboud JA, Silverberg D, Glaser DL, Ramsey ML, Williams GR. Arthroscopy effectively treats ganglion cysts of the shoulder. Clin Orthop Relat Res. 2006;444:129–33. https://doi.org/10.1097/01.blo.0000201155.44572.9b.
59. Hashiguchi H, Iwashita S, Ohkubo A, Takai S. SLAP repair with arthroscopic decompression of spinoglenoid cyst. SICOT J. 2016;2:1. https://doi.org/10.1051/sicotj/2015036.
60. Westerheide KJ, Dopirak RM, Karzel RP, Snyder SJ. Supras- capular nerve palsy secondary to spinoglenoid cysts: results of arthroscopic treatment. Arthroscopy. 2006;22:721–7.

61. Schroder CP, Skare O, Stiris M, Gjengedal E, Uppheim G, Brox JI. Treatment of labral tears with associated spinoglenoid cysts without cyst decompression. J Bone Joint Surg Am. 2008;90:523–30. https://doi.org/10.2106/JBJS.F.01534.
62. Pillai G, Baynes JR, Gladstone J, Flatow EL. Greater strength increase with cyst decompression and SLAP repair than SLAP repair alone. Clin Orthop Relat Res. 2011;469:1056–60.
63. Reineck JR, Krishnan SG. Subligamentous suprascapular artery encountered during arthroscopic suprascapular nerve release: a report of three cases. J Shoulder Elbow Surg. 2009;18:e1–3. https://doi.org/10.1016/j.jse.2008.08.007.

Index

A

Abductor digitiminimi (ADM) muscle, 9, 186
Abductor pollicislongus (APL), 2, 225
Adson's test, 235, 236
Agee device, 124, 125
Agee's single-portal technique, 45
American Academy of Electrodiagnostic Medicine (AANEM), 11
Amyotrophic lateral sclerosis (ALS), 3
Anterior interosseous nerve (AIN), 15, 16, 171, 172, 174, 176
Anterior scalenectomy, 242
Anterior sub-muscular transposition (ASMT), 146
Arcade of Fröhse, 196, 199, 202
Arthroscopic suprascapular nerve decompression, 268, 271, 272
Arthroscopic techniques, 268
Autologous vein graft, 248

B

Bishop's scoring system, 94
Brachial plexus neurolysis, 242
Brachial plexus tension test, 238
Brachioradialis (BR), 225

C

Carpal tunnel surgery complications
- anteriorinterosseous syndrome, 62
- brachial plexus abnormalities, 62
- cervical spine disorders, 62
- classification of, 62
- CRPS, 71
- early complications
  - Bedeschi sign, 65
  - distal TCL, 65
  - hematomas, 66
  - Phalen and Gilliatt and Wilson tests, 65
  - post-operative infection, 66, 67
  - postsurgicalpyodermagangrenosum, 67
  - proximal TCL, 65
  - pyodermagangrenosum, 67
  - thoracic outlet syndrome, 67
- flexor tendons, 69
- intraoperative complications, 62–64
- late postoperative complications, 67, 68
- loss of hand grip strength, 68
- OCTR and ECTR, 62
- painful cutaneous scar, 69, 70
- pillar pain, 70
- piso-triquetral pain syndrome, 70–71
- pronator syndrome, 62
- thoracic outlet syndrome, 62
- trigger finger, 68, 69

Carpal tunnel syndrome (CTS), 1–4, 6, 7, 9, 10, 210
- classic presentation, 27, 28
- compression test, 27
- CTS-6, 29
- definition, 27
- diabetes mellitus, 43
- diagnosis, 254
- diagnostic tools
  - CNAP, 30
  - CTS-6, 29
  - EMG/NCS, 29–31
  - Phalen test, 29
  - Tinel sign, 29
  - ultrasound, 31, 32
- epidemiology, 253
- etiology, 253
- hypothyreoidism, 43
- median nerve, 44
- physical examination, 28
- sarcoidosis, 43
- surgical techniques and complains, 44, 45
- Tinel sign, 27
- Tinel's and Phalen's sign, 43
- TSCAI, 45–51
- tumors/anatomic abnormalities, 43

Cervical radiculopathy
- diagnosis, 254
- epidemiology, 253
- etiology, 253
- treatment, 255

Charcot-Marie-Tooth (CMT) diseases, 1, 76
Cheiralgiaparesthetica, 225
Cicatrix, 247

D. G. Sotereanos, L. K. Papatheodorou (eds.), *Compressive Neuropathies of the Upper Extremity*,
https://doi.org/10.1007/978-3-030-37289-7

Complex regional pain syndrome (CRPS), 49, 71, 226
Compound muscle action potentials (CMAP), 5, 171
Coracoacromial ligament, 268
Costoclavicular compression syndrome, 232
Cubital tunnel syndrome (CUTS), 19, 23–25, 248, 251
adjunctive techniques, 163, 164
Adson forceps, 114
amniotic membrane nerve wrapping, 163
clinical outcomes, 163
clinical presentation, 103, 104
complications, 117, 118
electrodiagnostic studies, 106, 107
etiology, 161, 162
Guyon's canal, 111
history, 162
in situ decompression, 112
Adson toothed forceps, 112
anterior ulnar nerve transposition, 117
army-navy retractor, 112, 114
asymptomatic ulnar nerve, 116
cubital tunnel, 115
data supports transposition, 116
home passive motion program, 117
intraoperative ulnar nerve subluxation, 115
medialintermuscular septum, 112
medial intramuscular septum, 116
Osborne's ligament, 112
pre-operative education, 117
routine circumferential dissection, 114
Semmes Weinstein test, 117
skin incision, 112, 115
subcutaneous dissection, 112
superficial fascia, 113
intermittent or positional dysesthesias, 111
intrinsic wasting and dense numbness, 112
MABC, 114
McGowan classification system, 106
MRI, 107, 108
physical examination, 104–106, 162
plain radiographs, 107
porcine extracellular matrix wrap, 163
post-transpositional impingement, 115
primary surgery, 164
revision surgery, 162, 164
small distally based strip, 116
subcutaneous transposition, 165
submuscular transposition, 165
testing, 162
ulnar nerve wrapping, 163
ultrasonography, 107
vein grafts, 163
Wilson-Krout grade, 163
Cubital tunnel syndromes, 248, 251

D

De Quervain's tenosynovitis pain, 227
Dellon's classification, 126
Dellon's technique, 146
Disabilities of the Arm, Shoulder and Hand (DASH), 132
Distal latency, 5
Dorsal cutaneous branch of the ulnar nerve (DCBUN), 171
Dorsal ulnar hand (DSBUN), 148
Double crush syndrome, 257

E

Eelevated arm stress test, 237, 238
Electrodes, 6
Electrodiagnostic Studies, 255
Electrodiagnostic testing
abductorpollicisbrevis, 3
axon continuity, 1
C8 and T1 innervated muscles, 4
carpal tunnel syndrome, 3
EMG/NCV
above-elbow to below-elbow segment, 8
ADM muscle, 9
anastomoses of median, 9
APB muscle cells, 7
back firing, 5
chronic neurogenic process, 7
CMAP, 5, 9, 10
distal latency, 5
electrodes, 6
entrapment neuropathy, 4
F response, 5
individual muscles, 7
Martin-Gruber anastomosis, 9
measuring velocity, 4
median mixed motor/sensory nerve, 6
reinnervation, 7
SNAP, 5
ulnar nerve, 5, 7, 8
ulnar neuropathy, 8, 9
flexor carpi radialis, 3
flexordigitorumsuperficialis muscles, 3
flexorpollicisbrevis, 3
nerve trunks, 1
palmarislongus, 3
sensoryfibers, 3
spinal nerve roots, 1
Elevator technique, 13
Endoneurium, 1
Endoscopic assisted methods, 203
Endoscopic carpal tunnel release (ECTR) techniques, 44
Agee device, 124, 125
anatomy, 54
anterior transposition, 122
complications, 128
contraindications, 127
eye coordination and triangulation techniques, 129
hemostasis, 128
indications, 127
larger incision, 128
McGowen Grade 3, 129
postoperative protocol, 128
surgical technique, 127–128
ulnar nerve hypermobility, 129
childhood elbow fracture, 122

complication rates, 58
endoscopic visualization, 56
flexor carpi radialis, 55
flexor carpi ulnaris, 55
follow-up protocol, 58
indications for, 53, 54
intrinsic muscle wasting, 121
instrumentation, 54–55
local anaesthesia, 55
non-operative measures, 53
OCTR approach, 53
Osborne's ligament, 121
outcomes, 58, 59
positioning, 54
post-traumatic scarring, inflammatory arthropathy, 122
small right-angled blunt retractor, 57
ulnar nerve in-situ
Cannula technique, 123–124
complications, 125
contra-indications, 122
Dellon's classification, 126
elbow region, 126
indications, 122
postoperative protocol, 125
scar pain and superficial wound infection, 126
Storz equipment, 122–123
Storz instruments, 125
ulnar nerve subluxation, 122
U-shaped incision, 56
washboard effect, 56
Endoscopic ulnar nerve release, cannula technique, 124
Entrapment neuropathies, 247, 251
Entrapment neuropathy, 6, 201
Extensor carpi radialislongus (ECRL), 225
Extensor pollicisbrevis (EPB), 225

F
First dorsal interosseous (FDI) muscle, 9
Flexor carpi ulnaris (FCU), 55, 113, 121, 147, 171, 174, 186
aponeurosis, 133
muscle, 9
Flexor digitorumprofundis (FDP), 148, 171, 186
Flexor digitorumsuperficialis (FDS), 16, 21, 209
Flexor pollicis brevis (FPB), 171
Flexor pollicis longus (FPL) muscle, 209
Flexor-pronator mass, 146
Froment's sign, 105, 189, 190

G
Ganglion cyst, 94
Guyon's canal, 24, 86

H
Halsted maneuver, 238
Hepatocyte growth factor (HGF), 248
Horner syndrome, 98
Hunter's Test, 238
Hyperabduction syndrome, 232
Hypothenar fat pad flap (HTFPF)
carpalcana, 86
distalantebrachial fascia, 85
dysesthetic pain, 85
dysesthetic symptoms, 85
externalneurolysis, 86
Guyon's canal, 86
hypothenar and palmarisbrevis muscles, 86
latex-injectedhypothenar tissue, 86
layered skin closure, 87
postoperative development of adhesions, 85
tenosynovitis, 85
transverse carpal ligament, 85, 87
wrist motion, 87

I
Idiopathic cubital tunnel syndrome, 122
Indiana Tome, 38–41
Inflammatory pseudotumor of peripheral nerve (IPPN), 96–97
Interphalangeal joints (IPJs), 171

L
Lacertus syndrome, 212
Larger incision, 124
Lateral antebrachial cutaneous nerve (LABCN), 201
anatomy, 217–219
clinical presentation, 219, 220
definition, 217
diagnosis, 221
differential diagnosis, 221, 222
epidemiology, 220
pathophysiology, 221
risk factors, 221
socioeconomic effects, 220, 221
treatment
conservative, 222
operative, 222
Learmonth's technique, 146

M
Malignant peripheral nerve sheath tumors (MPNST), 98, 99
Martin-Gruber anastomosis, 9
McGowan classification system, 106, 148
Medial antebrachial cutaneous nerve (MABC), 112, 114, 133
Medial brachial and antebrachial cutaneous nerve (MABCN), 161
Medial distal arm (MBC), 148
Medial intermuscular septum (MIMS), 127

Median nerve (MN) compression, 87
high median neuropathy
AIN, 181
motor reconstruction, 181, 182
sensory reconstruction, 182
low median neuropathy
flexorpollicusbrevis, 179
motor reconstruction, 179–181
sensory reconstruction, 181
Metacarpophalangeal joints (MCPJ), 95, 171
Minimal incision carpal tunnel release (MICTR), 44
Minimal medial epicondylectomy
advantage, 155
clinical outcomes, 158
complications, 155, 158
indications, 155, 156
surgical technique
bone wax, 157
medialantebrachial cutaneous nerve, 156
Osborne's ligament and cubital tunnel, 156
osteotomy fragment, 157
skin incision, 156
subperiosteal dissection, 156, 157
subperiosteal flap closure, 157
Motor nerve action potential (MNAP), 30
Motor unit action potentials (MUAPs), 6, 7
Musculocutaneous nerve, 217
Myopathy radiculopathy, 6

N

Nerve conduction velocity (NCV), 148, 212
Nerve transfers
diagnosis, 170, 171
end to side transfer, 169
end-organ unresponsiveness, motor denervation, 170
median nerve compression
high median neuropathy, 181, 182
low median neuropathy, 179–181
nervecoaptation, 169
Oberlin transfer, 170
post-operative protocol, 170
SETS transfer, 170
ulnar nerve compression
AIN, 176
FCU, 171
FDP, 171
MCPJ, 171
motor reconstruction, 179
sensory reconstruction, 179
SETS transfer, 171–174
surgical technique, 174–178
Wartenberg's sign, 171
zone of injury, 170
Nerve transposition, *see* Ulnar nerve
Neuralgic amyotrophy, 201
Neuritis ossificans, 95, 96
Neurofibroma, 90
Neuromuscular ultrasound imaging
"electric cable" pattern, 14
"honeycomb" pattern, 14
median nerve (C6-T1), 13, 15
non-invasive technique, 11
optimization of, 12
peripheral nerve, 12, 13
transverse image, 14
ulnar nerve, 20, 23, 24

O

Oberlin procedure, 170
Omega (Ω) deformity, 137
Open carpal tunnel release (OCTR), 44, 53
distal volar forearm, 38
Indiana Tome, 38–41
palmar fascia, 37
skin incision, 37
tenosynovectomy, 38
Osborne's ligament, 121

P

Paget–Schroetter syndrome, 232
Paresthesia, 219–221
Parosteallipomas, 93
Parsonage-Turner syndrome, 212
Perineurium, 1
Peripheral neuropathy, 6
Phalen's test, 28
Posterior interosseous nerve compression syndrome (PINCS)
anatomy, 195, 196
anterior approach, 201, 202
BR and ECRL, 202
clinical outcomes, 203, 204
definition, 195
electrodiagnostic testing, 199, 200
endoscopic assisted methods, 203
etiology, 196
forearm pain, 197
mechanical constriction, 197
MRI, 198, 199
physical examination, 198
posterior approach, 202
transbrachioradialis, 202, 203
treatment, 200, 201
ultrasonography, 199
Pronator quadratus (PQ), 176
Pronator teres syndrome (PS)
anatomy, 209–211
bicipitalaponeurosis, 209
clinical manifestations, 210
diagnostic tests, 210–212
electromyography, 212, 213
imaging, 213
nerve conduction, 212, 213
treatment
nonsurgical management, 213
surgical management, 213, 214

R

Radial tunnel syndrome (RTS)
- anatomy, 195, 196
- anterior approach, 201, 202
- BR and ECRL, 202
- clinical outcomes, 203, 204
- definition, 195
- electrodiagnostic testing, 199, 200
- endoscopic assisted methods, 203
- etiology, 196
- magnetic resonance imaging, 198, 199
- mechanical constriction, 197
- physical examination, 197, 198
- posterior approach, 202
- transbrachioradialis, 202, 203
- treatment, 200, 201
- ultrasonography, 199

Raynaud's disease, 233
Recurrent carpal tunnel, 75
Reflex sympathetic dystrophy (RSD), 71
Revision carpal tunnel syndrome
- evaluation, 76
- hypothenar fat pad flap, 79, 80
- muscle flaps, 81
- principles of surgical treatment, 77
- recurrent carpal tunnel, 75
- remote pedicle/free flaps, 82
- repeat simple decompression, 77, 78
- synovial and tenosynovial flap, 78
- synthetic wraps, 81
- vascularizedfascial flaps, 81–82
- vein wrapping, 81
- WALANT technique, 83

Roos' test, 237, 238
Rule-of-Nine test, 197

S

Safety clip, 40
Scalenusanticus syndrome, 232
Schwannomas, 97
Scratch- collapse test, 211
Semmes Weinstein test, 117
Semmes-Weinstein monofilament test, 76, 189
Sensory nerve action potential (SNAP), 5, 30
Simple Shoulder Test (SST), 273
Soft tissue sarcomas (STS), 98
Spinoglenoid notch, 267
Subclavian venous thrombosis, 234
Subcutaneous anterior transposition
- biomechanicals, 132, 133
- complications, 141
- DASH score, 132
- fasciodermal sling technique, 136
- ligamentodermal sling, 137
- medial epicondyle, 131
- medialintermuscular septum, 135
- nerve decompression and transposition, 134
- outcomes of, 138, 140, 141
- superior ulnar collateral artery, 131
- techniques of
  - adipose flap, 136
  - fascial sling, 135
  - fasciodermal sling, 134–135
  - flexor carpi ulnaris, 133
  - *in situ* decompression, 133
  - ligamentofascial/ligamentodermal sling, 137
  - medialintermuscularseptal sling, 136, 137
  - omega (Ω) deformity, 137
  - Osborne's ligament, 133
  - subcutaneous pocket, 134
- ulnar nerve vascular supply, 132
- whole-arm ischemia, 132

"Supercharged" end to side transfers (SETS), 170
- AIN transfer, 171–174, 176
- curvilinear/Bruner-style incision, 174, 175
- fibrin glue, 176
- flexordigitorumprofundus, 176
- pronatorquadratus, 176
- sensory reconstruction, 176–178

Superficial branch of the radial nerve (SBRN), *see* Wartenberg's syndrome
Suprascapular nerve
- anatomy, 259, 261
- arthroscopic techniques, 267
- diagnostic injection, 266
- electromyography, 265
- ganglion cysts, 264
- nerve conduction velocity, 265
- radiological imaging, 265
- scapular notch compression, 263
- spinoglenoid ligament, 270
- spinoglenoid notch compression, 264

Suprascapular notch, 268
Synovial sarcomas, 99, 100

T

Tenosynovitis, 95
Tenosynovium, 39
Thoracic outlet syndrome (TOS)
- arterial TOS, 233, 234
- cervical ribs, 232
- costoclavicular space, 232
- definition, 231
- history, 232, 233
- interscalene triangle, 231, 232
- neurogenic TOS
  - Adson's test, 235, 236
  - classification, 233
  - diagnosis, 235
  - diagnostic studies, 238, 239
  - disputed, 235
  - electrodiagnostic testing, 239, 240
  - etiology, 234
  - Halsted maneuver, 238
  - Hunter's Test, 238
  - physical examination, 235
  - Roos' test, 237, 238
  - true, 234

Thoracic outlet syndrome (TOS) (*cont.*)
upper limb tension test, 238
Wright's hyperabduction test, 237
neurogenic type, 233
subcoracoid space, 232
treatment
anterior and middle scalenectomy, 242
anteriorscalenectomy, 240
anterior scalenotomy, 242
brachial plexus neurolysis, 242
comprehensive program, 240
first rib, 240
first rib resection, 242
incidence, 243
indications, 240
meta-analysis, 243
predictive factors, 243
psychological factors, 243
recurrent TOS, 243, 244
supraclavicular rib resection, 241, 242
transaxillary rib resection, 240, 241
vascular, 242
vascular type, 233
venous TOS, 234
Tinel's test, 104
Tinel's, Phalen's, Carpal compression test, 76
Transaxillary approach, 232
Transaxillary rib resection, 240, 241
Transbrachioradialis, 202, 203
Transcutaneous electrical nerve stimulation (TENS), 222
Transverse carpal ligament (TCL), 37, 186
Transverse scapular ligament (TSL), 261
Trigger finger (TF), 68, 69
Tumors and tumor like lesions
diagnostic approach, 89
differential diagnosis, 89–90
ganglion and synovial cysts, 94, 95
lipomas, 90
lipomatoustumors, 90–93
nervelipomatosis, 91, 93
parosteallipomas, 93
peripheral nerve compression and malignancy
lymph nodes and peripheral nerve lymphomatosis, 97–98
metastatic disease, 98
MPNSTs, 98, 99
STS, 98–100
peripheral nerve sheath tumors
neurofibromas, 97
schwannomas, 97
reactive and inflammatory lesions
IPPN, 96–97
neuritisossificans, 95, 96
tenosynovitis, 95
treatment, 90
Two small cross aligned incisions (TSCAI), 45–51

U
Ulnar nerve, 20, 23, 24
pathology, 145
stability, 145
submuscular transposition
clinical outcomes, 151, 152
comparative trials, 147, 148
curvilinear incision, 149
EMG and NCVs, 148
flexor-pronator mass, 150, 151
history, 146, 147
longitudinal septa, 150
nerve bed, 150
Osborne's ligament, 149
proximal and distal, 150
range of motion, 151
surgical indications, 148
tourniquet, 151
transposition, 145
Ulnar neuropathy, 8
Ulnar tunnel syndrome (UTS)
clinical findings, 189, 190
compressive neuropathy, 185
diagnostics, 190
distal ulnar tunnel, 186
eighth cervical (C8), 185
FCU, 186
FDP, 186
fibrous arch, 187
first thoracic (T1) nerve, 185
history, 185
Martin-Gruber anastomosis, 186
pathoetiology, 187–189
Riche-Cannieu anastomosis, 186
superficial branch, 187
superficial sensory branch and deep motor branch, 186
TCL, 186, 187
treatment, 190–192
ulnar artery, 186
VCL, 186, 187
Upper extremity peripheral neuropathies, 89
Upper limb tension test, 238

V
Vascular endothelial growth factor (VEGF), 248
Vasculitic neuropathy, 95
Vein wrapping
allograft, 247
autologous vein graft, 247
indications, 248, 249
surgicaltechhiniqe, 249, 250
Visual analog scale (VAS), 273
Volar carpal ligament (VCL), 186

W
Wartenberg sign, 104
Wartenberg's migrant sensory neuritis (WMSN), 227

Wartenberg's sign, 105, 171
Wartenberg's syndrome
  anatomy, 225, 226
  clinical presentation, 226, 227
  definition, 225
  differential diagnosis, 226, 227
  electrodiagnostic tests, 227, 228
  magnetic resonance imaging, 228
  pathophysiology, 226
  treatment, 226, 228, 229
  ultrasonography, 228
Wide Awake Local Anesthesia No Tourniquet (WALANT) technique, 83
Wright's hyperabduction test, 237

MIX
Papier aus verantwortungsvollen Quellen
Paper from responsible sources
FSC® C105338

If you have any concerns about our products,
you can contact us on
ProductSafety@springernature.com

In case Publisher is established outside the EU,
the EU authorized representative is:
Springer Nature Customer Service Center GmbH
Europaplatz 3, 69115 Heidelberg, Germany

Printed by Libri Plureos GmbH
in Hamburg, Germany